Mineral Trioxide Aggregate in Dentistry

Josette Camilleri
Editor

Mineral Trioxide Aggregate in Dentistry

From Preparation to Application

Springer

Editor
Josette Camilleri, BChD, MPhil,
PhD, FIMMM, FADM
Department of Restorative Dentistry
Faculty of Dental Surgery
Medical School, Mater Dei Hospital
University of Malta
Msida
Malta

ISBN 978-3-642-55156-7 ISBN 978-3-642-55157-4 (eBook)
DOI 10.1007/978-3-642-55157-4
Springer Heidelberg New York Dordrecht London

Library of Congress Control Number: 2014944739

Printed on acid-free paper

Springer is part of Springer Science+Business Media (www.springer.com)

This book is dedicated to the memory of Professor Thomas Pitt Ford.

Foreword

Mineral trioxide aggregate commonly known as MTA has been favourably received by the dental community for over two decades, due to its repertoire of clinical applications. However this versatile dental material owes its humble origins to civil engineering and the construction industry. The late Professor Thomas Pitt Ford was the veteran scientist and endodontist who supervised the doctoral research of the MTA inventor Dr. Mahmoud Torabinejad and the editor of this book Dr. Josette Camilleri. This scholarly overview represents the first attempt in bringing together a diverse group of academics and clinicians who have dedicated their research career on the development and understanding of this tricalcium silicate-based material.

The book discusses the advances in the manipulation of the material over the years, the chemical and physical properties of material in the non-hydrated and hydrated phases along with its biological properties. An evidenced-based discussion of the different clinical applications of MTA in endodontic treatments and complications, traumatic injuries, and management of the pulp in both dentitions is presented. However one must question if the biocompatibility properties apply to all the different presentations of the material.

Apart from presenting the latest research on MTA, the book cultivates an important balance between basic research and the clinical disciplines. The topics covered in his book highlight the need for thorough investigation using appropriate testing designed specifically for the material under study. Currently many of these specific testing designs are lacking for MTA. As such, techniques and standards used for other dental materials have been adopted and extrapolated for the study of MTA-type products. Some of these adopted techniques may have limitations and may not have been correctly used for investigation of calcium silicate-based materials.

An underlying theme of the book is that materials that are serving the profession well in a particular field of dentistry may be adopted for new applications in other dental disciplines. Thus, this book should be an important reference for both materials science and clinical researchers.

Msida, Malta

Nikolai Attard, BChD,
MSc Prosthodont (To), PhD (To)

Acknowledgements

The editor would like to acknowledge the following individuals and groups for their assistance with the following chapters:

Chapter 2: Composition and Setting Reaction

Ing James Camilleri, Mr. Lawrence Spiteri, Professor Franklin Tay, Dr. Adrienne Busuttil and students, collaborators and technical staff

Chapter 3: Properties of Hydrated Mineral Trioxide Aggregate

Dr. Raqueli Viapiana

Chapter 5: Reactivity and Environmental Factors

Dr. Mohammed Nekoofar

Chapter 6: Clinical Applications

Luis Gonzales Navarro

Chapter 9: Mineral Trioxide Aggregate and Evidence-Based Practice

The Knowledge Management Unit (KMU) of Iranian Center for Endodontic Research, Research Institute for Dental Sciences, Shahid Beheshti University of Medical Sciences, Professor S. M. Safavi, Professor M. J. Eghbal, Professor J. Ghoddusi, Dr. H. Torabzadeh, Dr. M. Fazlyab, Dr. A. Shirvani, Dr. L. Alim Marvasti, Dr. S. H. Yazdani, Dr. N. Davari Ardekani, Dr. S. Ehsani, Dr. R. Hasnizadeh, Ms. Z. Motlagh, Ms. L. Asgari, and Ms. M. Roshanzamir

Contents

Contributors

Saeed Asgary, DDS, MS Department of Endodontics, Iranian Center for Endodontic Research, Shahid Beheshti Dental School, Shahid Beheshti University of Medical Sciences, Tehran, Iran

Clóvis Monteiro Bramante, PhD Department of Dentistry, Endodontics and Dental Materials, Bauru Dental School, University of Sao Paulo, Bauru, SP, Brazil

Josette Camilleri, BChD, MPhil, PhD, FIMMM, FADM Department of Restorative Dentistry, Faculty of Dental Surgery, Medical School, Mater Dei Hospital, University of Malta, Msida, Malta

Gustavo De Deus, DDS, MSc, PhD Department of Endodontics, Grande Rio University (UNIGRANRIO), Rio de Janeiro, RJ, Brazil

Paul Dummer, BDS, MScD, PhD, DDSc, FDSRCS(Ed) School of Dentistry, College of Biomedical and Life Sciences, Cardiff University, Cardiff, Wales, UK

Jamileh Ghoddusi, DDS, MSc Department of Endodontics, School of Dentistry, Mashhad University of Medical Sciences, Mashhad, Iran

Juliane Maria Guerreiro-Tanomaru, PhD Department of Restorative Dentistry, Araraquara School of Dentistry, UNESP – São Paulo State University, Araraquara, SP, Brazil

Marco Antonio Hungaro Duarte, PhD Department of Dentistry, Endodontics and Dental Materials, Bauru Dental School, University of Sao Paulo, Bauru, SP, Brazil

Carolyn M. Primus, PhD Primus Consulting, Bradenton, FL, USA

Mario Tanomaru-Filho, PhD Department of Restorative Dentistry, Araraquara School of Dentistry, UNESP – São Paulo State University, Araraquara, SP, Brazil

Franklin R. Tay, BDSc (Hons), PhD Department of Endodontics, Georgia Regents University College of Dental Medicine, Augusta, GA, USA

1 Introduction to Mineral Trioxide Aggregate

Gustavo De Deus, Josette Camilleri,
Carolyn M. Primus, Marco Antonio Hungaro Duarte,
and Clóvis Monteiro Bramante

1.1 Introduction

The first reported use of Portland cement in dental literature dates to 1878, when Dr. Witte in Germany published a case report on using Portland cement to fill root canals [92]. At that time, he would have been using a new material, since Portland cement was invented in 1824. No records exist of others following Dr. Witte's success or a further description of the materials he used, although we can surmise that he used a locally made Portland cement. Over a century later, Dr. Mahmoud Torabinejad at Loma Linda University and his coinventor Dean White obtained two US patents [89, 90] for a Portland cement-based endodontic material, which became known as mineral trioxide aggregate (MTA). Since then, over 20 new patents have been issued in the USA and EU for materials that include Portland cement for dentistry.

The term mineral trioxide aggregate (MTA) was coined for a dental material containing Portland cement blended with a radiopaque powder [87]. The name is suitable first because Portland cement is made from primarily three oxides: calcia, silica and alumina (CaO, SiO_2 and Al_2O_3). Secondly, minerals are used as the sources for the oxides that are fired in a furnace (kiln) to create an aggregation of phases. Lastly, aggregate refers to the addition of the radiopaque powder, analogous to the concrete industry that refers to the additions of sand and gravel to Portland cement as aggregate. Furthermore, the powder particles of cement are aggregations of the cement phases described hereafter.

1.2 Portland Cement

Portland cement is primarily tricalcium and dicalcium silicate powder made by firing oxides in a kiln. The invention of Portland cement is attributed to Joseph Aspin in 1824 in England, but his son improved the properties by raising the firing temperature and creating the modern firing regimen for Portland cement. Many other

G. De Deus, DDS, MSc, PhD
Department of Endodontics, Grande Rio University (UNIGRANRIO), Av. Henrique Dodsworth 85 apto 808 Lagoa, Rio de Janeiro, RJ 22061-030, Brazil
e-mail: endogus@gmail.com

J. Camilleri, BChD, MPhil, PhD, FIMMM, FADM (✉)
Department of Restorative Dentistry, Faculty of Dental Surgery, Medical School, Mater Dei Hospital, University of Malta, Msida, MSD 2090, Malta
e-mail: josette.camilleri@um.edu.mt

C.M. Primus, PhD
Primus Consulting, 7046 Owl's Nest Terrace, Bradenton, FL 34203, USA
e-mail: cprimus@me.com

M.A. Hungaro Duarte, PhD • C. Monteiro Bramante, PhD
Department of Dentistry, Endodontics and Dental Materials, Bauru Dental School, University of Sao Paulo, Al Octavio Pinheiro Brisola 9-75, Bauru, SP 17012-901, Brazil
e-mail: mhungaro@fob.usp.br; bramante@fob.usp.br; clobra@uol.com.br

J. Camilleri (ed.), *Mineral Trioxide Aggregate in Dentistry*,
DOI 10.1007/978-3-642-55157-4_1, © Springer-Verlag Berlin Heidelberg 2014

inventors can be credited for their contributions to the development of Portland cement manufacturing processes [60]. Prior to Portland cement, Egyptian, Greek and Roman civilizations used slaked lime (calcium hydroxide) mixed with a fine form of silica, such as volcanic ash or fly ash, a mixture denoted as pozzolanic cement. The pozzolanic reaction, in Eq. 1.1, is the hydration and reaction of a reactive, hydrated silica with calcium hydroxide (Portlandite):

$$\mathrm{Ca(OH)_2 + H_4SiO_4 \rightarrow Ca^{2+} + H_2SiO_4{}^{2-} + 2H_2O \rightarrow CaH_2SiO_4 \cdot 2H_2O} \quad (1.1)$$

Portland cement differs from these ancient cements because it contains the pre-reacted hydraulic calcium silicate powders rather than hydration of CaO or $Ca(OH)_2$ with silica. Higher compressive strengths were achieved with Portland cements, which supplanted the use of pozzolanic cement by the 1900s. However, pozzolanic materials (fine silica-containing powders) are now added to Portland cement to reduce the cost of Portland cement, improve workability, retard the setting time or reduce the amount of water needed.

For Portland cement, the raw materials, the formula, the phase proportions and the firing and grinding methods vary depending on the local raw materials and are different in every cement factory around the world. The raw materials usually are calcium carbonate blended with silica- and alumina-containing minerals, such as (1) limestone, shells or chalk for calcium oxide; (2) shale, clay, sand, slag for silicon oxide and aluminium oxide; and (3) iron ore. Although the materials vary widely, local raw materials are preferred, particularly the limestone, to keep the costs as low as possible. Although the ternary (three) oxides are sufficient to make a Portland cement, usually 5 % or less of iron oxide or iron is present in the raw materials for reasons explained below. The iron forms a dark-coloured phase, which imparts the usual grey colour to cement. For white Portland cement, the iron content of the raw materials is less than 0.5 %. Chromium, manganese, titanium copper or vanadium or magnesium oxides are also capable of colouring Portland cement. Firing of white cement requires higher temperatures or the additions of fluxes other than iron oxide, such as alumina or sodium and potassium oxides.

The formula for Portland cement is not unique, but covers a range of silica, alumina and calcia compositions. Materials scientists use phase diagrams to illustrate the equilibrium phase relationships of materials, usually over a range of temperatures. Figure 1.1a is a ternary phase diagram for the primary components: silica, alumina and calcia showing the various compounds that can be formed by firing the three oxides in various proportions. The range of Portland cement compositions is the area denoted by "P" in Fig. 1.1b, which includes primarily di- and tricalcium silicate phases and less tricalcium aluminate. Note that monocalcium silicate ($CaSiO_3$, also known as wollastonite) is not a hydraulic (water reactive) phase and is not part of Portland cement in Fig. 1.1.

Many standards have been developed for the construction cement industry, from compositional requirements to testing methods and requirements. For instance, Standard Specifications for Portland Cement (ASTM C150) [5] or Cement: Composition, Specifications and Conformity Criteria for Common Cements (EN 197-1) [47] standards for cement compositions restrict the magnesium oxide to less than 5 %. Magnesium oxide is commonly found with calcium compound deposits, just as it is present in the human bone (<5 %) but can expand when hydrated. Barium oxide and phosphorous pentoxide are common trace oxides found with calcium carbonate mineral deposits. Other common accessory oxides in Portland cement are sodium oxide, potassium oxide, titanium oxide, manganese oxide, nickel oxide, phosphorous pentoxide, barium oxide, chromium oxide and fluoride, usually in amounts less than 0.5 % and many at less than 100 ppm. The sodium oxide, potassium oxide, sulphates (from the raw materials or the fuel) and fluoride act as fluxing agents, reducing the firing temperature for Portland cement, which also reduces the cost for making the cement.

The powdered raw materials for Portland cement are blended and usually formed into

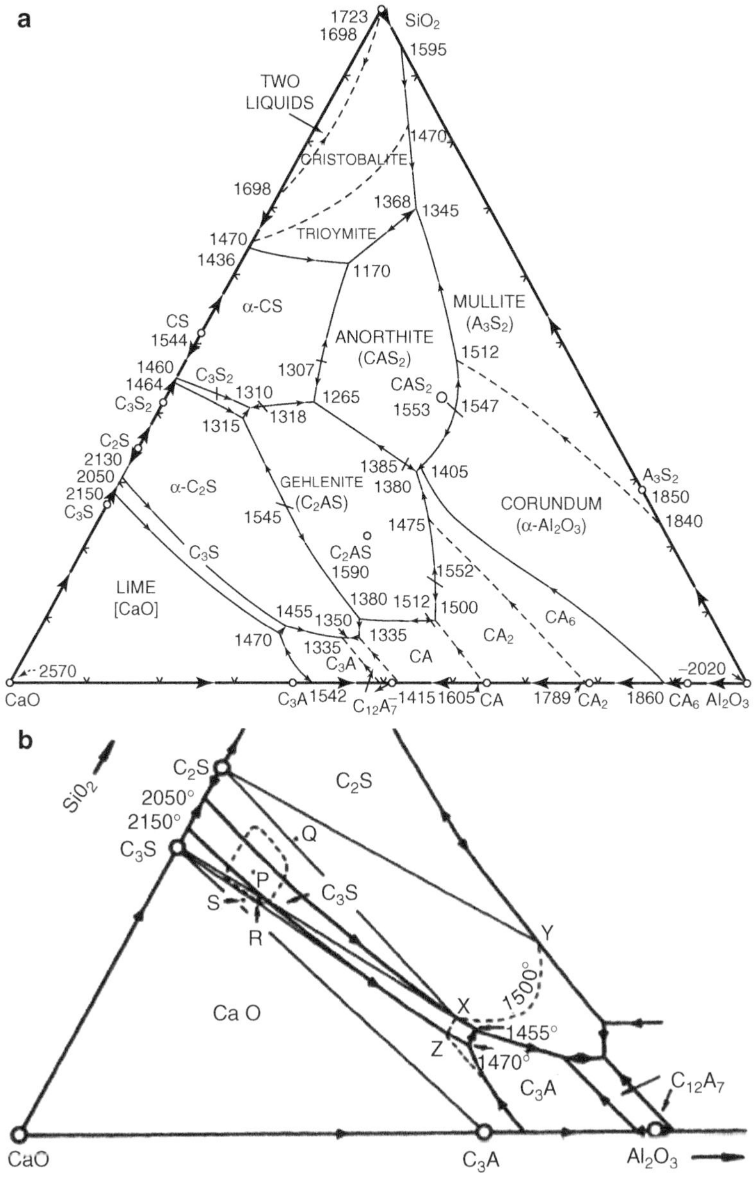

Fig. 1.1 (**a**) The ternary phase diagram for calcia, silica and alumina showing the many phases that can be formed by reaction of these three oxides at various temperatures (°F). Cement notation (abbreviations) is used for the phases. (**b**) Section of the ternary phase diagram in (**a**) showing the range of compositions *P* where Portland cement is formed of tricalcium silicate (C3S), dicalcium silicate (C2S) and tricalcium aluminate (C3A)

balls to feed into the kiln. Portland cement is economically manufactured in large furnaces called rotary kilns. During the first part of the firing process (up to about 850 °C), the calcium carbonate decomposes to calcium oxide releasing carbon dioxide, a process called calcining. The calcium oxide is retained in the powder mixture in the kiln and reacts with the silicate, alumina and iron oxide raw materials as the temperature is gradually raised to about 1,500 °C and new phases are formed: calcium silicates and aluminates. Figure 1.2 depicts a typical progression during firing from raw materials to formation of the cement phases. Some

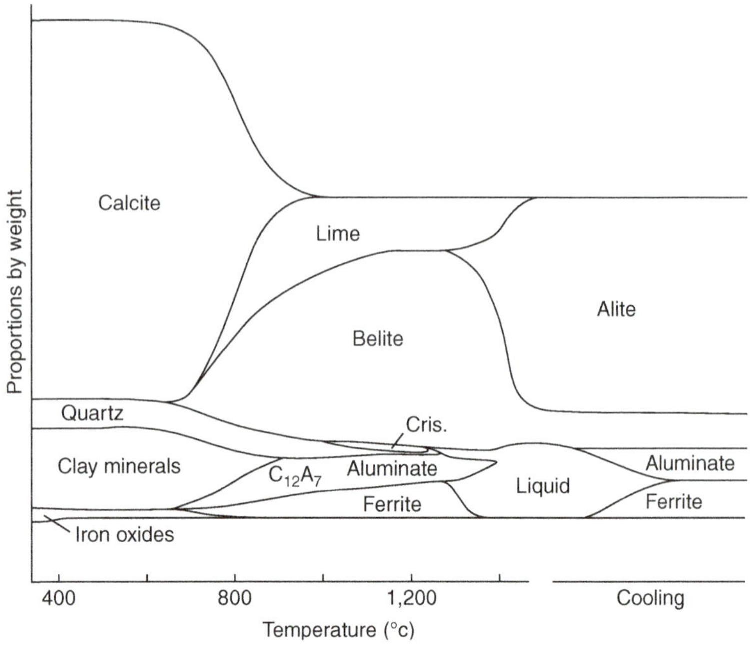

Fig. 1.2 In this diagram depicting firing of Portland cement, the formation of phases is depicted from the raw materials reacting and forming the calcium silicate, aluminate and ferrite phases

intermediate compounds are formed during firing, which react further as the temperature is increased. During firing, as much as 25 % liquid is formed in the material, which solidifies during cooling. This process, called liquid phase sintering, hastens reactions to form the calcium silicate phases and allows the firing temperature to be lower. The firing diagram depicts a starting material that included clay minerals and iron in the raw materials.

The reacted ceramic materials that exit the rotary kilns are large particles (>0.5 cm) called clinker, because of the sound they make when falling into a quenching bin after firing. The clinker nodules are porous and contain several ceramic phases as described below. Rapid cooling is preferred to prevent decomposition of alite to belite and lime (CaO) and to make the grinding easier. Air quenching is usually used to cool the clinker and ensure that only the beta phase of dicalcium silicate (β-C_2S) is formed thus preventing the formation of the gamma phase of dicalcium silicate ($\gamma - C_2S$). The beta phase is more hydraulic; that is, this crystalline form of the dicalcium silicate more readily forms hydrated C_2S, a benefit to the strength of Portland cement.

Keeping the energy and raw materials' costs low is the primary objective for Portland cement manufacturers, because it is a very price-sensitive commodity. Local materials, lower firing temperature, and minimal grinding are preferred which keep energy and transportation costs lower. Because of the price sensitivity, materials of lesser purity and lower quality fuels are used and grinding is minimized for manufacturing. For instance, worn out automobile tyres are added as a supplemental fuel in firing cement [30]. The raw materials and the fuels can contribute minor amounts of accessory oxides to the composition.

After firing, the clinker particles are crushed and ground to a powder so that most of the cement particles are smaller than 80 microns. Calcium sulphate as gypsum ($CaSO_4 \cdot 2H_2O$) is blended with the powder, usually by grinding the materials together (intergrinding). After grinding, the calcium sulphate may be present as the soluble anhydrite ($CaSO_4$) or hemihydrate $CaSO_4 \cdot ½H_2O$. Sometimes, other organic grinding aids or CaO are interground. The combined calcium silicate and calcium sulphate powder is called normal or "ordinary Portland cement" (OPC). The degree of grinding determines what type of cement is created; the types are defined in various cement standards including ASTM C150 [5]. Types I and III are the most common with Type III being a finer powder. The calcium sulphate is important for construction because it delays setting reactions in concrete as described below, which is very important for transporting mixed cement and for large concrete structure pouring.

1.3 Portland Cement Phases and Reactions

After manufacture, OPC contains several phases in the powder: alite (tricalcium silicate, C_3S), belite (dicalcium silicate, C_2S) and a lesser amount of tricalcium aluminate (C_3A) and calcium aluminoferrite (ferrite, C_4AF) phases. Free lime (CaO) may be present, but preferably in a minor amount, because lime is less hydraulically active. Cement scientists calculate the possible proportions of the cement phases from the raw materials using the Bogue calculation [86].

The alite crystals are very reactive with water and are usually present from 45 to 70 % of the OPC. Belite crystals are less reactive and the reaction is less exothermic; they usually constitute 5–30 % of an OPC powder. Tricalcium aluminate's hydration reaction is more exothermic than that of alite or belite. Ferrite also reacts with water, but weakly. The tricalcium aluminate and ferrite phases each typically constitute less than 10 % of an OPC. When observed microscopically, the alite crystals are elongated and hexagonal. Belite crystals are more rounded or equiaxed. Ferrite and aluminate phases are usually smaller and attached to alite or belite crystals. Free lime (CaO) forms thin hexagonal plates.

OPC reacts with water to form a solid mass of hydrated gel and unreacted cement particles via a complex and prolonged processes of exothermic setting and hardening reactions. The water to cement ratio is usually 0.3–0.7 by weight. Higher proportions of water generally increase porosity and permeability while decreasing the compressive strength. The reaction products of hydrated phases have been referred to as gels but are now referred to as amorphous reaction products. These processes are governed by the cement's phase composition, impurities in the phases, fineness of the powder and additions to the cement or water [86]. The cement literature describes the four stages of setting and hydration:

1. Preinduction, lasting a few minutes
2. Induction or dormant period, lasting a few hours
3. Acceleration, about 3–12 h after mixing
4. Post-acceleration from 12 h onwards

In Stage 1, the calcium sulphate, calcium aluminate and calcium aluminoferrite phases rapidly dissolve, and superficial hydration of the alite phase particles occurs. The calcium sulphate and calcium aluminate form ettringite, a hexacalcium aluminate trisulphate hydrate, of the general formula $(CaO)_6(Al_2O_3)(SO_3)_3 \cdot 32H_2O$, also written as $(CaO)_3(Al_2O_3)(CaSO_4)_3 \cdot 32H_2O$. Iron can substitute partially for the alumina, and carbonate can partially substitute for sulphate. These needle-like crystals grow in the liquid between particles. Without calcium sulphate, the tricalcium alumina hydrates rapidly, releasing heat, and the hydration causes the cement to become unworkable by quickly reacting with the water. This phenomenon is denoted as "flash setting". A similar phenomenon of false setting occurs when the sulphate is present as gypsum, not the anhydrite or hemihydrate. When hydration starts, the gypsum may start to precipitate quickly which gives the appearance of setting.

As the cement enters the acceleration stage, both the alite and belite react, as does the formation of ettringite. During Stage 1 or 2, the cement can be "remixed", which breaks up the nascent hydration structure. During Stage 2 the cement "sets", which is a gradual transition in cement from a fluid to a rigid state. Setting time is arbitrarily defined by laboratory testing procedures. Initial and final setting tests are described for cement, which are usually determined by using weighted needles to penetrate the cement surface, with either Vicat or Gillmore apparatus, as described later. This stiffening of the cement is a result of the water becoming part of the reaction products on the cement particles that begin to impinge on one another on the microscopic level.

Hydration of the alite crystals proceeds in Phase 3 reducing the free water, and more calcium hydroxide precipitates from the liquid. The hydration reaction for the tricalcium silicate phase that began in Phase 1 resumes following Eq. 1.2:

$$2Ca_3SiO_5 + 7H_2O \rightarrow 3CaO \cdot 2SiO_2 \cdot 4H_2O + 3Ca(OH)_2 \quad (1.2)$$

As the amount of non-hydrated material declines, hydration becomes a slower, diffusion-controlled process of the alite and belite particles. Some of the ettringite crystals dissolve to release tricalcium aluminate and calcium monosulphate ($3CaO \cdot Al_2O_3 + CaSO_4 \cdot 12H_2O$).

During Stage 4, the belite phase continues hydration following Eq. 1.3, forming the same surface reaction product as alite but releasing less portlandite:

$$2Ca_2SiO_4 + 5H_2O \rightarrow 3CaO \cdot 2SiO_2 \cdot 4H_2O + Ca(OH)_2 \quad (1.3)$$

Slow hydration continues at a decreasing rate, and the terminal amount of hydration is usually reached after about 4 weeks. Unreacted cement particles may remain in the solidified mass, each surrounded by a layer of hydrated reaction products. These hydration reactions occur minimally in the presence of moisture in the air. Hence, storing cement in bulk and protected from moisture is advantageous.

1.4 MTA and Portland Cement

MTA was invented by combining a grey Portland cement with bismuth oxide and used for endodontic applications [87, 90]. The original MTA materials contained the same tri- and dicalcium silicate major phases as Portland cement, with about 20 % bismuth oxide. Also, the original MTA products were expected to perform very similarly to OPC in setting, strengthening and hydrating, as was shown by Islam [58]. Unfortunately, the original description in the dental literature was erroneous and contained a description of MTA after reaction with water as [88]:

> calcium oxide and calcium phosphate .... The principle compounds present in this material are tricalcium silicate, tricalcium aluminate, tricalcium oxide, and silicate oxide. In addition, there are small amounts of a few other mineral oxides that are responsible for the chemical and physical properties of this aggregate. Bismuth oxide powder has been added to make the aggregate radiopaque. Electron probe microanalysis of MTA powder showed that calcium and phosphorous are the main ions present in this material.

This often quoted description is wrong from a chemical point of view because no compound exists known as tricalcium oxide, and silicate oxide is customarily written as silica or silicon oxide. As a result, this first article on the physical properties of MTA has confused other researchers who have examined MTA products [8]. Errors in the literature about the MTA material's compositions can be attributed to the researchers using only energy-dispersive spectroscopy (EDS) without confirmatory X-ray diffraction. EDS and energy-dispersive X-ray analysis (EDXA) (electron microprobe analysis) are techniques to identify the characteristic X-rays from the elements present in a material, but these techniques do not identify the compounds (phases). Frequently, researchers have reported the weight percentages of silicon oxide, calcium oxide, aluminium oxide and other metal oxides from EDS [61], EDXA [8], XRF or ICP tests but ignored the apportionment of the oxides into the crystalline phases such as tri- and dicalcium silicate, tricalcium aluminate or the presence of calcium carbonate. Although it is convenient to detect elements with an SEM equipped with EDS, the distribution of the phases by X-ray diffraction is equally important. Knowledge of the crystalline phases is essential because the phases determine the properties of the material and the body's response. Without knowing the compounds, a discussion of energy-dispersive X-ray spectroscopy (EDS) data is as erroneous as describing salt as sodium oxide and chlorine rather than sodium chloride. The X-ray diffraction analyses of MTA and the appropriate crystalline phases present have been reported [10, 19, 24, 57].

The initial reports from the MTA introduction period into the dental market stated that the material had a basic calcium and phosphorus composition [88]; currently, it is scientifically well established that MTA is comprised of about 80 % Portland cement, which has only trace amounts of phosphorous. The material's biocompatibility was regarded as a direct consequence of its chemical similarity with hard dental tissues [88]. However, later, it was correctly published that MTA was primarily comprised of tricalcium and dicalcium silicates [24], based on its composition including 80 % Portland cement.

In 1999, the *Journal of Endodontics* published an abstract of the study presented at the annual meeting of the American Association of Endodontists (AAE), in which MTA was experimentally compared to Portland cement [93]. In this study, MTA's and Portland's cement chemical composition and biocompatibility were analysed, and comparable results were found. This was the first time that MTA was scientifically compared to Portland cement. In the following year, Estrela et al. [45] published the first full study in which MTA was directly compared to Portland cement, concluding that both materials were chemically similar, apart from bismuth oxide (the radiopacifier agent) present in MTA. Moreover, Portland cement and MTA were reported to have similar pH and antibacterial capacity. In the following year, Holland et al. [51] also observed similar results between MTA and Portland cement on direct pulp protection of dog's teeth.

After initial reports, various studies were published comparing MTA with Portland cement. The main reasons behind these research efforts were the high price ($50 per gram) of the only MTA product, ProRoot® MTA from Dentsply Tulsa Dental, USA, and the possibility of developing a low-cost alternative repair cement. Spångberg [83] summarized the situation well in 2006, when he stated that "ProRoot MTA (Dentsply, Johnson City, TN) is a new material, but for practical purposes is not very different from Portland cement. The factor responsible for the beneficial effects in ProRoot is also found in Portland cement". At the same time, concerns arose about the possible toxic metal content of Portland cement and MTA. However, Spångberg [83] wrote that "Considering the number of uncontrolled toxic materials dentists are allowed to use clinically, such as formaldehyde, cresol, mercury, phenol, eugenol … to name a few, less than half a gram of Portland cement seems like an innocuous amount". Complaints about the poor handling, slow setting and high price persisted, and many articles were written comparing Portland cement with ProRoot MTA or MTA-Angelus products (Angelus, Londrina, Brazil). Chapter 7 describes the properties of these materials in more detail. Some tested the clinical use of Portland cement [38] as an apical plug in the treatment of an open apex tooth with apical radiolucency. The clinical and radiographic follow-up showed treatment success (Fig. 1.3a–d).

More than 150 studies compared MTA to Portland cement, reinforcing the similarities with the exception of bismuth oxide present in the first two MTA products. Thus, it can be concluded that MTA is a kind of Portland cement especially produced for dental use [8, 24, 45, 58]. Additionally, it was ascertained that MTA has less iron-3 (Fe_3) and aluminium compounds than Portland cement [34]. Another difference between the two materials is the particle size; MTA has smaller and more regular particles than common Portland cement [34, 59].

Several researchers have raised concerns about heavy metal contamination of both grey and white MTA, believing that the arsenic or lead levels exceeded those permitted in ISO 9917-1:2007 for powder/liquid acid–base dental cements [55], namely, 2 or 100 ppm of acid-extractable arsenic or lead. These concerns arise from comparisons to construction-grade Portland cements, which are known to contain metal oxides including arsenic. Various construction-grade Portland cements have been tested as a substitute for MTA products because MTA is expensive when compared to other dental cements [1, 7, 58]. MTA is claimed to be produced under controlled conditions, resulting in a pure and well-controlled hydraulic cement powder, composed of contamination-free biocompatible particles. This is an important issue, since repair cements are classified as permanent-contact implant devices with the potential of

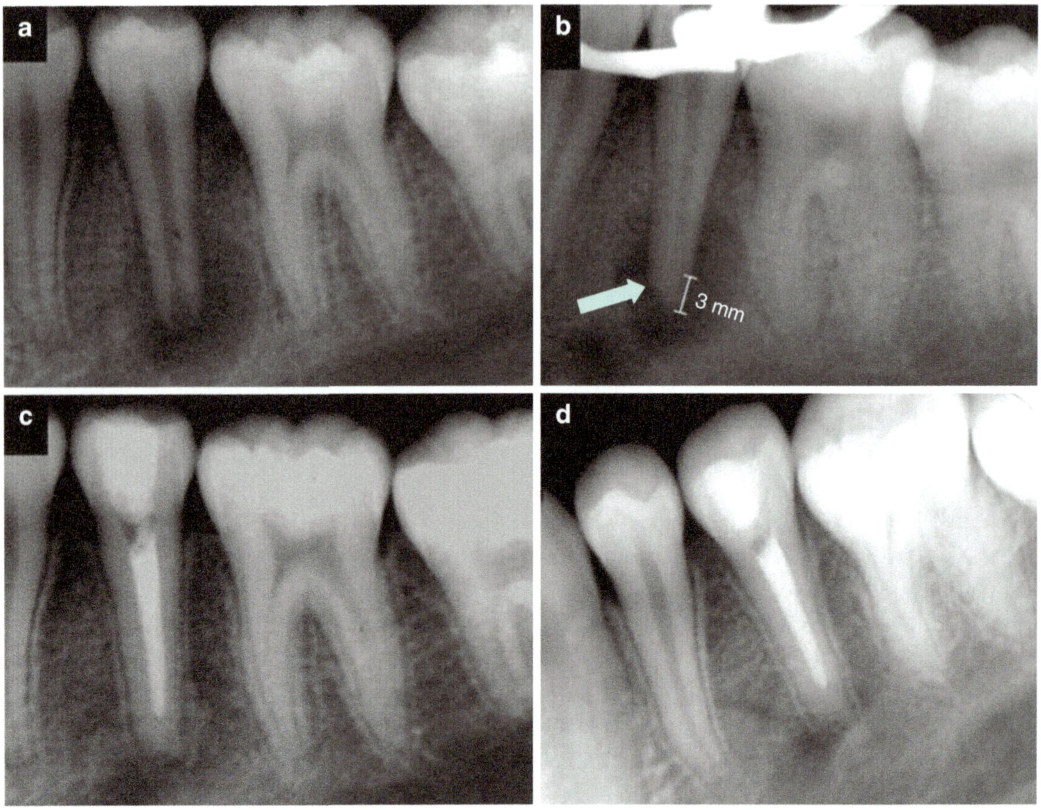

Fig. 1.3 Case report showing the use of white Portland cement as an apical plug in a tooth with a necrotic pulp and wide-open apex. (**a**) Preoperative radiograph of the mandibular left premolar. Note the wide-open apex and periapical radiolucent lesion. (**b**) Preoperative radiograph with WCP placed at the apical portion of the canal (approximately 3 mm). (**c**) Immediate postoperative radiograph with root canal filling and white Portland cement in the apical third. (**d**) One-year postoperative radiograph confirming healing of the periapical region

causing damage or irritation of the periapical tissue and delaying wound healing.

Studies have measured the total (not acid-extracted) arsenic (Table 1.1) in Portland cements and MTA products and found amounts that exceed the ISO 9917-1:2007 [55] limits. However, white Portland cement and white MTA have lower arsenic contents than their grey counterparts. Overall results of the heavy metals in both MTA and some Portland cement brands are negligible [81] and less than 10 ppm. Moreover, it must be understood that although hydraulic cements may have higher amounts of contaminants than those established by ISO 9917-1:2007 [55], leaching in solution is low (Table 1.2) [42, 81] as arsenic oxide is dissolved in the silicate and is relatively insoluble [39].

Table 1.1 Amount of arsenic in MTA and some commercial brands of Portland cement

Material	Arsenic (mg/kg) or (mg/g)
CPM	11.06
CPM sealer	10.30
MTA-Obtura	0.39
MTA-Experimental	10.13
White MTA-Angelus	1.03
Grey MTA-Angelus	5.91
ProRoot MTA	5.25
Grey Portland cement	34.27
White Portland cement	0.52

Adapted from Monteiro Bramante et al. [66]

Portland cement powder has insufficient radiopacity (<3 mm equivalent Al) [54] for dental materials as required in ADA 57 [4] and ISO

Table 1.2 Arsenic release (ppm) by MTA and some commercial brands of Portland cement

	Votoran		Ribeirão		Irajá branco		ProRoot		MTA Angelus	
P	3 h	168 h	3 h	168 h	3 h	168 h	3 h	168 h	3 h	168 h
M	0.0007	0.0003	0.0002	0.0002	0.0002	0.0002	0.0002	0.0002	0.0002	0.0002
DP	0.0006	0.0002	0	0	0	0	0	0	0	0

Adapted from Duarte et al. [42]

6876 [56] standard specifications. MTA's radiopacity was first achieved by blending bismuth oxide with the tricalcium silicate powder. ProRoot MTA has on average 7.5 mm Al [20], while MTA-Angelus has about 5.7 mm Al [17]. Lower radiopacity is attributed to less bismuth oxide in MTA-Angelus with the latter having 14 % bismuth oxide [27] as opposed to ProRoot MTA, which contains 20 % [10, 19]. Larger particle sizes or poorer dispersion also causes variations in radiopacity. The radiopacifier may affect the hydration and final properties of the cement. Bismuth oxide reduced compressive strength and increased porosity, as well as diminished the cellular growth [26, 32]. Leaching of bismuth in solution has also been reported [20]. Furthermore tooth discolouration has been associated with bismuth oxide in MTA [11]. Studies have tested the radiopacity imparted to raw Portland cement by higher molecular weight additions of gold and silver [20], zirconium oxide, calcium tungstate, zinc oxide, iodoform and barium sulphate [20, 54] (Table 1.3). Zirconium oxide has been studied as an alternative radiopacifing agent with the advantage of not affecting cement hydration as well as improving cement mixture homogeneity and consistency [22]. However, its atomic number is rather low compared to the usual dental radiopaque agents.

Similar results have been measured for the pH and calcium release by MTA and Portland cement [20, 58]. Portland cement demonstrates a higher calcium release ability than MTA due to the higher percentage of tricalcium silicate [18, 19, 73]. Moreover, it is important to note that biomineralization phenomenon (formation of hydroxyapatite in vivo) of both MTA and Portland cement has been demonstrated [76] (Fig. 1.4).

Table 1.3 Radiopacity (mm Al) of dentin and pure Portland cement and its association with different radiopacifing agents

Material	Average	SD
Portland cement + bismuth carbonate	3.25	± 0.38
Portland cement + iodoform	4.24	± 0.32
Portland cement + bismuth oxide	5.93	± 0.34
Portland cement + lead oxide	5.74	± 0.66
Portland cement + zinc oxide	2.64	± 0.02
Portland cement + zirconium oxide	3.41	± 0.19
Portland cement + barium sulphate	2.80	± 0.18
Portland cement + bismuth subnitrate	4.66	± 0.42
Portland cement + calcium tungstate	3.11	± 0.25
Pure Portland cement	1.01	± 0.01
Dentin	1.74	± 0.02

Adapted from Húngaro Duarte et al. [54]

The setting time of the original MTA products is too long for dental procedures. White versions of ProRoot MTA and MTA-Angelus have been reported to have initial and final setting times of about 40 and 140 min, and grey ProRoot, initial and final setting times of about 70 and 175 min [15, 16]. MTA-Angelus is believed to lack calcium sulphate, which is an effective setting retardant. In Portland cements, an initial and final setting time of about 70 and 170 min for the grey one has been observed, while white Portland cement requires 40 and 135 min for the initial and final setting time [58]. These differences may not be significant since there are interobservational differences for the subjective setting time test, as noted in the next section. All these times are significantly longer than other dental cements but shorter than some endodontic sealers. Calcium chloride has been added to MTA and Portland cement to shorten the initial setting time [58] and may increase sealing, pH and

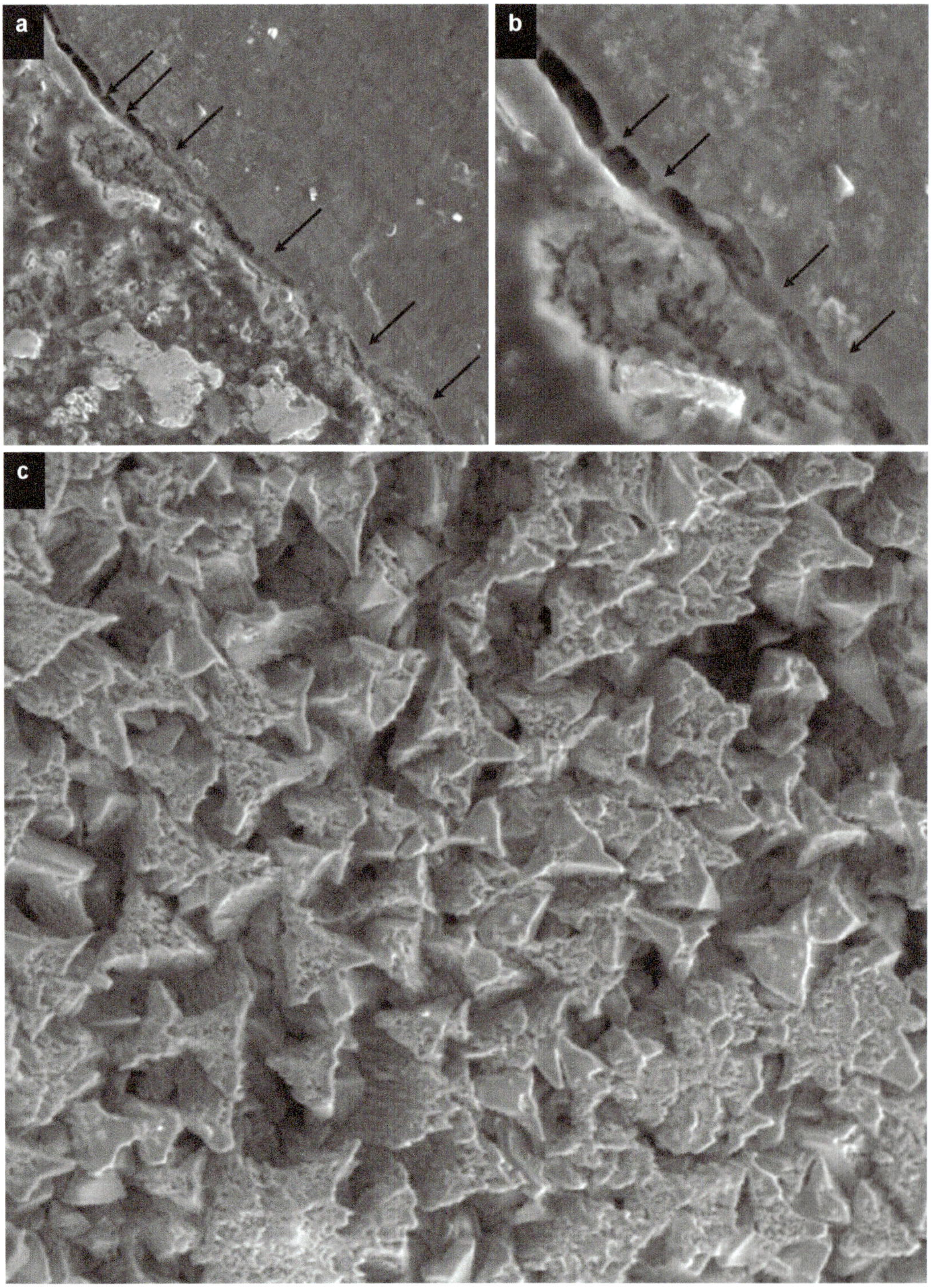

Fig. 1.4 Biomineralization (**a**, **b**) and superficial crystal formation (**c**) on white MTA-Angelus in phosphate buffered saline [76]

calcium release [14–16]. MTA solubility may be equal to or slightly less than Portland cements [21, 35, 58].

The sealability results show that Portland cement and MTA are quite comparable, even using different leakage models. Comparison of MTA and Portland cement sealability using a bacterial leakage model [40] and fluid transport [37, 41] exhibited similar results. This finding is in line with other results published on sealing ability of MTA and Portland cement [13, 82].

The biological responses of MTA and Portland cement have been compared by in vitro and in vivo assays. In vitro results from cell culture largely reported low cytotoxicity and no genotoxicity by MTA and Portland cements [77, 79, 80]. In subcutaneous tissue of mice, the tissue reactions were the same for MTA and Portland cement [52, 78], promoting calcium carbonate granule formation, even when iodoform was added as a radiopacifier agent [36]. In pulp capping and pulpotomy for dog's teeth, both MTA and Portland cement have shown similar results [51, 65]. Portland cement was successfully employed in vivo as an apical plug in the treatment of a wide-open apex tooth with apical lesion [38] and also in primary teeth pulpotomies.

1.5 Comparison of White and Grey MTA Products

The original MTA, dark grey in colour, was the first commercial product ProRoot® MTA (Dentsply, Tulsa Dental, Johnson City, TN, USA) in 1998. In 2002, the "tooth-colored ProRoot MTA" was introduced and later patented [75], a material often designated in the literature as white MTA. The grey and white versions of ProRoot MTA have similar compositions, but the tooth-coloured ProRoot MTA has less iron, roughly 5 versus 0.5 % iron oxide, respectively, as observed using energy-dispersive spectroscopy (EDS) [9, 24]. The white MTA was reported to have a finer particle size [9]. As described before iron oxide creates the calcium aluminoferrite phase during manufacture of Portland cement. The ferrite phase reduces the temperatures for cement manufacture. Regardless of the compositional differences, the biocompatibility of the grey and white versions are similar [26]. However, the first report for a prototype product of white ProRoot MTA exhibited less biocompatibility when tested using osteosarcoma cells than the grey version [72].

Portland cements are known for their dimensional stability over time. Grey MTA is believed to expand more than white MTA (1 vs. 0.1 %) in water or 0.7 versus 0.1 % in Hank's balanced salt solution [85]. In another test of grey and white ProRoot MTA materials, higher expansion was measured for the grey versus the white products (2.6 vs. 0.08 %), but varying the water/powder ratio did not affect the setting expansion [50].

No significant differences in microleakage have been reported between grey and white MTA as a root-end filling material [62] nor when used as apical barrier [84]. Conversely, grey MTA-Angelus product exhibited better sealing ability when used as an apical plug [31]. In a test of marginal adaptation, no significant differences were measured among white MTA, grey MTA and Portland cement [12]. Blood contamination has a detrimental effect on the surface micro-hardness of MTA. If blood or serum contamination is unavoidable, white MTA [68] may be preferred because it had higher surface hardness.

White and grey MTA materials have exhibited the same beneficial clinical outcome when used to treat pulpotomized primary molars [48] and as a pulp-capping agent in treatment of vital teeth [44, 70]: good biological response with no genotoxic effects [79]. Although there is evidence of a very good biological response with both types of MTA, grey MTA showed significantly higher percentage of dentine bridge formation than white MTA [28]. Histological assessment of grey and white MTA indicated that although both materials were well tolerated, supported cell attachment, proliferation and matrix formation [3, 91], more inflammation was associated with white MTA [71]. Addition of chlorhexidine to MTA resulted in tissue inflammation in the white MTA, but the grey was well tolerated [94]. Using MDPC-23 cells and XTT assay, two grey MTA products had higher cell viability than white MTA. In this test, grey and white MTA products had intracellular reactive oxygen species formation compared with untreated cells, although cells exposed to white MTA were not significantly different from untreated cells [43]. Both grey and white MTA were antimicrobial under aerobic conditions and damaged bacterial DNA [78]. *E. faecalis* and *S. sanguis* to MTA were more susceptible to damage by white MTA than grey MTA [2].

To date, the differences in colour were a result of a difference in iron oxide between grey and white MTA products under the brand names ProRoot and Angelus. By the end of 2013, more than a dozen new MTA-type products have been introduced that have various colours, particle sizes and formulas, as described in Chap. 8. The influence of the compositions on properties and performance is open for research. At this time, no one product or composition has shown superiority in all physical and in vivo performance.

1.6 Standards Used to Test Properties of MTA

International standards have been developed for many dental products, and committees exist to continually improve the suitability and the test methods for dentistry. Although MTA has been popular for root-end filling, no dental standard exists for root-end filling materials. Prior to MTA's introduction, materials for root-end filling were not unique; that is, amalgam or other zinc oxide eugenol-based restorative materials were used. MTA products are not used as restoratives, and most MTA products are not used as root canal sealers for which standards exist. This gap in testing standards has allowed researchers to apply any test from dental or cement standards to compare materials. This has also created a body of literature where comparisons are difficult because of the variety of test procedures. The slow setting and gradual strengthening of most MTA products over 4 weeks has also created new challenges for dental material methods to compare and evaluate MTA-type materials.

The International Standards Organization (ISO) or American Dental Association (ADA) specifications for root canal sealers do not require strength tests however, this relatively easy in vitro test has been used to compare MTA materials. Compressive strength has been measured but is not an essential property for root-end fillers because such materials are not subjected to occlusion or other dislodging forces. Compressive strength is commonly tested for restoratives, and also for Portland cements. Many researchers and manufacturers have used the ISO 9917-1 [55] compressive strength test. In this standard, the compressive strength testing method is performed after 1 day, which is much too short for the original MTA products so longer times are used. The results of compressive strength of MTA and tricalcium silicate-based materials are dependent on the same factors as Portland cement [25] including the liquid to cement ratio, the shape and size of the specimen, the sample preparation, the loading rate [25, 69] and condensation pressure during sample preparation [67]. When using cylindrical specimens, the flatness and parallelism of the ends are essential, otherwise the contact area between the specimen and the bearing plate is changed. The effect of changes in the water to powder ratio on the physical properties and hydration of MTA has been described above and also in Chapter 2. ISO 9917 [55] specifies the use of cylindrical specimens with a diameter of 4 and 6 mm high for compressive strength testing. These moulds have been used in various studies investigating the compressive strength of MTA [67, 88]. Other researchers have used different sized moulds (12 mm in length and 6 mm in diameter) [58]. Cylindrical specimens with a height to diameter ratio of 2 are commonly used in Portland cement research [25], because the strength of cylinders for height to diameter ratio of 2 is not influenced by the restraining effects of the loading plates, a phenomenon well understood in materials science. Values higher than 2 may lead to buckling of the specimens, and lower values require the use of a correction factor when calculating the compressive strength.

Setting of MTA products is quite different from other dental materials. The hydration process, particularly for dicalcium silicate phase in MTA, occurs over a period of about 4 weeks. No other dental material matures over such a long period of time. A second issue for testing the setting of MTA materials is the need for water during setting; drying conditions must be avoided. The current ISO 6876 standard for root canal sealer [56] specifies smaller diameter, shallower plaster moulds for sealers that require water to set versus sealers that do not require water, which complicates testing and comparisons.

The ISO 6876 [56] setting procedure also requires adding excess water to the sealers that require water for setting, a procedure that is necessary for traditional root canal formulas in vitro. Adding water is not suitable for MTA products because it changes the manufacturer's directions for use, and the physical properties of hydraulic cements depend on the water to cement ratio. Adding water diminishes the compressive strength and increases the setting time for MTA, while a low water to powder ratio, or drying conditions, will reduce strength and appear to cause setting by incomplete hydration. Factors that increase the suitable water to powder ratio include a high surface area of the powders, less radiopaque powder or radiopaque powder of a lower molecular weight [23]. Researchers who have created experimental powders and changed the radiopacifier to a much higher or lower molecular weight will note the changes in consistency of the mixtures. The usual radiopaque powders are non-cementitious and do not contribute to the kinetics of the hydration reaction. When MTA powders are mixed with excess liquid, usually the setting is slower, the mixture is less viscous, more pores will develop and the compressive strength will be lower [33].

Setting time determinations have been made by several methods, and the terms initial and final setting are also used. The ISO 6876 [56] and ISO 9917-1 standards [55] use flat cylindrical indenters of two sizes and two weights, but do not refer to an initial and a final setting time. The lighter weight and larger diameter needle is specified in ISO 6876 [56] for root canal sealers, and the heavier weight and smaller diameter needle is specified for water-based cements in ISO 9917-1 [55]. These setting time assessment tests are based on the visual inspection of a Gillmore needle's impression into a cement surface, which is subjective. Setting time comparisons are complicated by some authors using the heavier Gillmore weight for their tests [29, 53, 74], which necessarily will make the setting times longer than those who use the lighter weight Gillmore needle [63]. The quantity of material tested affects the results of setting time testing, which has also made comparison of data difficult since most investigators adapt moulds for testing rather than using the precise moulds specified by the particular standard [14, 49, 58, 64]. Automatic Vicat apparatus has been used by some, but the ability to use the device at 37 °C without dry-out has not been documented. Working time is defined based on flow under a weight for root canal sealers, which may be interpreted as an initial setting time. A student reviewing the literature must be alert to the test method used by the researcher; particularly the mould size, the needle diameter and the weight of the Vicat and Gilmore setting time apparatus referred to in the literature.

ASTM C266 [6] for Portland cements specifies the initial and final setting time to be determined with a lighter, larger diameter needle and then with a heavier, smaller diameter needle. However, this standard is designed for the cement industry and requires 1,650 g in a mould 100 by 5 mm thick, which is much larger than most dental samples. A Vicat apparatus is specified for cement in EN 196-3; 2005 [46] which uses two needles, weight for both being 300 g, and requires 400 g of cement.

Micro-hardness has been tested for MTA products, but is not required for endodontic materials in ISO or ADA standards. Micro-hardness testing is performed by applying a load to a material surface using a diamond indenter. The most common test is the Vickers, which uses a diamond-shaped indenter; others have used the Knoop indenter that has an elongated pyramidal shape. MTA is composed of multiple phases of varied hardness that adds variation to hardness measurements, depending on where the small diamond indenter is placed on the sample. Furthermore, some researchers have not followed good sample preparation procedures to create polished samples for indentation. Micro-hardness measures surface properties of materials and has not been shown to have clinical relevance to the performance of MTA-type products.

The dimensional stability of materials is predictive of shrinkage or expansion and has been specified for root canal sealers in ISO 6876 [56] to be less than 1 % shrinkage and less than 0.1 % expansion after 30 days. However, the newest version of ISO 6876: 2012 [56] eliminated this requirement. The earlier version of ISO 6876 and the ADA 57 test method specified the measurement of the change in length of cylindrical samples stored in water for 30 days. This method measures dimensional changes in one direction and assumes the material is isotropic. A novel method has been developed where by a linear variable displacement transducer (LVDT) for accurate measurement in the vertical direction is used, with horizontal restraint of the specimen in a metal mould [21, 85]. Large changes in dimensions are certainly unwanted in any endodontic material because of the potential for leakage or cracking of the root for shrinkage or expansion, respectively. The values measured for the MTA materials have attested to the small dimensional variations that are characteristic of their Portland cement "heritage".

Conclusions

Tricalcium silicate is the main constituent of MTA and was adopted for dentistry from construction-grade Portland cement. Radiopaque powders are a necessary addition to tricalcium silicate for dental products. In addition to tricalcium silicate, MTA products usually contain other cementitious phases including dicalcium silicate, with minor amounts of tricalcium aluminate, calcium sulphate or grey-coloured calcium aluminoferrite. This powdered material when mixed with water forms a hard, high pH, dimensionally stable material with remarkable biocompatibility. The hydration process is complex, and the strengthening of the tricalcium silicates continues over about 4 weeks. Both grey and white MTA products are available, analogous to construction-grade Portland cements. No definitive histological studies have shown a superiority of any one product or the grey versus the white versions. Ordinary Portland cement should not be used clinically, because a clinician would not know its purity, its particle size will be coarse and the material will not be sufficiently radiopaque. Despite the over 1,000 articles that have been written about MTA and root-end filling material, no dental standards exist for testing MTA specifically, accounting for its unique properties. Existing test methods for dental materials and cements have been adapted by researchers for evaluation of the MTA products and experimental alternatives.

References

1. Aguilar FG, da Fonseca Roberti Garcia L, Rossetto HL, Pardini LC, de Carvalho Panzeri Pires-de-Souz F. Radiopacity evaluation of calcium aluminate cement containing different radiopacifying agents. J Endod. 2011;37(1):67–71.
2. Al-Hezaimi K, Al-Shalan TA, Naghshbandi J, Oglesby S, Simon JH, Rotstein I. Antibacterial effect of two mineral trioxide aggregate (MTA) preparations against *Enterococcus faecalis* and *Streptococcus sanguis* in vitro. J Endod. 2006;32(11):1053–6.
3. Al-Rabeah E, Perinpanayagam H, MacFarland D. Human alveolar bone cells interact with ProRoot and tooth-colored MTA. J Endod. 2006;32(9):872–5.
4. American Dental Association. Council on Dental Materials. Specification nº 57 for endodontic filling material, Chicago, 2000.
5. American Standards for Testing Materials. ASTM C 150: Standard specification for Portland cement. West Conshohocken: ASTM International; 2012.
6. American Standards for Testing Materials. ASTM C266; Standard Test Method for time of setting of hydraulic-cement paste by Gillmore needles. West Conshohocken: ASTM International; 2013.
7. Asgary S, Eghbal MJ, Parirokh M, Ghoddusi J. Effect of two storage solutions on surface topography of two root-end fillings. Aust Endod J. 2009;35(3):147–52.
8. Asgary S, Eghbal MJ, Parirokh M, Ghoddusi J, Kheirieh S, Brink F. Comparison of mineral trioxide aggregate's composition with Portland cements and a new endodontic cement. J Endod. 2009;35(2):243–50.
9. Asgary S, Parirokh M, Eghbal MJ, Stowe S, Brink F. A qualitative X-ray analysis of white and grey mineral trioxide aggregate using compositional imaging. J Mater Sci Mater Med. 2006;17(2):187–91.

10. Belio-Reyes IA, Bucio L, Cruz-Chavez E. Phase composition of ProRoot mineral trioxide aggregate by X-ray powder diffraction. J Endod. 2009;35(6):875–8.
11. Belobrov I, Parashos P. Treatment of tooth discoloration after the use of white mineral trioxide aggregate. J Endod. 2011;37(7):1017–20.
12. Bidar M, Moradi S, Jafarzadeh H, Bidad S. Comparative SEM study of the marginal adaptation of white and grey MTA and Portland cement. Aust Endod J. 2007;33(1):2–6.
13. Borges AH, Pedro FL, Semanoff-Segundo A, Miranda CE, Pécora JD, Cruz Filho AM. Radiopacity evaluation of Portland and MTA-based cements by digital radiographic system. J Appl Oral Sci. 2011;19(3):228–32.
14. Bortoluzzi EA, Broon NJ, Bramante CM, Felippe WT, Tanomaru Filho M, Esberard RM. The influence of calcium chloride on the setting time, solubility, disintegration, and pH of mineral trioxide aggregate and white Portland cement with a radiopacifier. J Endod. 2009;35(4):550–4.
15. Bortoluzzi EA, Broon NJ, Bramante CM, Garcia RB, Moraes IG, Bernardineli N. Sealing ability of MTA and radiopaque Portland cement with or without calcium chloride for root-end filling. J Endod. 2006;32(9):897–900.
16. Bortoluzzi EA, Broon NJ, Duarte MAH, Demarchi ACCO, Bramante CM. The use of a setting accelerator and its effect on ph and calcium ion release of mineral trioxide aggregate and white Portland cement. J Endod. 2006;32(12):1194–7.
17. Bortoluzzi EA, Guerreiro-Tanomaru JM, Tanomaru-Filho M, Duarte MA. Radiographic effect of different radiopacifiers on a potential retrograde filling material. Oral Surg Oral Med Oral Pathol Oral Radiol Endod. 2009;108(4):628–32.
18. Camilleri J. Hydration mechanisms of mineral trioxide aggregate. Int Endod J. 2007;40(6):462–70.
19. Camilleri J. Characterization of hydration products of mineral trioxide aggregate. Int Endod J. 2008;41(5):408–17.
20. Camilleri J. Evaluation of the physical properties of an endodontic Portland cement incorporating alternative radiopacifiers used as root-end filling material. Int Endod J. 2010;43(3):231–40.
21. Camilleri J. Evaluation of the effect of intrinsic material properties and ambient conditions on the dimensional stability of white mineral trioxide aggregate and Portland cement. J Endod. 2011;37(2):239–45.
22. Camilleri J, Cutajar A, Mallia B. Hydration characteristics of zirconium oxide replaced Portland cement for use as a root-end filling material. Dent Mater. 2011;27(8):845–54.
23. Camilleri J, Gandolfi MG. Evaluation of the radiopacity of calcium silicate cements containing different radiopacifiers. Int Endod J. 2010;43(1):21–30.
24. Camilleri J, Montesin FE, Brady K, Sweeney R, Curtis RV, Ford TR. The constitution of mineral trioxide aggregate. Dent Mater. 2005;21(4):297–303.
25. Camilleri J, Montesin FE, Curtis RV, Ford TR. Characterization of Portland cement for use as a dental restorative material. Dent Mater. 2006;22(6):569–75.
26. Camilleri J, Montesin FE, Papaioannou S, McDonald F, Pitt Ford TR. Biocompatibility of two commercial forms of mineral trioxide aggregate. Int Endod J. 2004;37(10):699–704.
27. Camilleri J, Sorrentino F, Damidot D. Investigation of the hydration and bioactivity of radiopacified tricalcium silicate cement, Biodentine and MTA Angelus. Dent Mater. 2013;29(5):580–93.
28. Cardoso-Silva C, Barbería E, Maroto M, García-Godoy F. Clinical study of Mineral Trioxide Aggregate in primary molars. Comparison between Grey and White MTA – a long term follow-up (84 months). J Dent. 2011;39(2):187–93.
29. Charland T, Hartwell GR, Hirschberg C, Patel R. An evaluation of setting time of mineral trioxide aggregate and EndoSequence root repair material in the presence of human blood and minimal essential media. J Endod. 2013;39(8):1071–2.
30. Chen JH, Chen KS, Tong LY. On the pyrolysis kinetics of scrap automotive tires. J Hazard Mater. 2001;84(1):43–55.
31. Coneglian PZ, Orosco FA, Bramante CM, de Moraes IG, Garcia RB, Bernardineli N. In vitro sealing ability of white and grey mineral trioxide aggregate (MTA) and white Portland cement used as apical plugs. J Appl Oral Sci. 2007;15(3):181–5.
32. Coomaraswamy KS, Lumley PJ, Hofmann MP. Effect of bismuth oxide radiopacifier content on the material properties of an endodontic Portland cement-based (MTA-like) system. J Endod. 2007;33(3):295–8.
33. Cutajar A, Mallia B, Abela S, Camilleri J. Replacement of radiopacifier in mineral trioxide aggregate; characterization and determination of physical properties. Dent Mater. 2011;27(9):879–91.
34. Dammaschke T, Gerth HU, Züchner H, Schäfer E. Chemical and physical surface and bulk material characterization of white ProRoot MTA and two Portland cements. Dent Mater. 2005;21(8):731–8.
35. Danesh G, Dammaschke T, Gerth HU, Zandbiglari T, Schäfer E. A comparative study of selected properties of ProRoot mineral trioxide aggregate and two Portland cements. Int Endod J. 2006;39(3):213–19.
36. de Morais CA, Bernardineli N, Garcia RB, Duarte MA, Guerisoli DM. Evaluation of tissue response to MTA and Portland cement with iodoform. Oral Surg Oral Med Oral Pathol Oral Radiol Endod. 2006;102(3):417–21.
37. De-Deus G, Audi C, Murad C, Fidel S, Fidel R. Similar expression of through-and-through fluid movement along orthograde apical plugs of MTA Bio and white Portland cement. Int Endod J. 2008;41(12):1047–53.
38. De-Deus G, Coutinho-Filho T. The use of white Portland cement as an apical plug in a tooth with a necrotic pulp and wide-open apex: a case report. Int Endod J. 2007;40(8):653–60.

39. De-Deus G, de Souza MC, Sergio Fidel RA, Fidel SR, de Campos RC, Luna AS. Negligible expression of arsenic in some commercially available brands of Portland cement and mineral trioxide aggregate. J Endod. 2009;35(6):887–90.
40. De-Deus G, Petruccelli V, Gurgel-Filho E, Coutinho-Filho T. MTA versus Portland cement as repair material for furcal perforations: a laboratory study using a polymicrobial leakage model. Int Endod J. 2006;39(4):293–8.
41. De-Deus G, Reis C, Brandão C, Fidel S, Fidel RS. The ability of Portland cement, MTA and MTA Bio to prevent through-and-through fluid movement in repaired furcal perforations. J Endod. 2007;33(11): 1374–7.
42. Duarte MA, De Oliveira Demarchi AC, Yamashita JC, Kuga MC, De Campos FS. Arsenic release provided by MTA and Portland cement. Oral Surg Oral Med Oral Pathol Oral Radiol Endod. 2005;99(5):648–50.
43. Eid AA, Gosier JL, Primus CM, Hammond BD, Susin LF, Pashley DH, et al. In vitro biocompatibility and oxidative stress profiles of different hydraulic calcium silicate cements. J Endod. 2014;40(2):255–60.
44. Eskandarizadeh A, Shahpasandzadeh MH, Shahpasandzadeh M, Torabi M, Parirokh M. A comparative study on dental pulp response to calcium hydroxide, white and grey mineral trioxide aggregate as pulp capping agents. J Conserv Dent. 2011; 14(4):351–5.
45. Estrela C, Bammann LL, Estrela CR, Silva RS, Pécora JD. Antimicrobial and chemical study of MTA, Portland cement, calcium hydroxide paste, Sealapex and Dycal. Braz Dent J. 2000;11(1):3–9.
46. European Standards. Methods of testing cement. Determination of setting time and soundness. EN 196-3. London: British Standards Institutions; 2005.
47. European Standards. Cement composition, specifications and conformity criteria for common cements. EN 197-1. London: British Standards Institutions; 2011.
48. Frenkel G, Kaufman A, Ashkenazi M. Clinical and radiographic outcomes of pulpotomized primary molars treated with white or grey mineral trioxide aggregate and ferric sulfate – long-term follow-up. J Clin Pediatr Dent. 2012;37(2):137–41.
49. Gandolfi MG, Iacono F, Agee K, Siboni F, Tay F, Pashley DH, Prati C. Setting time and expansion in different soaking media of experimental accelerated calcium-silicate cements and ProRoot MTA. Oral Surg Oral Med Oral Pathol Oral Radiol Endod. 2009;108(6):e39–45.
50. Hawley M, Webb TD, Goodell GG. Effect of varying water-to-powder ratios on the setting expansion of white and grey mineral trioxide aggregate. J Endod. 2010;36(8):1377–9.
51. Holland R, de Souza V, Murata SS, Nery MJ, Bernabé PF, Otoboni Filho JA, Dezan JE. Healing process of dog dental pulp after pulpotomy and pulp covering with mineral trioxide aggregate or Portland cement. Braz Dent J. 2001;12(2):109–13.
52. Holland R, de Souza V, Nery MJ, Faraco Júnior IM, Bernabé PF, Otoboni Filho JA, Dezan Júnior E. Reaction of rat connective tissue to implanted dentin tube filled with mineral trioxide aggregate, Portland cement or calcium hydroxide. Braz Dent J. 2001;12(1):3–8.
53. Huang TH, Shie MY, Kao CT, Ding SJ. The effect of setting accelerator on properties of mineral trioxide aggregate. J Endod. 2008;34(5):590–3.
54. Húngaro Duarte MA, de Oliveira El Kadre GD, Vivan RR, Guerreiro Tanomaru JM, Tanomaru Filho M, de Moraes IG. Radiopacity of Portland cement associated with different radiopacifying agents. J Endod. 2009;35(5):737–40.
55. International Standards Organization. Dentistry – Water-based cements – Part 1: Powder/liquid acid-base cements. ISO 9917-1. Geneva: International Standards Organization; 2007.
56. International Standards Organization. Dentistry – Root canal sealing materials. ISO 6876. Geneva: International Standards Organizations; 2012.
57. Islam I, Chang HK, Yap AU. X-ray diffraction analysis of mineral trioxide aggregate and Portland cement. Int Endod J. 2006;39(3):220–5.
58. Islam I, Chng HK, Yap AU. Comparison of the physical and mechanical properties of MTA and Portland cement. J Endod. 2006;32(3):193–7.
59. Komabayashi T, Spångberg LW. Comparative analysis of the particle size and shape of commercially available mineral trioxide aggregates and Portland cement: a study with a flow particle image analyzer. J Endod. 2008;34(1):94–8.
60. Lea FM, Hewlett PC. Lea's chemistry of cement and concrete. 4th ed. London/New York: Arnold; 1998. Co-published in North, Central, and South America by J. Wiley.
61. Lendini M, Rigolone M, Tribaudino M, Zabetta FC, Mazza D, Berutti E. Caratterizzazione in microscopia SEM-EDS del cemento endodontico MTA: un confronto tra diversi prodotti. G Ital Endod. 2011;25(1): 33–40.
62. Lotfi M, Vosoughhosseini S, Saghiri MA, Rahimi S, Zand V, Reyhani MF, Samiei M, Ghasemi N, Mehrvarzfar P, Azimi S, Shokohinejad N. Effect of synthetic tissue fluid on microleakage of grey and white mineral trioxide aggregate as root-end filling materials: an in vitro study. Sultan Qaboos Univ Med J. 2012;12(3):323–9.
63. Loushine BA, Bryan TE, Looney SW, Gillen BM, Loushine RJ, Weller RN, et al. Setting properties and cytotoxicity evaluation of a premixed bioceramic root canal sealer. J Endod. 2011;37(5):673–7.
64. Massi S, Tanomaru-Filho M, Silva GF, Duarte MA, Grizzo LT, Buzalaf MA, Guerreiro-Tanomaru JM. pH, calcium ion release, and setting time of an experimental mineral trioxide aggregate-based root canal sealer. J Endod. 2011;37(6):844–6.
65. Menezes R, Bramante CM, Letra A, Carvalho VG, Garcia RB. Histologic evaluation of pulpotomies in dog using two types of mineral trioxide aggregate and regular and white Portland cements as wound dress-

ings. Oral Surg Oral Med Oral Pathol Oral Radiol Endod. 2004;98:376–9.
66. Monteiro Bramante C, Demarchi AC, de Moraes IG, Bernadineli N, Garcia RB, Spångberg LS, Duarte MA. Presence of arsenic in different types of MTA and white and gray Portland cement. Oral Surg Oral Med Oral Pathol Oral Radiol Endod. 2008;106(6):909–13.
67. Nekoofar MH, Adusei G, Sheykhrezae MS, Hayes SJ, Bryant ST, Dummer PM. The effect of condensation pressure on selected physical properties of mineral trioxide aggregate. Int Endod J. 2007;40:453–61.
68. Nekoofar MH, Oloomi K, Sheykhrezae MS, Tabor R, Stone DF, Dummer PM. An evaluation of the effect of blood and human serum on the surface microhardness and surface microstructure of mineral trioxide aggregate. Int Endod J. 2010;43(10):849–58.
69. Neville AM. Properties of concrete. 3rd ed. Essex: Longman Scientific and Technical; 1981.
70. Parirokh M, Asgary S, Eghbal MJ, Stowe S, Eslami B, Eskandarizade A, Shabahang S. A comparative study of white and grey mineral trioxide aggregate as pulp capping agents in dog's teeth. Dent Traumatol. 2005;21(3):150–4.
71. Parirokh M, Mirsoltani B, Raoof M, Tabrizchi H, Haghdoost AA. Comparative study of subcutaneous tissue responses to a novel root-end filling material and white and grey mineral trioxide aggregate. Int Endod J. 2011;44(4):283–9.
72. Pérez AL, Spears R, Gutmann JL, Opperman LA. Osteoblasts and MG-63 osteosarcoma cells behave differently when in contact with ProRoot MTA and White MTA. Int Endod J. 2003;36(8):564–70.
73. Petrucci ER. Concreto de cimento Portland. 13th ed. São Paulo: Editora Globo; 1998.
74. Porter ML, Berto A, Primus CM, Watanabe I. Physical and chemical properties of new-generation endodontic materials. J Endod. 2010;36(3):524–8.
75. Primus CM, inventor; DENTSPLY International, Inc., assignee. Dental material. United States Patent 7,892,342, 22 Feb 2011 Feb.
76. Reyes-Carmona JF, Felippe MS, Felippe WT. Biomineralization ability and interaction of mineral trioxide aggregate and Portland cement with dentin in a phosphate-containing fluid. J Endod. 2009;35(5):731–6.
77. Ribeiro DA, Duarte MA, Matsumoto MA, Marques ME, Salvadori DM. Biocompatibility in vitro tests of mineral trioxide aggregate and regular and white Portland cements. J Endod. 2005;31(8):605–7.
78. Ribeiro DA, Matsumoto MA, Duarte MA, Marques ME, Salvadori DM. Ex vivo biocompatibility tests of regular and white forms of mineral trioxide aggregate. Int Endod J. 2006;39(1):26–30.
79. Ribeiro DA, Sugui MM, Matsumoto MA, Duarte MA, Marques ME, Salvadori DM. Genotoxicity and cytotoxicity of mineral trioxide aggregate and regular and white Portland cements on Chinese hamster ovary (CHO) cells in vitro. Oral Surg Oral Med Oral Pathol Oral Radiol Endod. 2006;101(2):258–61.
80. Saidon J, Jianing H, Zhu Q, Safavi K, Spangberg L. Cell and tissue reactions to mineral aggregate and Portland cement. Oral Surg Oral Med Oral Pathol Oral Radiol Endod. 2003;95(4):483–9.
81. Schembri M, Peplow G, Camilleri J. Analyses of heavy metals in mineral trioxide aggregate and Portland cement. J Endod. 2010;36(7):1210–15.
82. Shahi S, Yavari HR, Rahimi S, Eskandarinezhad M, Shakouei S, Unchi M. Comparison of the sealing ability of mineral trioxide aggregate and Portland cement used as root-end filling materials. J Oral Sci. 2011;53(4):517–22.
83. Spangberg SW. Response to letter to the editor by Carolyn M. Primus. Oral Surg Oral Med Oral Pathol Oral Radiol Endod. 2006;101:418.
84. Stefopoulos S, Tsatsas DV, Kerezoudis NP, Eliades G. Comparative in vitro study of the sealing efficiency of white vs grey ProRoot mineral trioxide aggregate formulas as apical barriers. Dent Traumatol. 2008;24(2): 207–13.
85. Storm B, Eichmiller FC, Tordik PA, Goodell GG. Setting expansion of grey and white mineral trioxide aggregate and Portland cement. J Endod. 2008;34(1): 80–2.
86. Taylor HFW. Cement chemistry. 2nd ed. London: T. Telford; 1997.
87. Torabinejad M. Historical and contemporary perspectives on root-end filling materials. J Endod. 1993;19(8):432–3.
88. Torabinejad M, Hong CU, McDonald F, Pitt Ford TR. Physical and chemical properties of a new root-end filling material. J Endod. 1995;21:349–53.
89. Torabinejad M, White DJ. Tooth filling material and method of use. US Patent 5,415,547, 1993.
90. Torabinejad M, White DJ, inventors; Loma Linda University, assignee. Tooth filling material and method of use. United States Patent 5,769,638, 16 May 1995.
91. Vosoughhosseini S, Lotfi M, Shahi S, Baloo H, Mesgariabbasi M, Saghiri MA, Zand V, Rahimi S, Ranjkesh B. Influence of white versus grey mineral trioxide aggregate on inflammatory cells. J Endod. 2008;34(6):715–17. doi:10.1016/j.joen.2008.03.005.
92. Witte. The filling of a root canal with Portland cement. German Q Dent; J Central Assoc German Dent. 1878;18:153–4.
93. Wucherpfennig AL, Green DB. Mineral trioxide vs. Portland cement: two compatible filling materials. J Endod. 1999;25(4), Abstract PR 40;308.
94. Yavari HR, Shahi S, Rahimi S, Shakouie S, Roshangar L, Mesgari Abassi M, Khavas SS. Connective tissue reaction to white and gray MTA mixed with distilled water or chlorhexidine in rats. Iran Endod J. 2009;4(1): 25–30.

Composition and Setting Reaction

2

Josette Camilleri

2.1 Introduction

Mineral trioxide aggregate (MTA) has been introduced as a root-end filling material due to its hydraulic properties. Most dental materials exhibit a deterioration in physical properties upon contact with moisture. Thus, a hydraulic material used in the construction industry was introduced in order to counteract this problem. The first US patent [79, 80] drawn for MTA explains this invention saying 'Due to the presence of blood and moisture, the mouth is a less than ideal environment for many materials which could otherwise be useful as dental filling and sealing materials. For example, typical amalgams are sensitive to moisture and set less than adequately if care is not taken to minimize moisture. Not only is the cement of the present invention not adversely affected by moisture in the mouth, but such moisture actually plays an important role in the hydration reactions responsible for the hardening and sealing process'. The composition of MTA and the processes of hydration will be discussed in this chapter.

J. Camilleri, BChD, MPhil, PhD, FIMMM, FADM
Department of Restorative Dentistry,
Faculty of Dental Surgery, Medical School,
Mater Dei Hospital, University of Malta,
Msida MSD 2090, Malta
e-mail: josette.camilleri@um.edu.mt

2.2 Composition of Un-hydrated Material

MTA is composed of a mixture of Portland cement and bismuth oxide. The bismuth oxide is added to the cement to enhance the radiopacity of the material. The original MTA patent registered in 1995 [79] stated that 'MTA consists of 50–75 % (wt) calcium oxide and 15–25 % silicon dioxide. These two components together comprise 70–95 % of the cement. When these raw materials are blended, they produce tricalcium silicate, dicalcium silicate, tricalcium aluminate, and tetracalcium aluminoferrite'. The patent also stated that 'MTA is Type 1 Portland cement (American Society for Testing Materials), with a fineness (Blaine number) in the range of 4,500–4,600 cm^2/g. A radiopacifier (bismuth oxide) is added to the cement for dental radiological diagnosis'.

Calcium oxide and silicon dioxide are the raw materials used for the manufacture of Portland cement. When these oxides are sintered together with other raw materials, tricalcium silicate, dicalcium silicate, tricalcium aluminate and tetracalcium aluminoferrite are produced. The aluminoferrite phase is only present in the grey cement [64]. White MTA was introduced later (circa 2001). The current US patent for white MTA is dated 2011. This supersedes all previous applications. The white MTA uses the same formulation of the grey version patented in 1995; however, the 2011 patent specifies the use of white Portland cement with low levels of iron [69].

J. Camilleri (ed.), *Mineral Trioxide Aggregate in Dentistry*,
DOI 10.1007/978-3-642-55157-4_2, © Springer-Verlag Berlin Heidelberg 2014

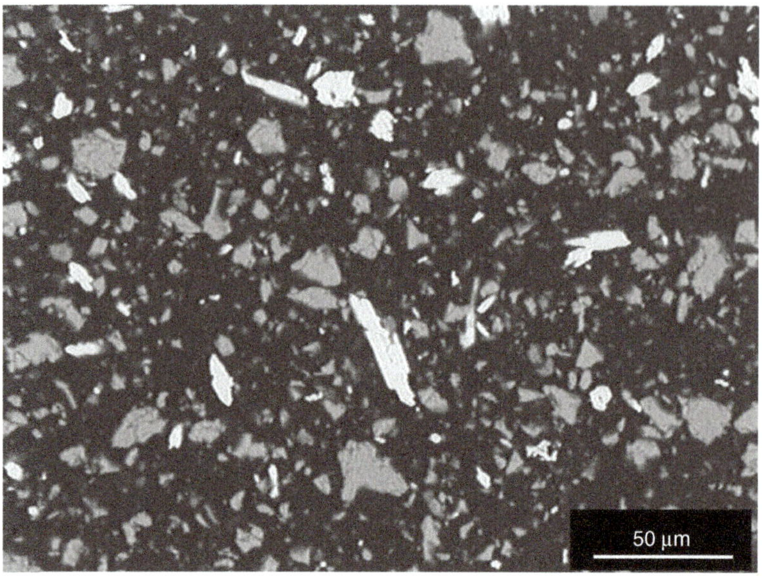

Fig. 2.1 Back-scatter scanning electron micrograph of polished surface of MTA powder (Reprinted with permission from Camilleri 2007 [21]. Copyright ©2007, John Wiley and Sons)

The US patent also states that the cement component is to be ASTM International Type 1 Portland cement with a specific Blaine fineness [2]. Portland cements used in industry are classified into different subcategories depending on their intended use. ASTM Type 1 Portland cements are common Portland cements that are intended for general purpose use, precluding contact with any chemical substances. The specified Blaine fineness is 4,500–4,600 cm^2/g indicating a very fine cement. In fact, the Colton Fast-Set brand was suggested for use.

The chemical composition and material microstructure of un-hydrated MTA have been investigated using various techniques. These techniques include scanning electron microscopy (SEM) [13, 17, 18, 21] and energy-dispersive spectroscopy (EDS) [5, 13, 17, 18, 21, 28, 30], X-ray fluorescence [17, 30] and X-ray diffraction (XRD) analysis [5, 7, 66] as well as XRD with Rietveld refinement [7, 17, 18]. The latter is valuable for quantitative analysis.

Scanning electron microscopy of polished sections of un-hydrated MTA embedded in resin shows distinctive cement grains and bismuth oxide particles, which are separated from one another. This feature indicates that the material is composed of a simple mixture of the two components (Fig. 2.1). The elemental composition of MTA as shown by EDS analysis indicates the presence of calcium, silicon and oxygen with minor peaks for aluminium, potassium, magnesium and bismuth. A semi-quantitative assessment of the elemental composition can be worked out using a cobalt standard assuming they are in the oxide form (Fig. 2.2). The oxide percentage composition depends on the mineralogy of the original cement. This can be quantitatively determined by X-ray fluorescence. The levels of silicon and calcium vary with the type of Portland cement used. Hence, these elemental levels are different for each brand of MTA.

The phases present in MTA are determined using X-ray diffraction analysis. Using this method of analysis, un-hydrated MTA exhibits peaks for tricalcium silicate, dicalcium silicate and bismuth oxide. Using a copper Kα tube, each phase has a particular pattern as shown in Fig. 2.3, which can then be searched and matched with data derived from the International Centre of Diffraction Data (ICDD) bank. Bismuth oxide (ICDD: 27-0053) exhibits typical peaks at 25.757, 26.906, 27.386, 28.010 and 33.229°2θ. Tricalcium silicate (ICDD: 86-0402) exhibits peaks at 29.414, 32.193, 32.504, 32.623, 34.355 and 41.298°2θ. Dicalcium silicate, usually exhibits a peak at 32.7°2θ,

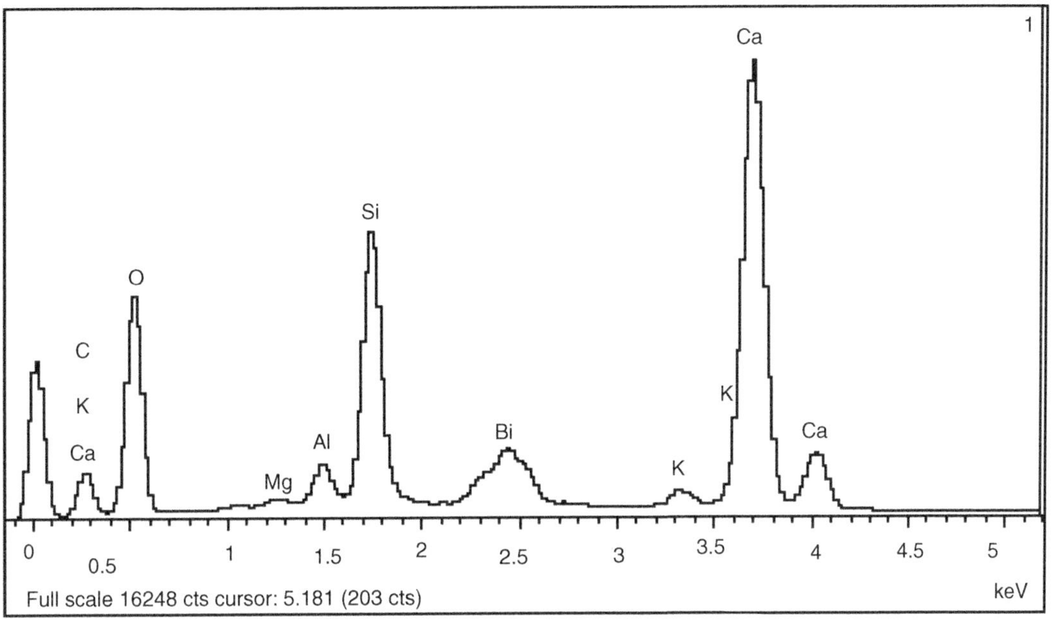

Element	Weight%	Atomic%	Compd%	Formula%
Mg K	0.53	0.56	0.88	MgO
Al K	2.16	2.06	4.08	Al_2O_3
Si K	12.04	13.80	32.18	SiO_2
K K	1.13	0.74	1.36	K_2O
Ca K	38.08	24.47	53.28	CaO
Bi M	7.37	0.91	8.21	Bi_2O_3
O	35.69	57.46		
Totals	100.00			

Fig. 2.2 Energy-dispersive spectroscopy of a typical MTA powder and semi-quantitative elemental composition

however such a peak is difficult to discern, due to its superimposition with the peaks present in the tricalcium silicate phase. Tricalcium aluminate is also present in un-hydrated MTA but in minimal quantities. X-ray diffraction analysis of MTA thus eliminates the myth that MTA is composed mainly of oxides. Thus, the term 'trioxide aggregate' is essentially a misnomer.

Quantitative phase analysis can be performed by Rietveld refinement using an internal standard such as rutile (titanium dioxide) added to the un-hydrated MTA. The principle of Rietveld analysis is to compare the experimental pattern with a pattern simulated based on the presumed amounts, crystal parameters and equipment parameters of a mixture of known phases. Rietveld refinement enables the amounts of different phases in anhydrous cementitious materials to be determined to a high degree of precision [71]. Quantitative assessment of ProRoot MTA (Dentsply Tulsa Dental, Johnson City, TN, USA) and MTA Angelus (Angelus, Londrina, Brazil) is shown in Table 2.1. Both cements exhibit different quantities of tricalcium silicate and dicalcium silicate when compared to Portland cement. The difference is due to variations in the manufacturing of Portland cement used as a raw material for preparing MTA. Phase analysis of ProRoot MTA has been published by Camilleri in 2008 [18] and has been validated by other researchers using Rietveld X-ray diffraction analysis [7] (Table 2.1). The main difference between the two

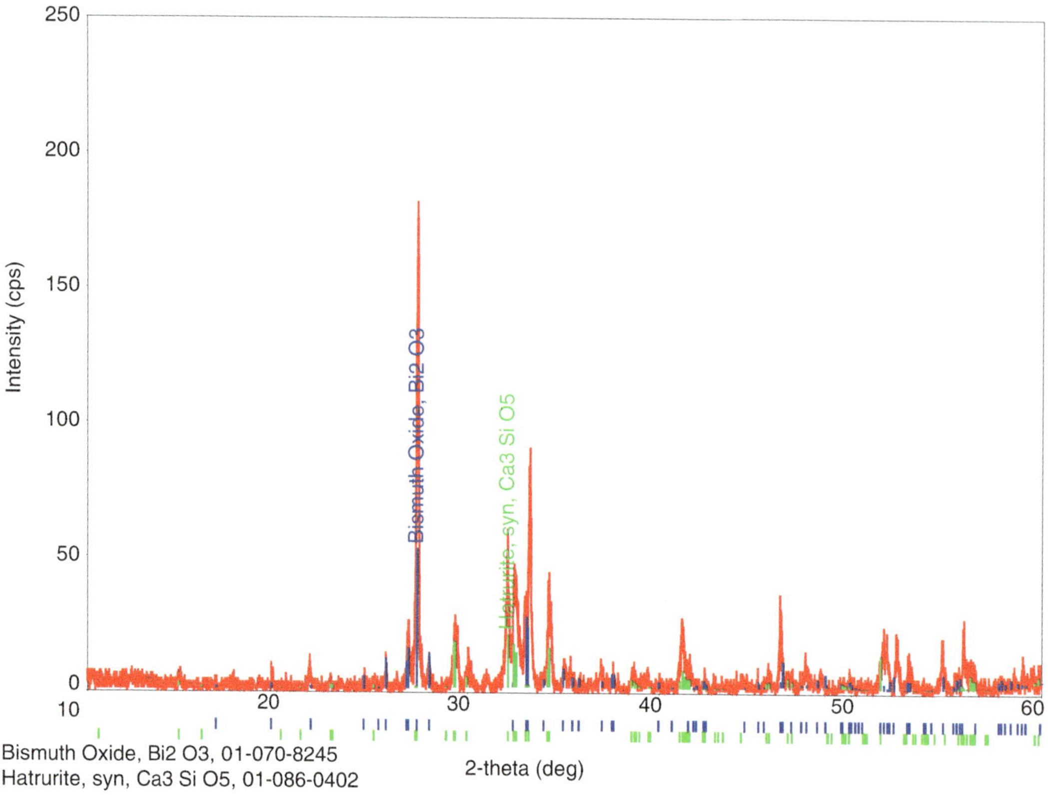

Fig. 2.3 X-ray diffractogram of un-hydrated MTA showing the main phases present

Table 2.1 Rietveld X-ray diffraction analysis of the phases present in un-hydrated Portland cement, ProRoot MTA and MTA Angelus

Phases identified	Material type in mass %		
	Portland cement	ProRoot MTA[a]	MTA Angelus[b]
Tricalcium silicate	74.7	53.1 (51.9)	66.1
Dicalcium silicate	7.4	22.5 (23.2)	8.4
Tricalcium aluminate	3.6	0.0 (3.8)	2.0
Gypsum	1.1	0.0	0.0
Hemihydrate	1.1	0.0	0.0
Anhydrite	2.7	1.5 (1.3)	0.0
Calcium carbonate	5.0	1.4	0.0
Calcium oxide	0.0	0.0	8.0
Bismuth oxide	0.0	21.6 (19.8)	14.0

Adapted from Camilleri [18], [a]Belío-Reyes et al. [7], [b]Camilleri et al. [17]

studies is the presence of tricalcium aluminate in ProRoot MTA in the latter study [7]. Lack of an aluminate phase was also evident in scanning electron microscopy of polished sections of ProRoot MTA powder [18]. The absence of tricalcium aluminate phase, low levels of anhydrite and absence of gypsum may infer that the cement component in ProRoot MTA may not be a commercial Portland cement manufactured in a kiln but a laboratory-made cement. The manufacturer of ProRoot MTA (Dentsply Tulsa Dental Specialties, Tulsa, OK, USA) in fact claims that ProRoot MTA does not utilise a commercial Portland cement but the raw materials are certified for purity by inductively coupled plasma (ICP) spectroscopy. In the same document, the manufacturer also disclaims the presence of phosphate, which was stated to be the main constituent of MTA in the original publication [78]. In that publication, MTA was purportedly reported to be composed of 'calcium oxide and calcium phosphate. Further analysis demonstrated that the former appeared as discrete crystals and the latter as an amorphous structure with no apparent crystal growth but a granular appearance. The mean value of the prisms was 87 % calcium and 2.47 % silica, the remainder being oxygen. In areas of amorphous structure, there seemed to be 33 % calcium, 49 % phosphate, 2 % carbon, 3 % chloride, and 6 % silica'.

Another calcium silicate-based cement, MTA Angelus, was found to contain tricalcium aluminate but no sulphate-containing phase (Table 2.1). The absence of the gypsum is claimed by the manufacturer to reduce the setting time of the material. In fact, MTA Angelus has been shown to set in less than 50 min [59], as opposed to ProRoot MTA which was reported to have a setting time of over 2 h [9, 10, 20, 25, 30, 78]. Furthermore, 8 % calcium oxide is present in MTA Angelus [17]. This calcium oxide is a result of a raw mix with poor combustibility and with an unstable thermal profile. ProRoot MTA exhibits a higher level of bismuth oxide when compared to MTA Angelus (Table 2.1). This accounts for the higher radiopacity of ProRoot MTA [15, 20].

2.3 MTA Fineness

The MTA patent [79, 80] specifies the brand of Portland cement used in the original MTA formulation (Colton Fast-Set brand: Blaine number in the range of 4,500–4,600 cm^2/g). The Blaine number is a numerical value which is calculated using the Blaine fineness measuring equipment. This is the industrial standard for measuring cement fineness. The Blaine method is specified by both European (EN 196-6) [34] and American (ASTM C204) [3] standards. Both standards specify an air permeability method wherein a bed of cement of known density is prepared; the resistance to a flow of air passing through the cement is measured and the fineness of the cement is calculated. This method measures cement fineness compared to standard cement. A range of 4,500–4,600 cm^2/g is considered a fine cement.

Other industrial methods for measuring cement fineness include the Lea and Nurse apparatus. This method is an absolute method for determining the fineness of a cement and is adopted by most cement manufacturers. The particle size distribution of MTA has been calculated using laser particle size analysis [14], optical methods which involve measuring particle sizes of cement on polished sections of cement powder [5, 30], flow particle image analyser [54, 55] and by using the BET (Brunauer–Emmett–Teller) gas adsorption method [12] to calculate the specific surface area of MTA [13, 17]. The latter method is an extension of the Langmuir theory, which is a theory for monolayer molecular adsorption to multilayers. This theory hypothesises that gas molecules physically adsorb on a solid in layers infinitely; as there is no interaction between each adsorption layer, the Langmuir theory may be applied to each layer. The BET method is widely used in materials and surface science for the calculation of surface areas of solids by physical adsorption of gas molecules. By application of the BET theory, it is even possible to determine the inner surface area of hardened cement paste.

Optical assessment of MTA shows that the cement contains more uniform and finer-sized particles than Portland cement [5, 30]. However, other researchers using the same method reported coarser and more irregularly shaped crystalline particles in MTA [5]. Optical assessment shows that MTA consists of particles with diameters ranging from less than 1 μm to approximately 30 μm, and occasionally up to 50 μm. Particles of bismuth oxide (10–30 μm) are numerous [30]. Flow particle image analyses of various calcium silicate-based hydraulic cements indicate that the cumulative percentages of particles ranging from 6 to 10 μm for grey ProRoot MTA, white ProRoot MTA, grey MTA Angelus, white MTA Angelus and Portland cement are 65, 73, 48, 53 and 70 %, respectively. Thus, MTA Angelus contains a larger number of small particles with relatively low circularity and a wider range of size distribution and is less homogeneous than ProRoot MTA. Furthermore, white MTA contains smaller particles with a narrower range of size distribution than grey MTA [54]. The cumulative percentage of particles that are between 0.5 and 3 μm in size was reported to be 88 % [55]. Laser granulometry of MTA confirmed that this cement has a smaller particle size when compared to Portland cement

[28]. Moreover, bismuth oxide, which is not present in Portland cement, exhibits a large particle size when examined microscopically [13] and with the use of laser granulometry [15].

ProRoot MTA and MTA Angelus were found to have a similar fineness when tested using the BET gas adsorption method [13, 17]. Both materials exhibit a specific surface area of approximately 1 m^2/g. A novel MTA (MTA Plus compounded by Prevest Denpro, Jammu, India, for Avalon Biomed Inc. Bradenton, FL, USA) has a specific surface area of 1,537 m^2/g [13], which is higher than the values obtained for MTA Angelus [17]. The higher specific surface area results in more surface available for cement reaction, which, in turn, results in a more rapid reaction rate.

2.4 Manipulation

Mineral trioxide aggregate is a water-based dental cement. It is usually supplied in pre-dosed powder and liquid that are mixed together to obtain a homogeneous paste. The recommended water/powder ratio is about 0.33. Changing the water/powder ratio affects the properties of MTA. The degree of solubility and the porosity of the cement increases when the water/powder ratio is increased. Cement pastes with a water/powder ratio higher than 0.33 are not viscous enough for clinical application. A ratio of 0.26 was the minimum that allowed a mix of putty consistency that can be manipulated [39]. Most MTA manufacturers supply prepacked 1 g powders with ampoules containing 0.33 g of water. Since the amount of material in each package is large enough for several applications, clinicians commonly estimate the amount of water and powder at the chairside, which results in using an unknown water/powder ratio. Variations in the water/powder ratio do not seem to affect the clinical performance of the material, No significant difference in material expansion [48] and no influence on the histological outcome was observed for MTA mixed at different water/powder ratios when used as a direct pulp-capping material on human healthy pulps [74]. When taking into consideration water/powder ratios in MTA, a distinction from water/cement ratio should be made. MTA contains 20 % bismuth oxide, which does not react with water. Thus effectively the water/cement ratio for MTA mixed at a water/powder ratio of 0.33 would be 0.41. Thus, comparison of properties of MTA with those of other systems using a different quantity or no radiopacifier or mineral additives is not possible since the effective water/cement ratio will vary depending on the quantity of additive. Modification of the water/cement ratio affects the properties of the set cement [29].

There have been a large number of reports on addition of various chemicals to the mixing liquid or replacement of the water by other liquids. The most popular is calcium chloride [1, 4, 10, 53, 56, 85], calcium nitrite/nitrate and calcium formate [85]. These chemical additions are also used in the industry to accelerate the setting of Portland cement. Setting accelerators affect the setting reaction of both tricalcium silicate and tricalcium aluminate [65].

Addition of water-soluble polymers [11, 14, 16, 19] increases material flow. ProRoot Endo Sealer is a commercial formulation using cement particles dispersed in a water-soluble polymer [49, 84]. The water-soluble polymer creates charges on the cement particles, resulting in repulsion of these charged particles with reduced flocculation and increased material flow at low water/cement ratios [65]. Propylene glycol has also been used to improve MTA flow [33]. Other polymers have been included to reduce washout of the unset cement. Anti-washout liquid is included in the MTA Plus formulation (compounded by Prevest Denpro, Jammu, India for Avalon Biomed Inc. Bradenton, FL, USA).

Other clinically available liquids have been added to MTA to improve its handling characteristics. These include local anaesthetic solution [40, 50, 53, 81, 83], sodium hypochlorite, chlorhexidine gluconate, saline and physiological solution [42, 50, 53], calcium lactate gluconate [51, 56] and citric acid [56]. The use of un-hydrated MTA as a root-end filling material has been reported [67]. Un-hydrated MTA will hydrate using the physiological fluid available at the root-end cavity. Non-specific and contradicting effects have been reported with the use of these chemicals. Physiological and synthetic tissue fluids contain chloride ions and glucose. The former is a cement hydration accelerator [65] while glucose is a hydration retarder. The combination of these effects may adversely alter the cement paste microstructure. Local anaesthetic solution contains both chloride and sulphate ions which again have a conflicting effect on cement hydration. A higher content of sulphate in the cement may lead to sulphate attack, whereby excessive expansion and cracking will be observed over time due to delayed ettringite deposition [64]. MTA is known to have low levels of sulphate ions and, although these ionic levels would alter the relative proportions of ettringite and monosulphate phases for a given degree of cement hydration, they are unlikely to create sulphate attack of the set cement. The chloride present in both synthetic tissue fluids and anaesthetic solutions may also alter the relative proportions of ettringite and monosulphate phases due to the formation of Friedel's salt (calcium chloroaluminate, $3CaO \cdot Al_2O_3 \cdot CaCl_2 \cdot 10H_2O$). The formation of Friedel's salt will change the lattice structure of hydrated cement monosulphate phases and can potentially lead to microcracking [64].

Other variations to the mixing liquid include replacement of the water by various resins. These modifications result in the development of light-activated MTA and resin-modified MTA for use as root canal sealer cement. Resin-modified MTA reduces the setting time and enhances the bonding to both dentine and overlying composite, thus purportedly reducing micro-leakage. The use of a number of resin systems has been reported, with the main ones being light-curing systems containing bisphenol A-glycidyl methacrylate (bis-GMA) and a biocompatible resin [45, 46] consisting of 2-hydroxyethyl methacrylate (HEMA), triethylene glycol dimethacrylate (TEGDMA), camphorquinone and ethyl-4-(dimethylamino)benzoate (EDMAB), with or without polyacrylic co-maleic acid [42, 43], bis-GMA and TEGDMA [36] and bis-GMA, pyromellitic acid diethylmethacrylate (PMDM) and HEMA [70]. Chemically cured resins have also been employed [26, 36]. Other resins were added with the aim of increasing material flow, thus making MTA suitable to be used as a sealer cement [45, 46]. One such formulation is marketed by Angelus (Angelus, Londrina, Brazil) as MTA Fillapex. The latter is composed of MTA, a salicylate resin (methyl salicylate, butylene glycol and colophony) and other additives. Other proprietary brands such as MTA Obtura and Endo CPM Sealer exist. These sealer cements contain other additives to the MTA formula, that enhance material flow. Other experimental epoxy resin-based systems that incorporate MTA as fillers have also been reported as sealer cements [57].

Classically, MTA is mixed by manipulating the powder and liquid components on a mixing pad. Alternative mixing techniques such as the use of an amalgamator have been investigated [6, 63, 73]. MM MTA™, manufactured by MICRO-MEGA (Besançon Cedex, France), is supplied as MTA capsules that enable the MTA to be mixed using an amalgamator. Ultrasonic agitation has also been employed for mixing MTA [6, 63, 73]. The effectiveness of mechanical mixing and ultrasonic agitation is not clear, although mechanical mixing was shown to enhance the compressive strength of the set material, while ultrasonic agitation was found to improve the compressive strength of the material regardless of the mixing technique [6]. In addition to enhanced material micro-hardness [63], other research has shown that the various mixing methods have no significant effects on the resultant MTA mixtures [73]. Application of a condensation pressure of 1.68 MPa results in enhanced compressive strength. Higher condensation pressures result in fewer voids and micro-channels, while specimens prepared with lower condensation pressures exhibit distinctive crystalline structures [62].

2.5 Washout

One of the drawbacks of MTA is washout after it is placed in situ. Washout refers to the tendency of a freshly prepared cement paste to 'disintegrate upon early contact with blood or other fluids' [82]. Washout can be measured using different methods. Most methods involve immersion of the unset cement in a liquid [24, 52, 58]. Agitation [82] or freeze drying [52] is then employed to disrupt the cement; alternatively the cement is sprayed with air from a specified distance [68]. The amount of material lost is then determined using photography [68] or quantified using a gravimetric method [52, 82]. One of the latest reported methods [37] includes a setup based on Specification CRD-C 661-06 [75] which was scaled down to allow testing of dental materials. When the results were compared to a metered water spray, they were found to yield quantitative, objective and reproducible results [37]. In the same study, MTA Plus and MTA Angelus exhibited washout when compared to Intermediate Restorative Material (IRM, Dentsply Caulk, Milford, Delaware, USA) and dental amalgam. The addition of anti-washout gel manufactured by Avalon Biomed Inc. reduced washout considerably [38].

2.6 Setting Reaction

Mineral trioxide aggregate hydrates when it comes in contact with water and undergoes two main reactions. The tricalcium silicate and dicalcium silicate react with water to form calcium silicate hydrate and calcium hydroxide. The tricalcium aluminate reacts with water and, in the presence of calcium sulphate, produces ettringite initially. When the sulphate-containing phases are depleted, a monosulphate phase is formed [21]:

$$\begin{array}{l}2(3CaO.SiO_2) + 6H_2O \rightarrow 3CaO.2SiO_2.3H_2O + 3Ca(OH)_2 \\ \text{Tricalcium silicate} + \text{Water} \quad \text{calcium silicate hydrate} + \text{Calcium hydroxide}\end{array} \tag{2.1}$$

$$\begin{array}{l}2(2CaO.SiO_2) + 4H_2O \rightarrow 3CaO.2SiO_2.3H_2O + Ca(OH)_2 \\ \text{Dicalcium silicate} + \text{Water} \quad \text{calcium silicate hydrate} + \text{Calcium hydroxide}\end{array} \tag{2.2}$$

$$\begin{array}{l}3CaO.Al_2O_3 + CaSO_4 + H_2O \rightarrow 3CaO.Al_2O_3.3CaSO_4.31H_2O \\ \text{Tricalcium aluminate} + \text{Gypsum} + \text{Water} \quad \text{Ettringite}\end{array} \tag{2.3}$$

The reactions that occur in MTA after hydration are the same reactions that are seen in Portland cement. During the initial stages of reaction, calcium silicate hydrate is formed; coating the cement particles with calcium silicate hydrate prevents further reaction. Tricalcium aluminate dissolves and reacts with the calcium and sulphate ions present in the liquid phase to produce ettringite that also precipitates on the cement particle surface. The initial phase is followed by a dormant period wherein the hydrate coating on the cement grains prevents further hydration. The dormant period lasts for 1–2 h, and is a period of relative inactivity when the cement is plastic and workable. Following the completion of the dormant period, setting of the cement proceeds to the acceleration stage wherein the hydration process accelerates again. The rate of tricalcium silicate hydration increases and more calcium silicate hydrate gel is formed. Hydration of dicalcium silicate also increases at this stage. Sulphate ions are depleted and monosulphate forms from ettringite. Crystalline calcium hydroxide also precipitates from the liquid phase.

The hydration progress can be monitored using calorimetry. The heat flux released by the chemical reaction is monitored over time and enables estimation of the beginning of setting and the rate of increase of the mechanical performance of the cement paste. Both MTA Angelus and MTA Plus present an initial endothermic peak followed by an exothermic peak (Fig. 2.4). The first 2 h correspond to an induction period followed by initial setting and then hardening of the material. The initial endothermic peak is due

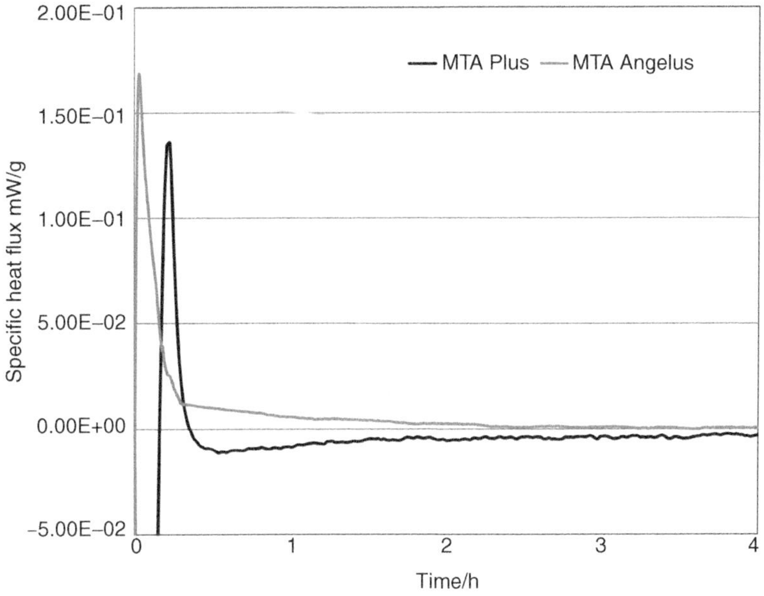

Fig. 2.4 Graphical representation of heat flux generated with time for MTA Plus and MTA Angelus

to the wetting of the surface. The first part of the exothermic peak is correlated with the very rapid and very exothermic hydration [13, 17]. It is interesting to note that MTA Angelus exhibits a higher exothermic peak, which occurs ahead of that of MTA Plus. This is caused by reaction of the calcium oxide present in MTA Angelus with water [17].

2.7 Characterisation of Set MTA

A combination of microscopy, elemental analysis and phase analysis has been used to characterise and evaluate the hydration mechanisms of MTA [13, 17, 18, 21]. The X-ray diffractograms are useful as MTA materials are mostly crystalline and individual mineral phases can be identified. Scanning electron microscopy allows observation of material microstructure and surface visualisation. Moreover, characterisation by X-ray energy dispersive analysis provides qualitative information of the elemental constitution of the test materials. Other useful methods have been employed for characterisation of MTA, including Fourier transform infrared spectroscopy (FT-IR) and Laser Raman spectroscopy. Laser Raman spectroscopy is largely complementary to infrared spectroscopy, but spectral interpretation is simpler [8]. The major components of Portland cement give distinctive Raman spectra [41, 44]. Both FT-IR and Raman spectroscopy have been used to investigate the interaction of calcium silicate cements with physiological solutions [27, 47, 76, 77]. These techniques are an adjunct to phase analysis by XRD and aid to verify the phases identified when peak overlap exists; which is the main disadvantage associated with the use of XRD to analyse Portland cement-based materials. This problem may be addressed by using the Rietveld method [71], which allows standardisation of powder diffraction analysis through the use of calculated reference diffraction patterns based upon crystal structure models.

Reaction by-products produced upon hydration of the cement are deposited around the periphery of the un-hydrated cement particles. As hydration proceeds, there is evidence of more reaction by-products. The hydration reaction takes several years to complete, although the cement mass would have achieved the final hardening and

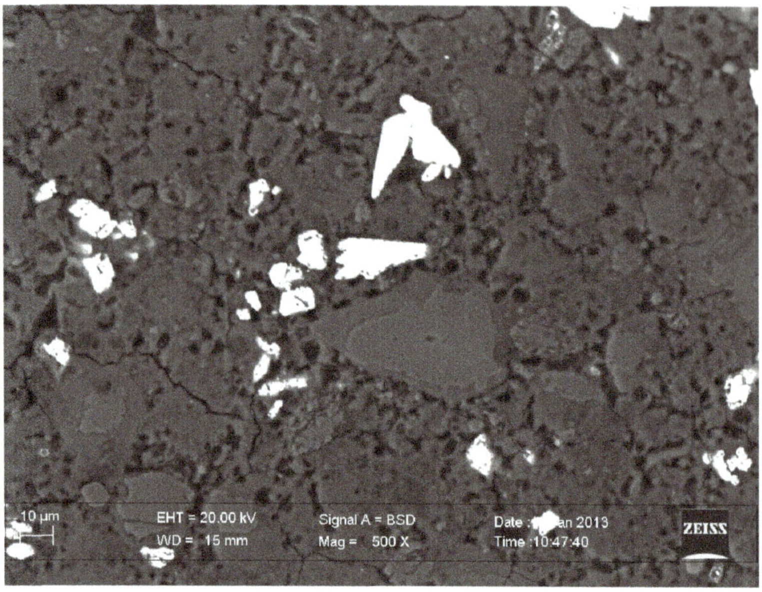

Fig. 2.5 Back scatter scanning electron micrograph of hydrated MTA after immersion in water for 28 days showing un-hydrated cement particle enclosed by a reaction rim. *Shiny particles* are bismuth oxide (×500 mag.)

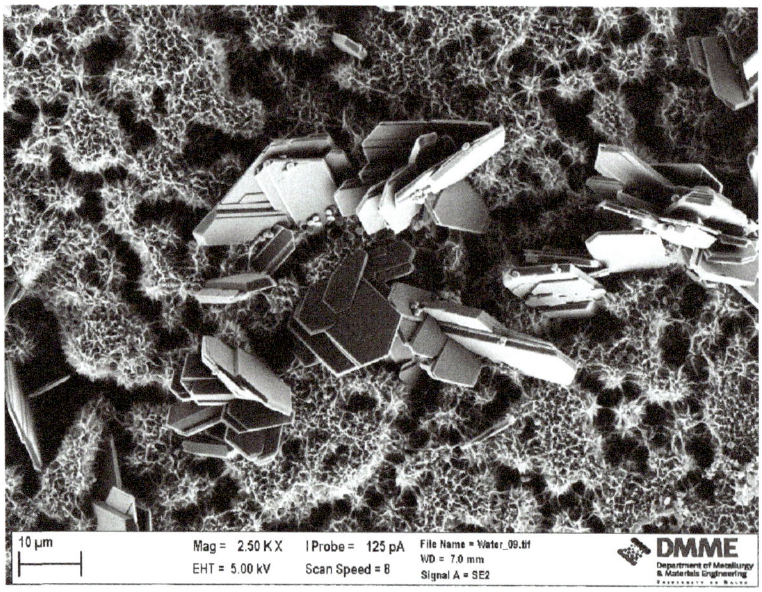

Fig. 2.6 Secondary electron scanning electron micrograph of MTA surface showing calcium silicate hydrate (*honeycomb appearance*) and calcium hydroxide (*hexagonal plates*) deposited on its surface (×2,500 mag.)

maximum physical and mechanical properties by 28 days. Hydrating MTA can be observed on back-scatter scanning electron micrographs of polished cement specimens (Fig. 2.5). The formation of cement by-products can be monitored by scanning electron microscopy in secondary electron mode. Calcium silicate hydrate exhibits a typical honeycomb appearance, while calcium hydroxide is deposited in the form of hexagonal plates (Fig. 2.6). The surface deposits are evident on the cement surface and may be measured by optical profilometry [35] (Fig. 2.7). The composition of the surface deposits in turn can be assessed using XRD analysis with the glancing angle modification. Phase analysis is usually performed by powder diffractometry using the Bragg–Brentano principle and thus moving both the X-ray source and the detector at a specified angle and speed.

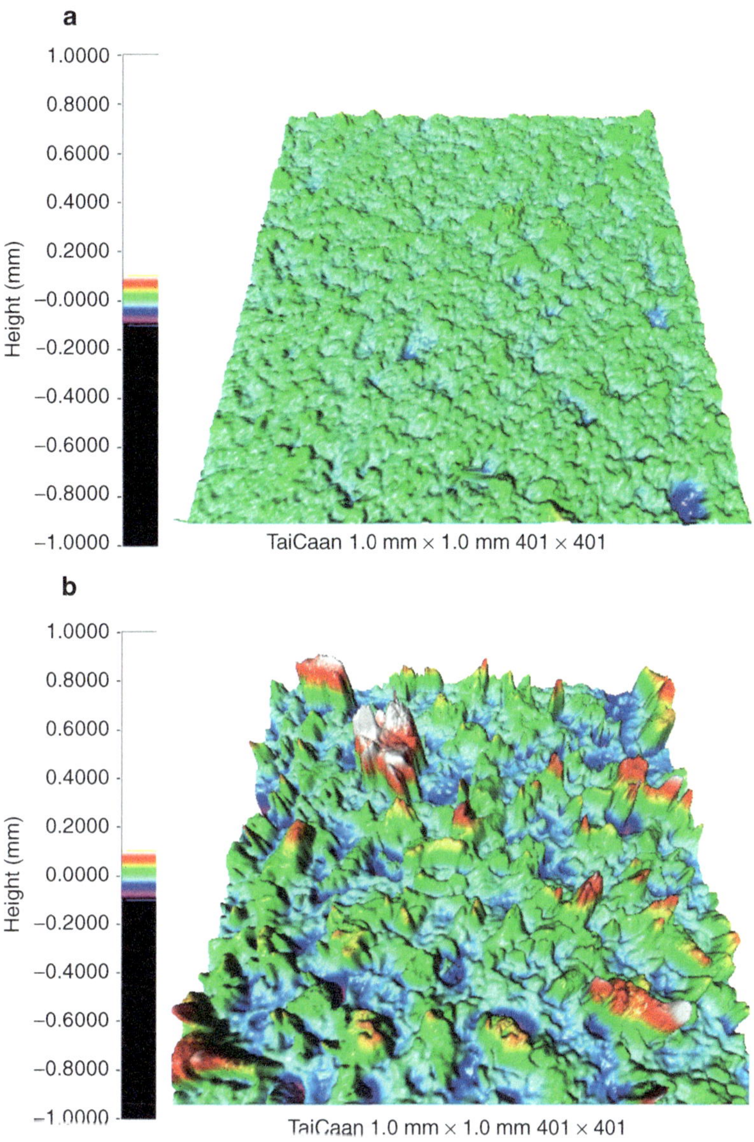

Fig. 2.7 Surface noncontact profilometry of MTA surface (**a**) before and (**b**) after immersion in Hank's balanced salt solution (Reprinted from Formosa et al. [35], copyright 2012, with permission from Elsevier)

With the glancing angle technique, the surface analysis is greatly enhanced by reducing the interference from the sample substrate and increasing the absorption path of the incident beam within the layer itself. An X-ray diffractogram of the MTA surface deposits exhibited a definite peak for beta-calcium phosphate when MTA was immersed in a physiological solution, whereas no peaks were visible when the material was immersed in water (Fig. 2.8).

Leaching of calcium hydroxide in solution may be monitored by inductive-coupled plasma mass spectroscopy (ICP-MS). High levels of calcium ions have been demonstrated in solution. If MTA is left exposed to the environment, the calcium hydroxide reacts with the atmospheric carbon dioxide resulting in deposition of calcium carbonate on the cement surface. These deposits are commonly mistaken to be an integral part of the cement microstructure.

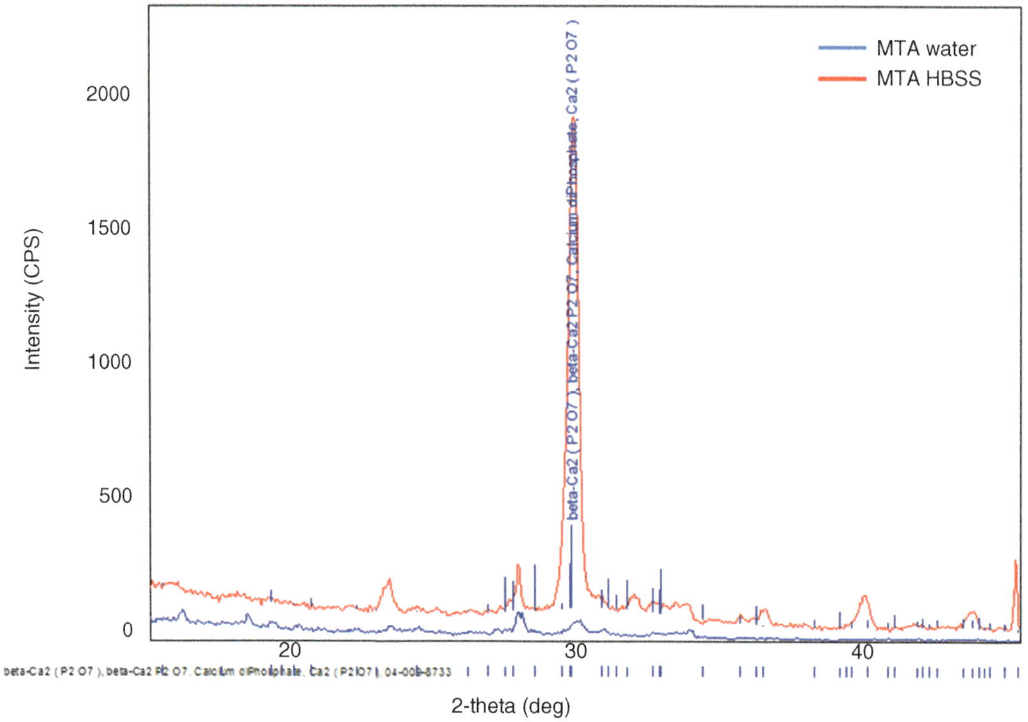

Fig. 2.8 Glancing angle X-ray diffractogram of MTA analysing surface deposits on MTA after immersion in water and Hank's balanced salt solution (HBSS) for 28 days

Calcium silicate hydrate is amorphous and thus cannot be detected by X-ray diffraction analysis. However, the other cement components and bismuth oxide are crystalline. As hydration progresses, a rise in calcium hydroxide peak (ICDD: 44-1481) is seen at 18.008 and 34.102°2θ using a copper Kα X-ray radiation. The un-hydrated tricalcium silicate phase (ICDD: 86-0402) at 29.414, 32.193, 32.504, 32.623, 34.355 and 41.298°2θ usually decreases in intensity (Fig. 2.9). Quantitative measurements of the different phases of MTA may be performed using Rietveld refinement of X-ray diffraction plots (Table 2.2). This quantitative assessment verifies the reduction in tricalcium silicate and dicalcium silicate levels of the un-hydrated cement as hydration proceeds, with the formation of calcium silicate hydrate. Calcium hydroxide and low levels of ettringite are also produced.

Table 2.2 Rietveld X-ray diffraction analysis of the phases present in un-hydrated and hydrated ProRoot MTA

	Material type in mass %	
Phases identified	Un-hydrated	Hydrated
Tricalcium silicate	53.1	10.6
Dicalcium silicate	22.5	14.9
Tricalcium aluminate	0.0	0.0
Gypsum	0.0	0.0
Hemihydrate	0.0	0.0
Anhydrite	1.5	0.0
Calcium hydroxide	0.0	14.4
Calcium silicate hydrate	0.0	49.5
Ettringite	0.0	2.1
Bismuth oxide	21.6	8.4

Reprinted with permission from Camilleri [18]. © 2008 *International Endodontic Journal*

Energy-dispersive spectroscopy gives the elemental distribution of particular elements in the hydrated MTA. A series of X-ray spectra are collected and quantified using suitable mineral standards. The data plotted in a standard format shows atomic ratios of silicon and calcium (Si/Ca) plotted against aluminium and calcium ratios (Al/Ca). These atomic ratio plots are used in

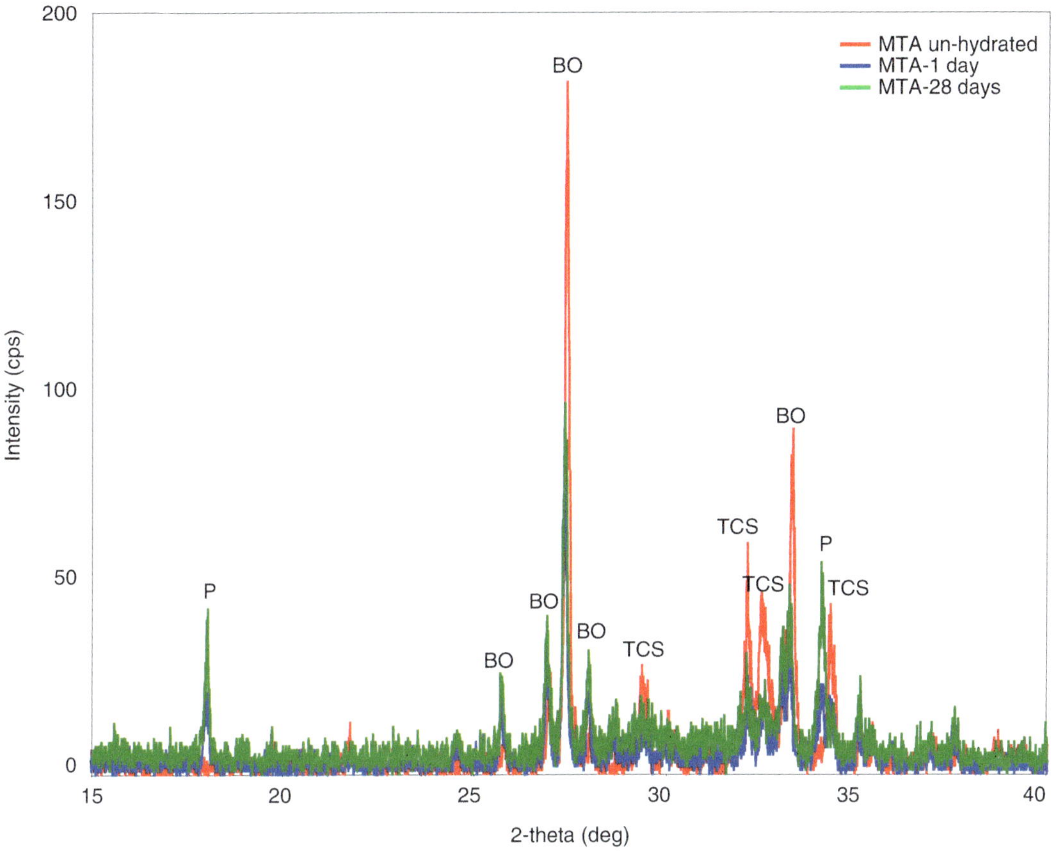

Fig. 2.9 X-ray diffractogram of un-hydrated and hydrated MTA after 1 and 28 days showing the main phases present. The tricalcium silicate peaks are more pronounced in the un-hydrated MTA compared to the hydrated forms. Portlandite is only present in the hydrated MTA. *BO* bismuth oxide, *P* portlandite or calcium hydroxide, *TCS* tricalcium silicate

scanning electron microscopy and X-ray energy-dispersive analyses (SEM/EDS) studies of cementitious materials and enable the principal hydration products to be differentiated. An atomic ratio plot for MTA's main constituents is shown in Fig. 2.10a. The atomic ratio plots of MTA show a mixture of calcium hydroxide and calcium silicate hydrate.

Infrared and Raman spectra also exhibit distinctive features for MTA [36, 44, 76]. Typical FT-IR plots for un-hydrated MTA and hydrated material before immersion and after immersion in solution for 28 days are shown in Fig. 2.11. The un-hydrated MTA displays a tricalcium silicate peak at ~875 cm^{-1}. Tricalcium silicate (peaking at ~875 cm^{-1}) is also identified in all the set cements with the peak reduced in intensity when compared to the un-hydrated material. The set MTA exhibits a characteristic set of bands at 973–981 cm^{-1} which are attributed to tricalcium silicate hydrate. These are the most intensive bands in all the spectra and can be assigned to Si–O stretching. In addition, very weak bands at 821–842 cm^{-1} also assigned to Si–O stretching vibrations are also present. The splitting of the band in the 1,000–850 cm^{-1} region results from the presence of silicate phases. The bands in the region of 1,640 cm^{-1} are due to H–O–H bending vibrations of H_2O molecules. Calcium hydroxide, which is a by-product of hydration of tricalcium silicate cement, also exhibits bands in the region of 1,600–1,400 cm^{-1}. The bands at 1,600–1,300 cm^{-1}

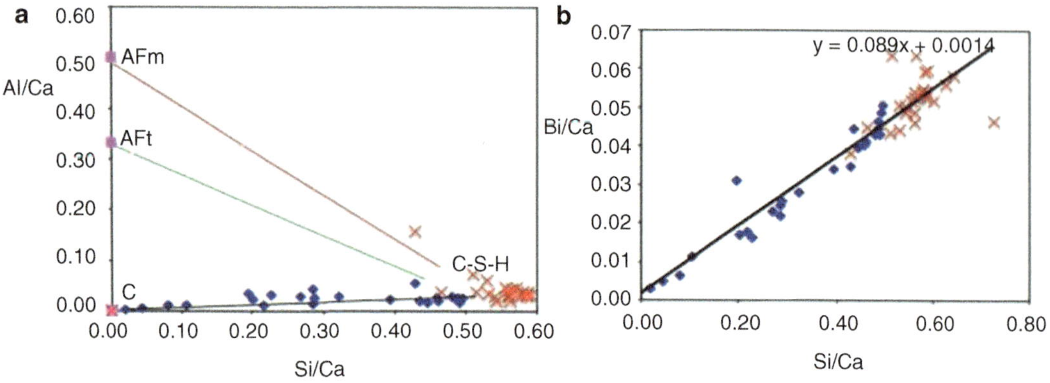

Fig. 2.10 (**a**, **b**) Atomic ratio plots of (**a**) Al/Ca versus Si/Ca indicating a mixture of calcium hydroxide and calcium silicate hydrate. *C* calcium hydroxide, *C–S–H* calcium silicate hydrate, *AFm* monosulphate, *AFt* ettringite and (**b**) Bi/Ca and Si/Ca demonstrating the relationship of bismuth and calcium silicate hydrate gel of MTA mixed with water and cured in different environmental conditions (*blue dots* are in the core region, while *red* crosses in the periphery) (Reprinted with permission from Camilleri [21]. Copyright ©2007, John Wiley and Sons)

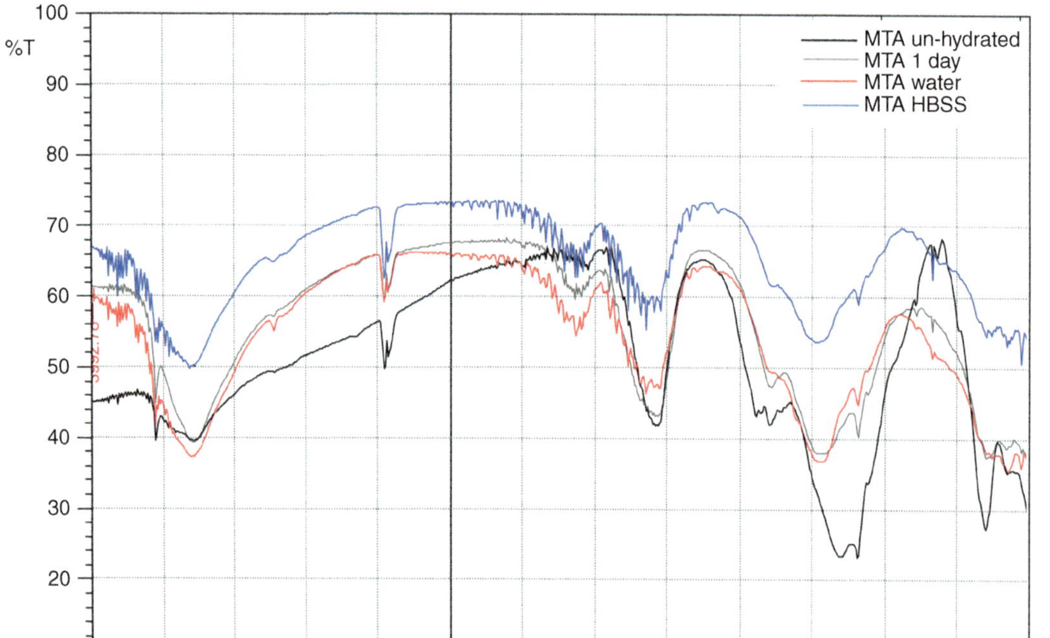

Fig. 2.11 Fourier transform infrared (FT-IR) spectroscopy of un-hydrated MTA, hydrated MTA and hydrated MTA stored in water and Hank's balanced salt solution (HBSS) for 28 days

correspond to the asymmetric stretching of CO_3^{2-}. Calcium carbonate is formed from the surface carbonation of cements by reaction of the calcium hydroxide with the atmospheric carbon dioxide.

Bismuth oxide is added to MTA to act as a radiopacifying agent since Portland cement is not sufficiently radiopaque. Quantitative X-ray diffraction analysis (Table 2.2) identifies a reduction of bismuth oxide after cement hydration, with 8.4 % present in the hydrated cement as opposed to the 21.6 % in the un-hydrated material [18]. Atomic ratio plots of Bi/Ca versus Si/Ca demonstrate a linear relationship between bismuth and silicon; the result infers that bismuth is replacing silicon in the calcium silicate hydrate structure (Fig. 2.10b).

2.8 Trace Elements

Since the main constituent of MTA is Portland cement, some concerns have been raised about the inclusion of trace elements in MTA. Portland cement is manufactured from naturally occurring raw materials in a kiln. Sometimes, waste materials are used as raw materials in the manufacturing of Portland cement for the construction industry. Additionally, waste materials are also used as replacement for primary fuels in order to keep the manufacturing costs low. This potentially leads to the inclusion of trace elements in the final product. Traces of arsenic, lead and chromium have been reported in both grey and white MTA [22, 23, 31, 32, 60, 61, 72]. Although the levels of acid-extractable trace elements are high, the amounts leached in solution are negligible. The inclusion of heavy metals in Portland cement has raised concerns regarding its use as a base material for MTA, since the latter is applied in contact with both hard and soft human tissues.

Conclusions

Mineral trioxide aggregate is composed of Portland cement and bismuth oxide radiopacifier. The cement component is in turn composed of tricalcium and dicalcium silicate and tricalcium aluminate which on reaction with water form calcium silicate hydrate and calcium hydroxide from the reaction of tri- and dicalcium silicate and ettringite and monosulphate from the reaction of tricalcium aluminate with water in the presence of gypsum. Addition of chemical and mineral oxides, cement fineness and incorporation of anti-washout gel can modify the setting time, workability, washout characteristics and reaction kinetics of the cement. Un-hydrated and set MTA can be characterised by a variety of techniques including SEM and EDS analysis, XRD with and without Rietveld correction, FT-IR and laser Raman techniques. A combination of techniques is always advisable.

References

1. Abdullah D, Ford TR, Papaioannou S, Nicholson J, McDonald F. An evaluation of accelerated Portland cement as a restorative material. Biomaterials. 2002;23(19):4001–10.
2. American Standards for Testing Materials. ASTM C150/C150M – 12; Standard specification for Portland cement. West Conshohocken: ASTM International; 2011.
3. American Standards for Testing Materials. ASTM C204 – 11 Standard Test Methods for fineness of hydraulic cement by air-permeability apparatus. West Conshohocken: ASTM International; 2011.
4. Antunes Bortoluzzi E, Juárez Broon N, Antonio Hungaro Duarte M, de Oliveira Demarchi AC, Monteiro Bramante C. The use of a setting accelerator and its effect on pH and calcium ion release of mineral trioxide aggregate and white Portland cement. J Endod. 2006;32(12):1194–7.
5. Asgary S, Parirokh M, Eghbal MJ, Stowe S, Brink F. A qualitative X-ray analysis of white and grey mineral trioxide aggregate using compositional imaging. J Mater Sci Mater Med. 2006;17(2):187–91.
6. Basturk FB, Nekoofar MH, Günday M, Dummer PM. The effect of various mixing and placement techniques on the compressive strength of mineral trioxide aggregate. J Endod. 2013;39(1):111–4.
7. Belío-Reyes IA, Bucio L, Cruz-Chavez E. Phase composition of ProRoot mineral trioxide aggregate by X-ray powder diffraction. J Endod. 2009;35(6):875–8.
8. Bensted J. Uses of Raman spectroscopy in cement chemistry. J Am Ceram Soc. 1976;59:140–3.
9. Ber BS, Hatton JF, Stewart GP. Chemical modification of ProRoot MTA to improve handling characteristics and decrease setting time. J Endod. 2007;33(10):1231–4.

10. Bortoluzzi EA, Broon NJ, Bramante CM, Felippe WT, Tanomaru Filho M, Esberard RM. The influence of calcium chloride on the setting time, solubility, disintegration, and pH of mineral trioxide aggregate and white Portland cement with a radiopacifier. J Endod. 2009;35(4):550–4.
11. Bryan TE, Khechen K, Brackett MG, Messer RL, El-Awady A, Primus CM, Gutmann JL, Tay FR. In vitro osteogenic potential of an experimental calcium silicate-based root canal sealer. J Endod. 2010;36(7): 1163–9.
12. Brunauer S, Emmett P, Teller E. Adsorption of gases in multimolecular layers. J Am Chem Soc. 1938;60:309–19.
13. Camilleri J, Formosa L, Damidot D. The setting characteristics of MTA Plus in different environmental conditions. Int Endod J. 2013;46(9):831–40.
14. Camilleri J, Gandolfi MG, Siboni F, Prati C. Dynamic sealing ability of MTA root canal sealer. Int Endod J. 2011;44(1):9–20.
15. Camilleri J, Gandolfi MG. Evaluation of the radiopacity of calcium silicate cements containing different radiopacifiers. Int Endod J. 2010;43(1):21–30.
16. Camilleri J, Mallia B. Evaluation of the dimensional changes of mineral trioxide aggregate sealer. Int Endod J. 2011;44(5):416–24.
17. Camilleri J, Sorrentino F, Damidot D. Investigation of the hydration and bioactivity of radiopacified tricalcium silicate cement, Biodentine and MTA Angelus. Dent Mater. 2013;29(5):580–93.
18. Camilleri J. Characterization of hydration products of mineral trioxide aggregate. Int Endod J. 2008;41(5): 408–17.
19. Camilleri J. Evaluation of selected properties of mineral trioxide aggregate sealer cement. J Endod. 2009;35(10):1412–7.
20. Camilleri J. Evaluation of the physical properties of an endodontic Portland cement incorporating alternative radiopacifiers used as root-end filling material. Int Endod J. 2010;43(3):231–40.
21. Camilleri J. Hydration mechanisms of mineral trioxide aggregate. Int Endod J. 2007;40(6):462–70.
22. Camilleri J, Kralj P, Veber M, Sinagra E. Characterization and analyses of acid-extractable and leached trace elements in dental cements. Int Endod J. 2012;45(8):737–43.
23. Chang SW, Baek SH, Yang HC, Seo DG, Hong ST, Han SH, Lee Y, Gu Y, Kwon HB, Lee W, Bae KS, Kum KY. Heavy metal analysis of ortho MTA and ProRoot MTA. J Endod. 2011;37(12):1673–6.
24. Chen CC, Lai MH, Wang WC, Ding SJ. Properties of anti-washout-type calcium silicate bone cements containing gelatin. J Mater Sci Mater Med. 2010;21(4):1057–68.
25. Chng HK, Islam I, Yap AU, Tong YW, Koh ET. Properties of a new root-end filling material. J Endod. 2005;31(9):665–8.
26. Chung H, Kim M, Ko H, Yang W. Evaluation of physical and biologic properties of the mixture of mineral trioxide aggregate and 4-META/MMA-TBB resin. Oral Surg Oral Med Oral Pathol Oral Radiol Endod. 2011;112(5):e6–11.
27. Coleman NJ, Awosanya K, Nicholson JW. A preliminary investigation of the in vitro bioactivity of white Portland cement. Cem Conc Res. 2007;37:1518–23.
28. Comin-Chiaramonti L, Cavalleri G, Sbaizero O, Comin-Chiaramonti P. Crystallochemical comparison between Portland cements and mineral trioxide aggregate (MTA). J Appl Biomater Biomech. 2009;7(3): 171–8.
29. Cutajar A, Mallia B, Abela S, Camilleri J. Replacement of radiopacifier in mineral trioxide aggregate; characterization and determination of physical properties. Dent Mater. 2011;27(9):879–91.
30. Dammaschke T, Gerth HU, Züchner H, Schäfer E. Chemical and physical surface and bulk material characterization of white ProRoot MTA and two Portland cements. Dent Mater. 2005;21(8):731–8.
31. De-Deus G, de Souza MC, Sergio Fidel RA, Fidel SR, de Campos RC, Luna AS. Negligible expression of arsenic in some commercially available brands of Portland cement and mineral trioxide aggregate. J Endod. 2009;35(6):887–90.
32. Duarte MA, De Oliveira Demarchi AC, Yamashita JC, Kuga MC, De Campos FS. Arsenic release provided by MTA and Portland cement. Oral Surg Oral Med Oral Pathol Oral Radiol Endod. 2005;99(5): 648–50.
33. Duarte MA, Alves de Aguiar K, Zeferino MA, Vivan RR, Ordinola-Zapata R, Tanomaru-Filho M, Weckwerth PH, Kuga MC. Evaluation of the propylene glycol association on some physical and chemical properties of mineral trioxide aggregate. Int Endod J. 2012;45(6):565–70.
34. European Standards. BS EN 196-6:2010. Methods of testing cement. Determination of fineness. London: British Standards Institutions; 2010.
35. Formosa LM, Mallia B, Bull T, Camilleri J. The microstructure and surface morphology of radiopaque tricalcium silicate cement exposed to different curing conditions. Dent Mater. 2012;28(5):584–95.
36. Formosa LM, Mallia B, Camilleri J. The chemical properties of light- and chemical-curing composites with mineral trioxide aggregate filler. Dent Mater. 2013;29(2):e11–9.
37. Formosa LM, Mallia B, Camilleri J. Mineral trioxide aggregate with anti-washout gel – properties and microstructure. Dent Mater. 2013;29(3):294–306.
38. Formosa LM, Mallia B, Camilleri J. A quantitative method for determining the antiwashout characteristics of cement-based dental materials including mineral trioxide aggregate. Int Endod J. 2013;46(2): 179–86.
39. Fridland M, Rosado R. Mineral trioxide aggregate (MTA) solubility and porosity with different water-to-powder ratios. J Endod. 2003;29(12):814–7.
40. Gandolfi MG, Perut F, Ciapetti G, Mongiorgi R, Prati C. New Portland cement-based materials for endodontics mixed with articaine solution: a study of cellular response. J Endod. 2008;34(1):39–44.

41. Gandolfi MG, Shah SN, Feng R, Prati C, Akintoye SO. Biomimetic calcium-silicate cements support differentiation of human orofacial mesenchymal stem cells. J Endod. 2011;37(8):1102–8.
42. Gandolfi MG, Taddei P, Siboni F, Modena E, Ciapetti G, Prati C. Development of the foremost light-curable calcium-silicate MTA cement as root-end in oral surgery. Chemical-physical properties, bioactivity and biological behavior. Dent Mater. 2011;27(7):e134–57.
43. Gandolfi MG, Taddei P, Siboni F, Modena E, De Stefano ED, Prati C. Biomimetic remineralization of human dentin using promising innovative calcium-silicate hybrid "smart" materials. Dent Mater. 2011;27(11):1055–69.
44. Gandolfi MG, Van Landuyt K, Taddei P, Modena E, Van Meerbeek B, Prati C. Environmental scanning electron microscopy connected with energy dispersive x-ray analysis and Raman techniques to study ProRoot mineral trioxide aggregate and calcium silicate cements in wet conditions and in real time. J Endod. 2010;36(5):851–7.
45. Gomes-Filho JE, de Faria MD, Bernabé PF, Nery MJ, Otoboni-Filho JA, Dezan-Júnior E, de Moraes Costa MM, Cannon M. Mineral trioxide aggregate but not light-cure mineral trioxide aggregate stimulated mineralization. J Endod. 2008;34(1):62–5.
46. Gomes-Filho JE, de Moraes Costa MT, Cintra LT, Lodi CS, Duarte PC, Okamoto R, Bernabé PF, Nery MJ, Cannon M. Evaluation of alveolar socket response to Angelus MTA and experimental light-cure MTA. Oral Surg Oral Med Oral Pathol Oral Radiol Endod. 2010;110(5):e93–7.
47. Han L, Okiji T, Okawa S. Morphological and chemical analysis of different precipitates on mineral trioxide aggregate immersed in different fluids. Dent Mater J. 2010;29:512–7.
48. Hawley M, Webb TD, Goodell GG. Effect of varying water-to-powder ratios on the setting expansion of white and gray mineral trioxide aggregate. J Endod. 2010;36(8):1377–9.
49. Huffman BP, Mai S, Pinna L, Weller RN, Primus CM, Gutmann JL, Pashley DH, Tay FR. Dislocation resistance of ProRoot Endo Sealer, a calcium silicate based root canal sealer, from radicular dentine. Int Endod J. 2009;42(1):34–46.
50. Jafarnia B, Jiang J, He J, Wang YH, Safavi KE, Zhu Q. Evaluation of cytotoxicity of MTA employing various additives. Oral Surg Oral Med Oral Pathol Oral Radiol Endod. 2009;107(5):739–44.
51. Ji DY, Wu HD, Hsieh SC, Teng NC, Chen CC, Ke ES, Lin YC, Lee SY, Yang JC. Effects of a novel hydration accelerant on the biological and mechanical properties of white mineral trioxide aggregate. J Endod. 2011;37(6):851–5.
52. Kai D, Li D, Zhu X, Zhang L, Fan H, Zhang X. Addition of sodium hyaluronate and the effect on performance of the injectable calcium phosphate cement. J Mater Sci Mater Med. 2009;20(8):1595–602.
53. Kogan P, He J, Glickman GN, Watanabe I. The effects of various additives on setting properties of MTA. J Endod. 2006;32(6):569–72.
54. Komabayashi T, Spångberg LS. Comparative analysis of the particle size and shape of commercially available mineral trioxide aggregates and Portland cement: a study with a flow particle image analyzer. J Endod. 2008;34(1):94–8.
55. Komabayashi T, Spångberg LS. Particle size and shape analysis of MTA finer fractions using Portland cement. J Endod. 2008;34(6):709–11.
56. Lee BN, Hwang YC, Jang JH, Chang HS, Hwang IN, Yang SY, Park YJ, Son HH, Oh WM. Improvement of the properties of mineral trioxide aggregate by mixing with hydration accelerators. J Endod. 2011;37(10):1433–6.
57. Lee SJ, Chung J, Na HS, Park EJ, Jeon HJ, Kim HC. Characteristics of novel root-end filling material using epoxy resin and Portland cement. Clin Oral Investig. 2013;17(3):1009–15.
58. Lin Q, Lan X, Li Y, Yu Y, Ni Y, Lu C, Xu Z. Anti-washout carboxymethyl chitosan modified tricalcium silicate bone cement: preparation, mechanical properties and in vitro bioactivity. J Mater Sci Mater Med. 2010;21(12):3065–76.
59. Massi S, Tanomaru-Filho M, Silva GF, Duarte MA, Grizzo LT, Buzalaf MA, Guerreiro-Tanomaru JM. pH, calcium ion release, and setting time of an experimental mineral trioxide aggregate-based root canal sealer. J Endod. 2011;37(6):844–6.
60. Matsunaga T, Tsujimoto M, Kawashima T, Tsujimoto Y, Fujiwara M, Ookubo A, Hayashi Y. Analysis of arsenic in gray and white mineral trioxide aggregates by using atomic absorption spectrometry. J Endod. 2010;36(12):1988–90.
61. Monteiro Bramante C, Demarchi AC, de Moraes IG, Bernadineli N, Garcia RB, Spångberg LS, Duarte MA. Presence of arsenic in different types of MTA and white and gray Portland cement. Oral Surg Oral Med Oral Pathol Oral Radiol Endod. 2008;106(6):909–13.
62. Nekoofar MH, Adusei G, Sheykhrezae MS, Hayes SJ, Bryant ST, Dummer PM. The effect of condensation pressure on selected physical properties of mineral trioxide aggregate. Int Endod J. 2007;40(6):453–61.
63. Nekoofar MH, Aseeley Z, Dummer PM. The effect of various mixing techniques on the surface microhardness of mineral trioxide aggregate. Int Endod J. 2010;43(4):312–20.
64. Neville AM, editor. Properties of concrete. 4th ed. Upper Saddle River: Prentice Hall; 2005. p. 2–8.
65. Paillere AM, Ben Bassat M, Akman S. Applications of admixtures for concrete. RILEM Technical Committees. New York: E & FN Spon, an imprint of Chapman & Hall; 1992.
66. Park JW, Hong SH, Kim JH, Lee SJ, Shin SJ. X-ray diffraction analysis of white ProRoot MTA and Diadent BioAggregate. Oral Surg Oral Med Oral Pathol Oral Radiol Endod. 2010;109(1):155–8.

67. Pelliccioni GA, Vellani CP, Gatto MR, Gandolfi MG, Marchetti C, Prati C. Proroot mineral trioxide aggregate cement used as a retrograde filling without addition of water: an in vitro evaluation of its microleakage. J Endod. 2007;33(9):1082–5.
68. Porter ML, Bertó A, Primus CM, Watanabe I. Physical and chemical properties of new-generation endodontic materials. J Endod. 2010;36(3):524–8.
69. Primus CM, inventor; DENTSPLY International, Inc., assignee. Dental material. United States Patent 7,892,342. 22 Feb 2011.
70. Profeta AC, Mannocci F, Foxton R, Watson TF, Feitosa VP, De Carlo B, Mongiorgi R, Valdré G, Sauro S. Experimental etch-and-rinse adhesives doped with bioactive calcium silicate-based micro-fillers to generate therapeutic resin-dentin interfaces. Dent Mater. 2013;29(7):729–41.
71. Rietveld HM. A profile refinement method for nuclear and magnetic structure. J Appl Cryst. 1967;2:65–71.
72. Schembri M, Peplow G, Camilleri J. Analyses of heavy metals in mineral trioxide aggregate and Portland cement. J Endod. 2010;36(7):1210–5.
73. Shahi S, Rahimi S, Yavari HR, Samiei M, Janani M, Bahari M, Abdolrahimi M, Pakdel F, Aghbali A. Effects of various mixing techniques on push-out bond strengths of white mineral trioxide aggregate. J Endod. 2012;38(4):501–4.
74. Shahravan A, Jalali SP, Torabi M, Haghdoost AA, Gorjestani H. A histological study of pulp reaction to various water/powder ratios of white mineral trioxide aggregate as pulp-capping material in human teeth: a double-blinded, randomized controlled trial. Int Endod J. 2011;44(11):1029–33.
75. Specification CRD-C 61-89ACRD-C 661-06. Specification for antiwashout admixtures for concrete, section 16, Test method for determining the resistance of freshly mixed concrete to washing out in water. Washington, DC: Chemical Research and Development Center, U.S. Army; 2006.
76. Taddei P, Tinti A, Gandolfi MG, Possi PML, Prati C. Ageing of calcium silicate cements for endodontic use in simulated body fluids: a micro-Raman study. J Raman Spectrosc. 2009;40:1858–66.
77. Tay FR, Pashley DH, Rueggeberg FA, Loushine RJ, Weller RN. Calcium phosphate phase transformation produced by the interaction of the Portland cement component of white mineral trioxide aggregate with a phosphate-containing fluid. J Endod. 2007;33(11):1347–51.
78. Torabinejad M, Hong CU, McDonald F, Pitt Ford TR. Physical and chemical properties of a new root-end filling material. J Endod. 1995;21(7):349–53.
79. Torabinejad M, White DJ, inventors; Loma Linda University, assignee. Tooth filling material and method of use. United States Patent 5,415,547. 16 May 1995.
80. Torabinejad M, White DJ, inventors; Loma Linda University, assignee. Tooth filling material and method of use. United States Patent 5,769,638. 23 June 1998.
81. Vanderweele RA, Schwartz SA, Beeson TJ. Effect of blood contamination on retention characteristics of MTA when mixed with different liquids. J Endod. 2006;32(5):421–4.
82. Wang X, Chen L, Xiang H, Ye J. Influence of anti-washout agents on the rheological properties and injectability of a calcium phosphate cement. J Biomed Mater Res B Appl Biomater. 2007;81(2):410–8.
83. Watts JD, Holt DM, Beeson TJ, Kirkpatrick TC, Rutledge RE. Effects of pH and mixing agents on the temporal setting of tooth-colored and gray mineral trioxide aggregate. J Endod. 2007;33(8):970–3.
84. Weller RN, Tay KC, Garrett LV, Mai S, Primus CM, Gutmann JL, Pashley DH, Tay FR. Microscopic appearance and apical seal of root canals filled with gutta-percha and ProRoot Endo Sealer after immersion in a phosphate-containing fluid. Int Endod J. 2008;41(11):977–86.
85. Wiltbank KB, Schwartz SA, Schindler WG. Effect of selected accelerants on the physical properties of mineral trioxide aggregate and Portland cement. J Endod. 2007;33(10):1235–8.

Properties of Hydrated Mineral Trioxide Aggregate

3

Mario Tanomaru-Filho
and Juliane Maria Guerreiro-Tanomaru

3.1 Introduction

MTA has been currently commercialized in two different forms, the gray (GMTA) and the white version (WMTA). In particular, the white MTA was developed due to the potential discoloration promoted by the gray version of the cement. The chemical composition of the MTAs is very similar to that of Portland cement despite the addition of components containing bismuth in the MTA's cements [91, 128], which aims to confer radiopacity to the materials [34]. The mixture of the MTA powder with distilled water results in the formation of by-products, such as calcium hydroxide and calcium silicate hydrate gel [27, 28] as discussed in Chap. 2. The particular mechanism of hydration and the structure of the set material result in particular properties displayed by the set MTA.

The initial pH of the MTA is approximately 10.2, but it increases to 12.5 after 3 h immersed in solution [177]. MTA has the ability to sustain high values of pH during long periods [75]. The high pH values exhibited by MTA are attributed to the constant release of calcium and the formation of calcium hydroxide.

M. Tanomaru-Filho, PhD (✉)
J.M. Guerreiro-Tanomaru, PhD
Department of Restorative Dentistry,
Araraquara School of Dentistry, UNESP – São Paulo State University, Rua Humaitá 1680, Araraquara, SP 14801-903, Brazil
e-mail: tanomaru@uol.com.br; jutanomaru@uol.com.br

Several studies had reported release of calcium from MTA [12, 74, 131]. The calcium ion release is enhanced when calcium chloride is added as an accelerator to MTA [12]. Moreover, when MTA was placed into the root canals of teeth with simulated radicular resorption, a greater calcium ion release was detected in comparison to teeth not filled with MTA [131].

3.2 Setting Time

The hydration of the MTA powder produces a colloidal gel, which solidifies and results in a solid structure. MTA is prepared by mixing the powder with distilled water using a ratio of 3:1 (powder/distilled water) [184]. It presents longer setting time (2 h and 45 min) in comparison to other retrograde materials, such as amalgam, super ethoxy benzoic acid (super EBA), and intermediate restorative material (IRM, Dentsply Caulk, Milford, Delaware, USA) [177].

GMTA presents initial and final setting times that are higher than the WMTA [92]. In comparison, WMTA exhibits a lower setting time than Portland cement. This can be attributed to the lower levels of tricalcium aluminate and sulfur in the WMTA [53]. The long setting time makes MTA unsuitable for most of the clinical applications.

When evaluated in the presence of human blood and minimal essential media, MTA (Dentsply Maillefer, Tulsa, OK) set faster than EndoSequence Root Repair Material (ESRRM; Brasseler, Savannah, GA, USA) [44]. Different

J. Camilleri (ed.), *Mineral Trioxide Aggregate in Dentistry*,
DOI 10.1007/978-3-642-55157-4_3, © Springer-Verlag Berlin Heidelberg 2014

powder-to-water ratios also exert influence on MTA's properties, promoting longer setting time, higher pH levels, and calcium ion release when a greater volume of water was used [41].

3.3 Compressive and Flexural Strength

After 24 h of mixing, MTA exhibited lower compressive strength (40 MPa) when compared to super EBA and IRM. However, the compressive strength values of the materials became statistically similar after 21 days [177]. This increase in compressive strength in the aged material is likely related to the hydration rate of the dicalcium silicate, which is slower than the tricalcium silicate [53]. Other researchers reported the maximum compressive strength of MTA being achieved after few days of mixing [164]. Studies analyzing the compressive strength of different MTAs in comparison to Portland cement after 3 and 28 days demonstrated that white MTA exhibited lower values when compared to the gray version [92]. Although some studies suggested that bismuth oxide promotes deterioration of the mechanical resistance of the cement when different ratios were added to the Portland cement [155], the strength of the resultant material was not affected when compared with pure white Portland. The reported deterioration was caused by a gradual increase in porosity of Portland-based cement [49].

The in vitro compressive tests used to evaluate the strength of dental materials are relative and just predict the clinical behavior. Experimental models proposed to evaluate the fracture resistance of immature bovine teeth with intra-radicular reinforcement and treated with MTA [23] indicated that the association of cast post and MTA increased the resistance to fracture of weakened teeth. In another study with immature teeth, the obturation of the samples with gutta-percha, MTA, and a calcium phosphate-based cement promoted significant radicular reinforcement [40].

The influence of a calcium hydroxide intra-canal dressing on the fracture resistance of immature teeth filled with MTA has also been tested, and the results showed that the intra-canal dressing was not able to increase the fracture resistance of these teeth [10]. On the other hand, the use of the intra-canal dressing with time-frames from 2 weeks up to 1 year in teeth obturated with MTA presented greater resistance to fracture when compared to those filled with calcium hydroxide after a year. The authors also observed the presence of a metalloproteinase-2 (TIMP-2) inhibitor only in the MTA samples, and they attributed the greater fracture resistance of these teeth to the inhibitory effect promoted by TIMP-2 on collagen destruction [83].

3.4 Bond Strength

The bond strength analysis of a reparative material used to seal dental perforation is important due to the fact that the material can suffer displacement under occlusal forces which might result in sealing failure. The bond strength values for ProRoot MTA ranged from 4.7 MPa after 72 h covered with a moist cotton pellet which increased to 7 MPa after immersion in solution for 2 months [139] to 3 MPa increasing to 10 MPa after 21 days [76]. The presence of moisture promoted greater MTA bond strength [76]. MTA is a hydraulic cement; thus, it improves its properties in the presence of moisture. When MTA is stored in a humid environment, the material bond strength increases with time [53]. Also, the MTA bond strength is significantly increased when the material is stored in synthetic body fluids, such as phosphate-buffered saline or Hank's balanced salt solution. These solutions have the ability to promote biomineralization which can exerts a positively influence on bond strength. The effects of the biomineralization process on bond strength of the ProRoot MTA (Dentsply Tulsa Dental, Tulsa, OK, USA), white MTA (Angelus Soluções Odontológicas, Londrina, PR, Brazil), MTA BIO (Angelus Indústria de Produtos Odontológicos Ltda., Londrina, PR, Brazil), and Portland cement with or without calcium chloride has been studied [139], and the samples immersed in phosphate-buffered saline exhibited greater resistance to displacement when compared to the samples that remained in contact with a moistened piece of cotton.

The surrounding pH is another factor that can affect the MTA adhesion. A study with radicular slices of teeth filled with WMTA immersed in neutral (pH 7.4) or alkaline (pH 8.4, 9.4 or 10.4) synthetic tissue fluids (STF) was performed, and the greatest and the lowest bond strength values were obtained after exposing the samples to pH 8.4 and 10.4, respectively. These results confirm the hypothesis that the WMTA adhesion is directly affected by an alkaline pH [152]. The opposite had also been tested. The influence of an acid environment on WMTA bond strength was evaluated using the same methodology. The samples filled with WMTA remained in contact with gauze soaked with neutral phosphate-buffered saline solution (pH 7.4) or with acid solutions (pH 4.4, 5.4 and 6.4). The highest bond strength values of the WMTA were verified with samples exposed to pH 7.4, and these values decreased with lower pH values, proving that acid environments also lead to lower MTA adhesion [162].

The physical or chemical treatment of the dentin surface using diode laser and MTAD™ (Dentsply, Tulsa Dental Specialities, Tulsa, Oklahoma) also may decrease the MTA adhesion [150]. MTA also demonstrated lower bond strength values when compared to IRM or super EBA after contacting whitening substances, such as sodium perborate in saline solution, Superoxol, or sodium perborate mixed with Superoxol [107]. Furthermore, nano-modification of the cement particles enhanced the push-out bond strength of the MTA [149].

3.5 Microhardness

The MTA microhardness values were reported to be 37.54 [79] and 53.56 [120, 151]. A variety of factors such as surrounding pH [101, 120], material thickness [112], mixing techniques [122], condensing pressure [121], powder particle size [146], etching [96], blood and serum contamination [123], and temperature [151] can affect MTA microhardness. An acidic environment [120], blood and serum contamination [123], and low temperatures [151] reduced the microhardness of MTA. Alternatively, MTA microhardness was improved by reducing the particle size of the MTA powder which increased the surface area of the material [146]. Apical plugs 5 mm thick were considered to be more resistant than thinner ones (2 mm thick) [112]. Acid treatment of the dentin prior to restorative procedures can negatively affect the compressive strength and the microhardness of MTA. Therefore, it is reasonable to perform restorative procedures only 96 h after placing MTA [96]. The authors suggest that the changes promoted by acids over MTA surface might potentially improve the adhesion of resinous materials. Layering of different materials over the MTA surface when it is used to seal perforations with cyanoacrylate, glass ionomer cement, or castor oil did not improve the microhardness and/or the sealing ability of MTA [26].

3.6 Dimensional Stability

The dimensional stability of dental materials can be influenced by several factors which include the conditions for setting and the solubility levels of the material. MTA exhibits hygroscopic expansion when in contact with tissue fluids [30, 168] and shrinkage if allowed to dry out [30]. The expansion of the material after setting [92] may enhance the sealing ability of MTA [45].

3.7 Solubility

The literature reports that MTA has low or no solubility [54, 177]. However, it has been observed in some studies that the solubility increases with time [75] and it is influenced by powder-to-water ratio; when a greater amount of water is added to the mixture, a material with higher porosity and solubility is produced [74]. Comparing white and gray MTAs, the white version of the cement exhibited greater solubility [92]. Although bismuth oxide is an insoluble substance, the presence of this substance in the composition of MTA may be responsible by the solubility of the cement due to the fact that bismuth oxide causes a deterioration of the mechanical strength and it increases the relative porosity of the material [49].

Initially, the immersion of white MTA in distilled water resulted in a decrease in weight, followed by an increase in weight after 30-day of immersion in physiologic solution. The loss weight has been attributed to the release of calcium hydroxide, while the increase in weight is likely related to the deposition of apatite crystals on the material surface [161].

3.8 Porosity

The influence of water-to-powder ratio on MTA porosity had been studied; the solubility and the porosity levels of the material increased with higher water-to-powder ratio [74]. The influence of the surrounding pH on MTA porosity levels has also been evaluated. White Portland and white MTA were submitted to two different environments, an acid medium with pH 4.4 and another with pH close to neutral (7.4). The porosity analysis revealed that the pore volume of white MTA was lower than those of white Portland at both pH values [147]. As described before, in the solubility section, the addition of bismuth oxide as radiopacifier in MTA cements is responsible for mechanical strength deterioration which likely is related to the gradual increase on porosity, which demonstrated a direct correlation between bismuth oxide amount and porosity [49].

3.9 Sealing Ability

The success of a root canal repair material depends on its sealing ability, since the post-endodontic treatment failure is usually due to the sealing failure. The sealing ability of MTA has been evaluated since its development. A sealing ability study with amalgam, super EBA, and mineral trioxide aggregate (MTA) as root-end filling materials showed that MTA leaked significantly less than amalgam and super EBA [184]. When the same materials were evaluated in root-end cavities contaminated by blood, MTA also demonstrated significantly lower leaking levels when compared to amalgam, super EBA, and IRM [175]. In addition, MTA presented better bacterial sealing than amalgam, super EBA, and intermediate restorative material (IRM) as root-end filling material [182]. The marginal adaptation of mineral trioxide aggregate (MTA) as a root-end filling was assessed by scanning electron microscopy (SEM), and MTA exhibited better adaptation compared to amalgam, super EBA, and IRM [183]. Therefore, MTA was shown to be superior to amalgam and comparable with super EBA in preventing microleakage when used as a root-end filling [17].

A literature review evaluating the sealing ability and biocompatibility of MTA from November 1993 up to September 2009 demonstrated that MTA presents an adequate sealing and it is a biocompatible material [180].

A variety of studies had been performed to evaluate MTA cements in comparison to other conventional cements in order to assess the sealing ability of these materials used as root-end fillers. Several methods have been employed to compare MTA to other materials that have been established as root-end filing materials in order to assess their sealing ability. The sealing ability of IRM Caps (IRM), Fuji IX Capsules (Fuji IX)(GC Europe, Leuven, Belgium), and ProRoot MTA tooth-colored formula (MTA) in human teeth was studied using the fluid transport method and capillary flow porometry. The conventionally setting glass ionomer cement Fuji IX showed the best results when used as a root-end filling material [56]. Using a bacterial leakage model with Streptococcus salivarius, Resilon (Pentron Dental Products, Wallingford Center, Connecticut, USA) and MTA leaked significantly less than super EBA [109]. In comparison to Portland cements, both white and gray MTA showed comparable sealing ability when tested using dye leakage [160]. A number of sealers, namely, Sealer 26 (Dentsply, Addlestone, United Kingdom) and Endo CPM Sealer (EGEO SRL, Argentina, Buenos Aires), were compared to white MTA and zinc oxide eugenol-based cements demonstrating comparable sealing ability when materials were all used as root-end filling materials [172].

MTA has also been compared to EndoSequence Bioceramic Root-end Repair (Brasseler, Savannah, Georgia, USA), and it could be observed that Endosequence exhibited equivalent sealing ability to white MTA when used as root-end filling material [119]. On the other hand, another study used a bacterial leakage model with Enterococcus faecalis demonstrated that the Endosequence putty leaked significantly more than MTA [85].

The sealing ability promoted by mineral trioxide aggregate (MTA Bio) when mixed with antibacterial vehicles, such as chlorhexidine and doxycycline, was compared to the conventional mixture with water. Both antibacterial mixtures did not affect the sealing properties of MTA Bio [13]. The sealing ability of MTA, glass ionomer cement, or resin composite when used to repair large pulp chamber floor perforations was assessed using a bacterial leakage method with *Enterococcus faecalis*. The resin composite leaked significantly more than MTA and glass ionomer cements. Also, it was observed that bacteria could penetrate into dentin even at a distance from the perforation filling [106]. The sealing of wide-open apices with apical plugs of white MTA Angelus, MTA Bio, ProRoot MTA, and Portland cement all cements allowed fluid movement [58].

In addition to assessing the sealing ability of MTA and comparing it to other materials, other factors affecting the sealing ability of the test materials were also evaluated. The effect of storage temperature on sealing ability and solubility of MTA was studied in root-end cavities filled with white MTA stored at 4, 25, or 40 °C. The highest microleakage and solubility rates were observed in 4 °C followed by samples submitted to 25 and 40 °C. Based on these findings, the storage temperature appears to play an important role in the properties and hence clinical outcomes of MTA [148].

The influence of different apicoectomy angles and root-end cavities prepared with different instruments on amalgam and gray MTA sealing ability was also evaluated. The only factor that seemed to affect microleakage significantly was the retrofilling material used to seal the cavities, with MTA exhibiting less leakage than amalgam [137]. Following this research, the sealing ability promoted by ProRoot MTA and MTA Angelus in retrograde cavities prepared with low-speed burs, ultrasonic or Er, Cr: YSGG laser was compared using fluid-filtration methodology. The results showed the less microleakage level with cavities prepared with Er, Cr: YSGG laser for all the tested materials, with no significant statistical difference between the materials [98].

If the root-end cavity preparation does not seem to exert any influence on material's sealing ability, the condensation technique may have some influence on sealing. Root-end cavities were filled with ProRoot MTA® using ultrasonic vibration or sonic vibration in comparison to the control group (no vibration) and immersed in rhodamine B and assessed for leakage by tracing the fluorescent dye showed that sonic vibration promoted the lowest leakage values and may be considered an efficient aid to improve MTA sealing ability in root-end fillings [20].

Another factor that seems to affect MTA sealing ability is water-to-powder ratio. The apical dye leakage in teeth retro-filled with white ProRoot MTA, using 0.28, 0.33, and 0.40 water-to-powder ratios of MTA and packed with plugger or wet cotton, was evaluated. The results showed that packing with moist cotton pellet in lower-liquid-to-powder ratios of MTA as well as packing with a plugger in higher-liquid-to-powder ratio decreased apical dye leakage [129].

Another factor that could influence the sealing ability of MTA is the irrigation regime employed during treatment of furcal perforations. Sodium hypochlorite and sodium hypochlorite in addition to ethylene diamine tetraacetic acid (EDTA) and MTAD were assessed by the fluid-filtration method after 1 day and 1 week. Leakage was not affected by the material used to seal the perforation, but the use of chelating solutions (EDTA and MTA) in association with NaOCl affected sealing [187]. Corroborating these findings, an apical microleakage study with teeth obturated with MTA showed that the apical microleakage is less when the smear layer is present than when it is absent [195]. The cavity thickness had no influence in bacterial leakage of the MTA retro-fillings. In addition, the authors suggested that removing smear layer may not be necessary in root-end cavities filled with MTA [194].

3.10 Antibacterial Properties

The antimicrobial evaluation of dental materials requires knowledge of antimicrobial methodologies. The most used methodologies to evaluate the antimicrobial property of dental materials are the agar diffusion test and the direct contact test. The agar diffusion test depends on the diffusion ability of the tested material, which may not reflect the true antimicrobial action while the direct contact test is based on the effects promoted by the material on bacterial population when the material under investigation is placed in direct contact with the tested microorganism.

Microorganism choice should take into consideration the most important species involved in the development of periapical disease. For antimicrobial effect evaluation of endodontic materials, the use of *Enterococcus faecalis* is important because this is a microorganism commonly associated with endodontic treatment failures. However, other microorganisms such as fungi and anaerobic microorganisms are also implicated in endodontic infections. One factor that may influence the results is the microorganism organization. Microorganism can be studied in planktonic form or organized in biofilms. In the planktonic form, the cells are in suspension and they are more sensitive, since they are not protected as in the biofilm form, which is a cluster formation protected by an extracellular lipopolysaccharide matrix highly resistant to the action of antibiotics and disinfectants. Due to the differences between methodologies, the types of the microorganisms, and their organization, variation in the results of antimicrobial activity studies of dental materials may be observed.

Since MTA's introduction in 1993, numerous studies have been published regarding various aspects of this material. The antibacterial and antifungal properties of MTA have been evaluated. Several investigations reported that MTA has limited antimicrobial effect against some microorganisms. A literature review regarding the chemical, physical, and antibacterial properties of MTA with published papers from November 1993 up to September 2009 related that MTA possesses some antibacterial and antifungal properties, depending on its powder-to-liquid ratio [133].

The antibacterial effects of amalgam, zinc oxide-eugenol, super EBA, and MTA on nine facultative bacteria and seven strict anaerobic bacteria were evaluated. Mineral trioxide aggregate had antibacterial effect on some of the facultative bacteria and no effect on any of the strict anaerobic bacteria. Zinc oxide-eugenol and super EBA pastes had some antibacterial effects on both types of bacteria tested [179]. Another study showed that the antimicrobial activity of the calcium hydroxide paste was superior to MTA and Portland cement for all microorganisms tested [68], and no antimicrobial activity was observed against *E. faecalis* [115], while MTA was effective on other strains (*E. coli* (ATCC 10538), *C. albicans* (ATCC 10231), *Actinomyces viscosus* (ATCC 15987), and *S. mutans* (ATCC 25175) [82]. ProRoot MTA demonstrated no antimicrobial activity against *S. aureus*, *E. faecalis*, *C. albicans*, *S. mutans*, and *Streptococcus sanguinis* [193]. Some investigations had suggested that MTA has antifungal effect against *C. albicans* when freshly mixed [9].

Different root-end filling materials and root canal sealers (Sealer 26, Sealapex [Kerr, Orange, California, USA] with zinc oxide, zinc oxide and eugenol, white and gray Portland cement, white and gray MTA Angelus, and gray ProRoot MTA [Dentsply/Tulsa Dental, Tulsa, Oklahoma, USA]) were evaluated against *Kocuria rhizophila* (*Micrococcus luteus*) (ATCC 9341), *S. aureus* (ATCC6538), *E. coli* (ATCC10538), *P. aeruginosa* (ATCC27853), *C. albicans* (ATCC 10231), and *E. faecalis* (ATCC 10541). All materials were shown to possess antimicrobial activity [174]. The antimicrobial effects of four mineral trioxide aggregate preparations, two white colored (WMTA-1, WMTA-2) and two gray colored (GMTA-1, GMTA-2), against *C.*

albicans and *E. faecalis* were assessed in vitro, and the origin of MTA as well as the type of preparation may affect its antimicrobial characteristics [8]. The gray MTA required lower concentrations than WMTA to exert the same antibacterial effect against each of the microorganisms tested [7].

Other materials that had the antibacterial properties compared to MTA (ProRoot MTA) were the amalgam, intermediate restorative material (IRM), Super Bond (Sun Medical, Shiga, Japan), Geristore (Denmat Holdings, Lompoc, California, USA), Dyract (Dentsply Caulk, Milford, Delaware, USA), Clearfil APX (Kuraray, Hattersheim am Main, Germany), and Protect Bond (Kuraray, Hattersheim am Main, Germany). These materials were examined using direct contact test (DCT) with *S. aureus*, *E. faecalis*, and *P. aeruginosa*. IRM and ProRoot MTA were generally more potent inhibitors of bacterial growth than the other tested materials [63]. The antimicrobial effect of MTA Dentsply (Tulsa Dental, Tulsa, Oklahoma, USA), MTA Angelus, calcium hydroxide, and Portland cement against *P. aeruginosa*, *E. coli*, *Bacteroides fragilis*, and *E. faecalis* was also evaluated. MTA Dentsply, MTA Angelus, and Portland cement inhibited the growth of *P. aeruginosa*. Under anaerobic conditions, the materials failed to inhibit *E. faecalis* and *E. coli* [141].

Some changes in the composition of the MTA are proposed to increase its antimicrobial property. The antimicrobial activity of MTA and calcium-enriched mixture (CEM) mixed with different concentrations of chlorhexidine were evaluated against *E. faecalis*, *S. mutans*, *C. albicans*, *Actinomyces* species, *E. coli*, and a mixture of these microorganisms. The results demonstrated that the mixture of MTA and CEM with different concentration of chlorhexidine significantly increased the antibacterial activity [21]. The use of 0.12 % chlorhexidine gluconate as vehicle to mix MTA enhanced the antimicrobial activity of tooth-colored ProRoot mineral trioxide aggregate (MTA) against *Actinomyces odontolyticus* (ATCC17982), *F. nucleatum* (ATCC2586), *S. sanguis* (ATCC10556), *E. faecalis* (ER3/2S), *E. coli* (SM10lambdapir), *S. aureus* (ATCC6538), *P. aeruginosa* (UME), and *C. albicans* (ATCC10261). MTA/chlorhexidine showed significantly larger zones of inhibition than MTA/water [169]. Two percent chlorhexidine was shown to be the most effective concentration even against *E. faecalis* [89]. Iodine potassium iodide in combination with MTA did not significantly increase the antimicrobial activity of MTA [145]. However, the addition of silver zeolite to MTA showed that the incorporation of silver zeolite may enhance the antimicrobial activity of MTA [126].

The hypothesis that the antimicrobial activity of gray and white MTA is related to the induction of reactive oxygen species (ROS) was evaluated. Both cements showed antimicrobial activity under aerobic conditions. On the other hand, both cements were not able to induce any bacterial inhibition under anaerobic conditions, suggesting that the inhibitory action is a result of ROS production [143].

3.11 Radiopacity

Mineral trioxide aggregate includes 20 % bismuth oxide which is added to enhance the radiopacity of the material [185]. The radiopacity of MTA depends on the quantity of bismuth oxide added. ProRoot MTA exhibits a radiopacity of around 8 mm aluminum thickness [29, 32, 92, 177]. The radiopacifier loading of ProRoot MTA is 21.6 % [18, 28]. MTA Angelus has less bismuth oxide (14 %) than ProRoot MTA [38] and exhibits lower radiopacity values [32, 38, 41, 190]. An assessment of the amount of bismuth oxide necessary to confer the necessary radiopacity to MTA showed that 15 % addition of bismuth oxide was an adequate amount [25].

The analysis of the radiopacity and biocompatibility of MTA, Portland cement, and Portland cement plus bismuth oxide suggested a positive correlation between the concentration of the radiopacifying agent and radiopacity values. Moreover, the histological evaluation suggested that all materials were biocompatible after 7 and 60 days [50]. However, the increase of bismuth oxide concentration is related to further deterioration of the material mechanical strength and increase in porosity [49].

The radiopacity of other retrograde materials, such as MTA Bio, light-cured MTA, Sealapex, and Portland cement clinker with bismuth oxide and calcium sulfate, had been compared to white MTA and all the retrograde materials met the minimum radiopacity standards of 3 mm Al except the light-cured MTA [190].

3.12 Color Stability

Endodontic materials might be responsible for tooth discoloration, which may compromise aesthetic outcomes. MTA has been used in several clinical procedures such as retro-fillings, repair of perforations, direct pulp cappings, and pulpotomies and as apical plugs in teeth with necrosis and incomplete apex formation [134]. However, this material presents some disadvantages, among which is tooth discoloration. Clinical reports describe the discoloration promoted by gray MTA on marginal gingiva when it was used to seal a perforation in upper incisors [22]. In this case, the treatment for tooth discoloration consisted in the replacement of gray MTA by white MTA. It is also reported that white MTA promoted tooth discoloration after pulpotomy [19], but when MTA was removed, significant color change of the dental crown was observed. The teeth remained vital and the formation of a dentinal bridge was clinical and radiographically confirmed. The authors suggested that the use of white MTA in aesthetic zone should be revised.

Many factors contribute to tooth discoloration in the presence of white MTA. Contamination with blood [71, 102] and contact of MTA with sodium hypochlorite [31] and presence of light and oxygen levels within the root canal [188, 189] result in MTA and tooth discoloration. Some alternative treatments had been attempted to prevent crown discoloration promoted by MTA. Dentin bonding agent has been applied before placing white or gray MTA in endodontically treated teeth, and it has showed an ability to prevent tooth discoloration [5].

A literature review about tooth discoloration promoted by endodontic procedures demonstrated that there is limited data about the discoloration promoted by endodontic materials currently available [99]. The authors suggested that the endodontic therapy should be focused not only on biological and functional aspects but also on the aesthetic condition. Therefore, further researches are required aiming to develop new endodontic materials that do not promote tooth discoloration.

3.13 Trace Elements

The amount of heavy metals present in MTA-based materials and Portland cements is a general concern among clinicians with respect to clinical employment. Several studies identified the presence of these chemical elements, especially arsenic. The limit of arsenic recommended by the International Standards Organization (ISO) in water-based cements is 2 mg/kg of material. Some studies investigated the presence of arsenic on several types of MTA and Portland cement. Only MTA-Obtura (Angelus Indústria de Produtos Ontológicos Ltda., Londrina, PR, Brazil), white MTA (Angelus), and white Portland demonstrated arsenic levels below to the limit established by ISO 9917-1 [90].

Arsenic levels had been measured in two types of gray Portland, one white Portland and two MTAs (ProRoot MTA and MTA Angelus). The levels of arsenic identified in Portland cements and MTAs were similar and much lower than those considered harmful [116]. MTA and Portland cements presented low amounts of arsenic, suggesting that these materials can be considered safe for clinical use [61]. In another study, the levels of arsenic, lead, and chromium were quantified in hydrated gray and white Portland cement, ProRoot MTA, and MTA Angelus. All cements displayed higher levels of chromium release in comparison to arsenic and lead. White Portland and the two types of MTA exhibited low release levels for all metallic ions. Moreover, both Portland cements and the MTAs showed evidences of heavy metals in the acid-soluble form [157]. The amount of arsenic released from other brands of MTA and Portland had also been compared. Gray MTA (Angelus,

Londrina, PR, Brazil), gray ProRoot MTA (Tulsa/Dentsply, Tulsa, OK), and Portland cement (Brasilatex Ltda, Diadema, SP, Brazil) have displayed no traces of arsenic [59].

A consecutive and more complex research investigated the levels of ten different heavy metals (arsenic, bismuth, cadmium, chromium, copper, iron, lead, manganese, nickel, and zinc) in two versions of Portland cements (gray and white) and in the two versions of MTA (gray and white). The concentrations of arsenic and lead were higher in the gray Portland which exhibited a higher amount of seven heavy metals when compared to the other materials. The MTAs presented higher purity levels when compared to the Portland cements, especially with respect to the arsenic amount [43].

A literature review about the composition of a Portland cement also dedicated especial attention for arsenic levels. The findings demonstrated that Portland cement is not cytotoxic and exhibits low levels of arsenic release. Furthermore, this cement has the ability to induce the deposition of reparative dentin, and it also allows cellular adhesion and proliferation [57]. Another investigations about arsenic release from gray and white MTA also demonstrated that the concentration of arsenic released by both MTAs were lower than 2 ppm [111], which is the limit suggested by ISO [90]. The arsenic levels released by MTA and Portland cements were also evaluated concomitantly to hydrogen potential and electrical conductivity [80]. These authors also verified insignificant levels of arsenic in both materials.

Lately, a variety of MTA-based materials were introduced in endodontics, and the levels of heavy metals have also been a concern in these materials. Thus, the levels of arsenic, chromium, hexavalent chromium, and lead between ProRoot MTA and Ortho MTA (BioMTA, Seoul, Korea) (MTA-based materials) were compared, and both materials demonstrated to be in accordance with ISO 9917–1 specifications with respect to arsenic and lead levels [42].

Calcium silicate-based materials have also been investigated with respect to arsenic release. Pure tricalcium silicate, Biodentine, and Bioaggregate were compared to conventional Portland and MTA cements. All the materials displayed higher arsenic content than the level specified by ISO 9917–1 (2007) [90]. On the other hand, the levels of lead were considered acceptable [33].

3.14 Biocompatibility

In vitro studies have been conducted to evaluate the MTA biocompatibility. The general survey of studies indicates that MTA is a biocompatible material. A review of literature on the constituents and biocompatibility of mineral trioxide aggregate (MTA) using papers published from November 1993 to August 2005 demonstrated that cytological evaluation was the most widely employed biocompatibility test, and these studies have shown that MTA is biocompatible [37]. The review of properties, biocompatibility, and the clinical outcomes involving the use of mineral trioxide aggregate in endodontic treatment was performed using papers from January 1990 to August 2006. The results show that MTA is biocompatible and has excellent potential to be use in endodontics [144].

A systematic review investigated whether the use of mineral trioxide aggregate for repair of an endodontic-periodontal communication leads to regeneration of the adjacent periodontal tissues. The databases MEDLINE-PubMed, Cochrane-CENTRAL, and EMBASE were searched up to July 2012, and in vivo studies reporting the histological response of the periodontium to MTA were selected. Within the limitations of the selected papers, the findings were consistent with regard to MTA's biocompatibility and cementogenic ability. Experimental studies with animals showed that MTA can promote healing towards regeneration [95]. Other literature reviews presented a variety of articles regarding the biocompatibility of MTA. The review of the literature was performed using electronic and hand-searching methods from November 1993 to September 2009. Based on available evidence it also appears that MTA is a biocompatible material [180].

In vitro studies on the biocompatibility of MTA, investigating the cellular proliferation and viability, using different cell lines in direct and/or indirect contact, have been performed, and MTA exhibited no cellular toxicity [130]. Several cell lines have been employed, and the use of biological markers aids in the assessment of material biocompatibility. MTA encourages cell proliferation and cytokine production [81]. Cells formed a monolayer over the material surface [197]. Cell morphology is mostly assessed by scanning electron microscopy [15, 197] or by MTT (3-[4,5-dimethylthiazol-2-yl]-2,5 diphenyl tetrazolium bromide) assay [35]. The assessment of the cellular metabolic function and proliferation of both the material and elution has been assessed and showed no toxic leachables from the gray or white MTA and accelerated Portland cement. Furthermore, the addition of bismuth oxide did not interfere with the material biocompatibility [35] although bismuth oxide itself does not encourage cell growth and proliferation [36].

The genotoxicity and cytotoxicity of gray and white mineral trioxide aggregate (MTA) was assessed and compared with Portland cements by the comet assay and trypan blue test. The cements and neither the compounds produced genotoxic effects or cellular death [140, 142].

The addition of various accelerators did not impair MTA biocompatibility. Hydration accelerators such as calcium chloride ($CaCl_2$), citric acid (CA), and calcium lactate gluconate solution (CLG) added to MTA showed favorable biocompatibility after 1 day. However, the association of MTA with 10 wt% $CaCl_2$ showed the lowest cell viability and poor cell attachment [94]. In addition, the effects of various additives on setting time and cell attachment on gray MTA (GMTA) were studied using osteoblasts and L929 mouse fibroblasts. Osteoblasts and fibroblasts attached and spread over GMTA mixed with additives similarly to GMTA mixed with water, suggesting that MTA is biocompatible when mixed with the tested additives [6]. The biocompatibility of gray mineral trioxide aggregate (MTA) mixed with other accelerants, such as calcium chloride ($CaCl_2$), calcium nitrite/nitrate (CaN/N), or calcium formate (CaF), had been also evaluated after implantation into rat mandibles. Corroborating the finding in other studies, the results indicated that MTA mixed with these accelerants may be a biocompatible alternative when a rapid set is indicated clinically [113].

Moreover, the cytotoxic effect and the tissue reaction induced by MTA and Portland cement implanted in the mandibles of guinea pigs demonstrated bone healing and minimal inflammatory response adjacent to ProRoot and Portland implants, suggesting that both materials showed biocompatibility when evaluated in vitro and in vivo [153]. The effectiveness of MTA as a pulp capping material has led to the investigation of its effect on human dental pulp stromal cells with assessment of cell surface morphology the levels of gene expression and secretion of vascular endothelial growth factor. MTA promoted cell survival and proliferation in human dental pulp stromal cells. The results support the biocompatible nature of MTA and the possible mechanism of dentin bridge formation along with tissue repair [132].

Histological evaluation of tissue reaction to MTA has been evaluated by subcutaneous and intraosseous implantation of the materials in animals. In vivo tests as retrograde filling and perforation repair material can also be verified in the scientific literature. Tissue reaction of implanted super EBA and the original MTA formulation in the mandibles of guinea pigs showed that MTA exhibited better tissue reaction than super EBA [178]. Other MTA formulations exhibited a similar response [24, 100].

At the tissue level gray MTA exhibited a better biological response than white MTA or amalgam after 1 week of tissue contact, but no difference was demonstrated after 3 weeks [159]. The tissue response of MTA and apatite which is postulated to be responsible for material bioactivity was assessed by subcutaneous tissue implantation in dorsal connective tissue of rats. The results suggested a possible role of apatite formation on the mineralization induction characteristics of WMTA, which indicated a definite effect on biocompatibility [55].

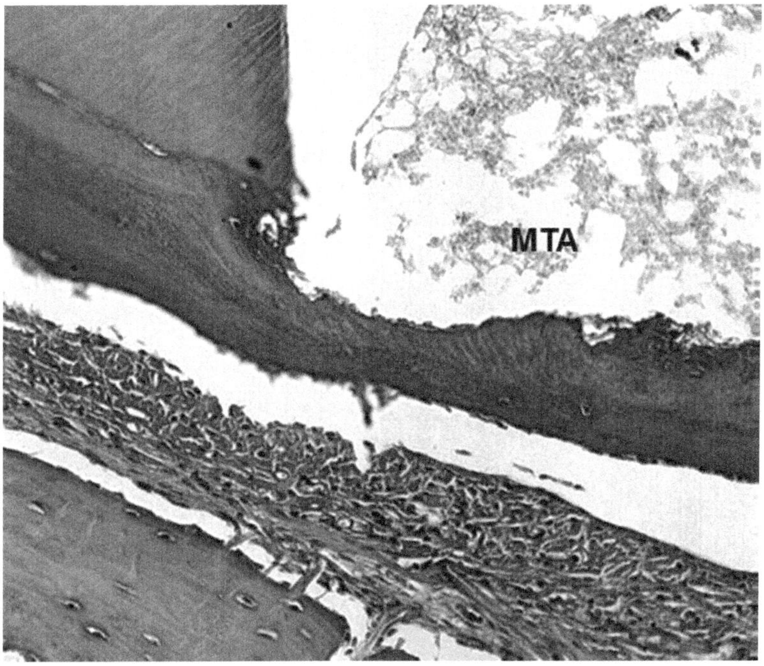

Fig. 3.1 Retrograde cavity filled with Mineral Trioxide Aggregate (MTA) showing the formation of mineralized tissue close to the filling material and periapical repair. Original magnification × 100. H&E (Reprinted from Tanomaru-Filho et al. [173] copyright 2006, with permission from Elsevier)

Laboratory tests using animals, such as monkey and dogs, as subjects have been conducted to investigate periapical response to cements uses as root-end fillings. The tissue response to MTA and amalgam as root-end fillings have been tested in monkeys, and no periradicular inflammation adjacent to five of six root ends filled with MTA was demonstrated. Also, MTA showed a complete layer of cementum covering the root-end filling. In contrast, all root ends filled with amalgam showed periradicular inflammation and no formation of cementum over the root-end filling material [181]. The periapical repair following retrograde fillings with Sealer 26, Sealapex plus zinc oxide, or MTA (Fig. 3.1) was evaluated after endodontic surgery in dogs' teeth, and the histopathologic analysis revealed similar periapical repair promoted by the materials [173].

The periapical tissue response of other retrofilling materials such as intermediate restorative material (IRM), thermoplasticized gutta-percha, reinforced zinc oxide cement (super EBA), and mineral trioxide aggregate (MTA) was studied in a dog model. Better reestablishment of the periapical tissues was observed with IRM and MTA. New hard tissue formation was observed directly over the material surface only in the MTA sections. MTA exhibited the most favorable periapical tissue response (Fig. 3.2) when comparing the biocompatibility with other tested materials [192].

MTA has also been designed to seal communication between pulp cavity and periodontium, and the histologic response to intentional perforation in the teeth's furcations of dogs repaired immediately with amalgam or MTA showed that MTA is more suitable than amalgam for perforation repair, particularly when it is used immediately after perforation [73]. The periradicular tissue response to MTA exhibited less periradicular inflammation and more fibrous capsules adjacent to MTA in comparison to amalgam. In addition, the presence of cementum over the MTA surface was observed [176]. The healing process of intentional lateral root perforation repaired with mineral trioxide aggregate (MTA) was observed in dogs' teeth (Fig. 3.3) showing no inflammation and deposition of cementum over MTA [88]. The biological response of the periodontium adjacent to furcation perforations in rat molars filled

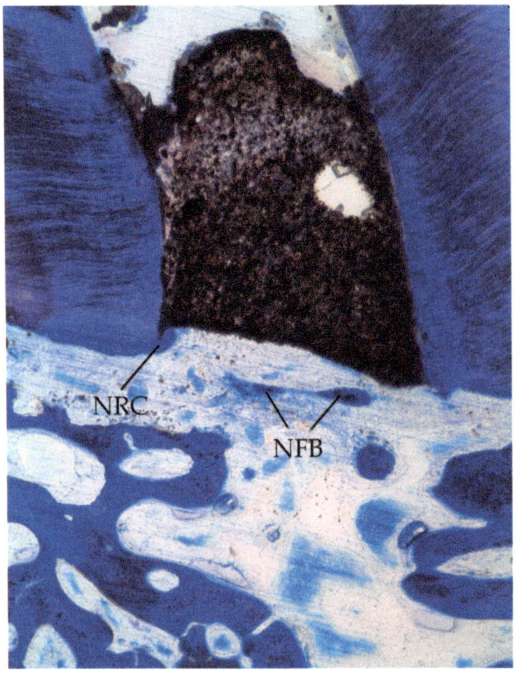

Fig. 3.2 Histologic section (magnification × 4) of a retrograde cavity filled with MTA in dog's teeth shows newly formed cement (*NRC*) growing from the periphery over the mineral trioxide aggregate surface and islands of newly formed bone (*NFB*) in close vicinity to the mineral trioxide aggregate surface (Reprinted from Wälivaara et al. [192] copyright 2012, with permission from Elsevier)

with Endo CPM Sealer, MTA Angelus, or zinc oxide-eugenol cement has also been evaluated. The greatest number of inflammatory cells was observed at 7 days, especially in the zinc oxide-eugenol (ZOE) group where the inflammatory process was related to a significant increase in the number of osteoclasts and, thereby, in an increase in the width of the periodontal space. At 60 days, no significant differences in osteoclast numbers among Endo CPM Sealer, MTA, and control groups were evident. The periodontal space was also significantly reduced in the experimental groups in comparison with the initial periods. The periodontium adjacent to perforations filled with MTA and Endo CPM Sealer exhibited clear evidence of reestablishment and thus demonstrated better biocompatibility than zinc oxide-eugenol (Fig. 3.4) [51]. Contaminations of lateral perforations can impair the healing process. Regardless the use of MTA, contaminated lateral root perforations immediately sealed with MTA presented worse repair than the non-contaminated ones [87].

The systemic toxic effect of gray ProRoot Mineral trioxide aggregate (MTA) on the liver and kidney of rats was evaluated after 7 and 30

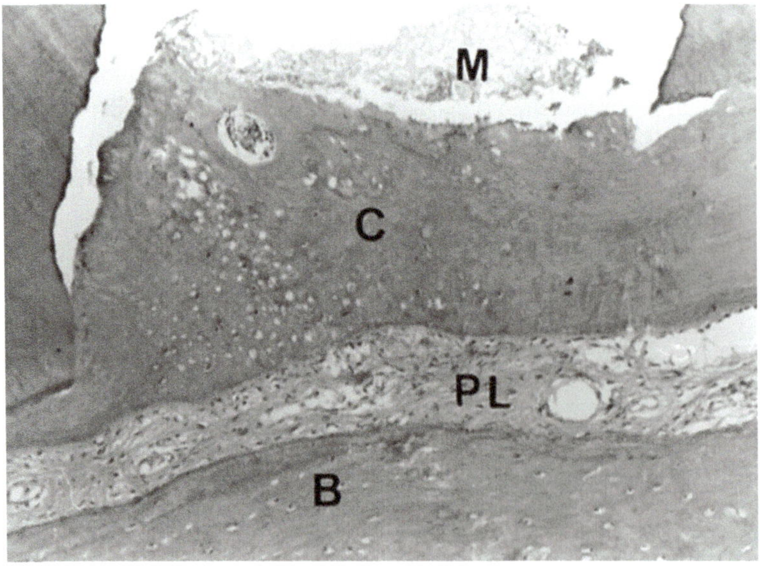

Fig. 3.3 Lateral root perforation repaired with mineral trioxide aggregate (MTA) in dogs' teeth. Cementum (*C*) over the filling material (*M*), periodontal ligament (*PL*), and bone (*B*). Hematoxylin and eosin; original magnification 3100 (Reprinted from Holland et al. [88] copyright 2001, with permission from Elsevier)

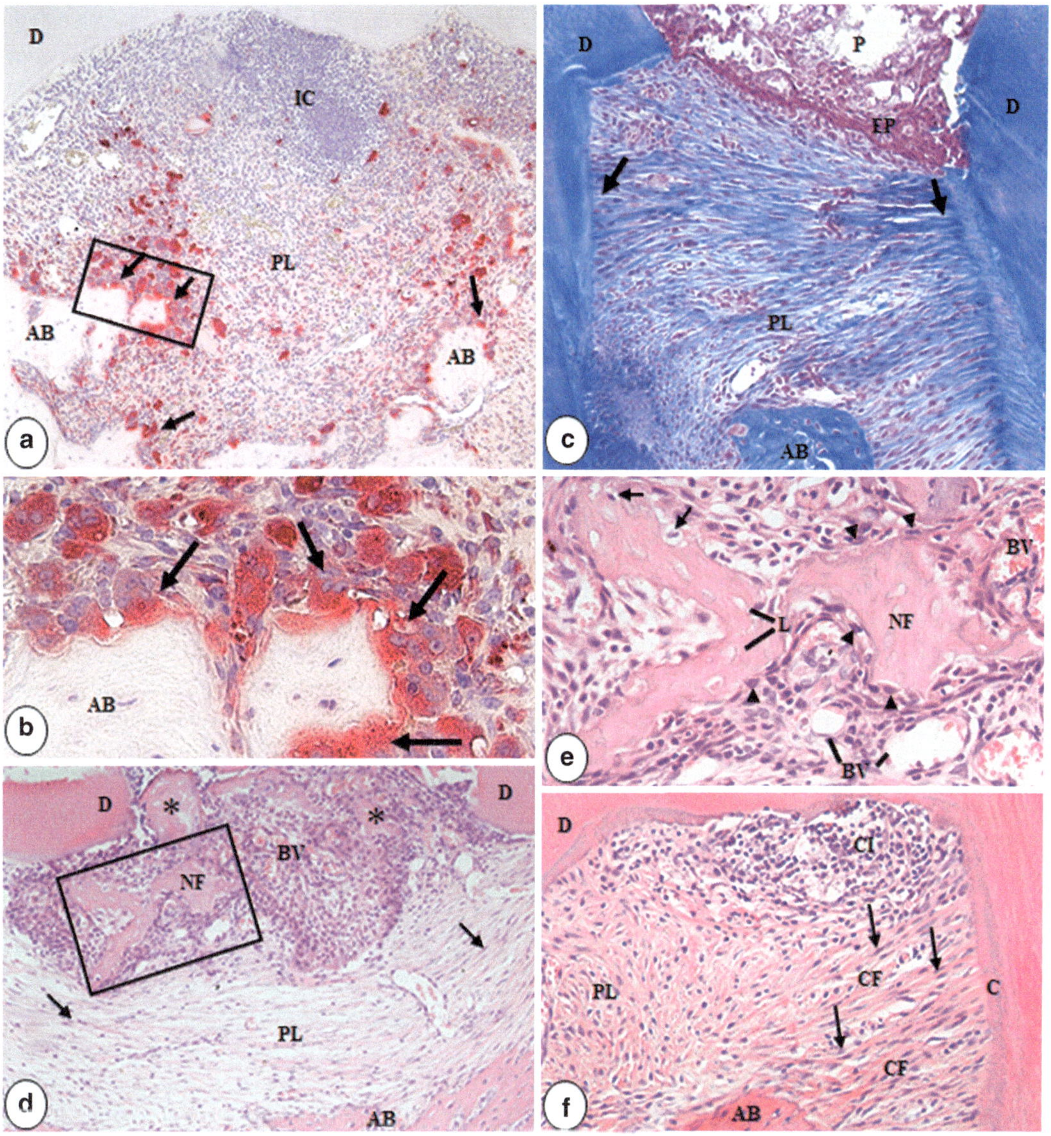

Fig. 3.4 Light micrographs of furcation region of molar teeth perforated and filled with MTA and examined after 7 (**a**, **b**), 15 (**c**), 30 (**d**, **e**), and 60 days (**f**). In (a), numerous inflammatory cells (*IC*) are present in the wide periodontal space. Tartrate-resistant acid phosphatase (TRAP)-positive osteoclasts (*arrows*) are next to the alveolar bone (*AB*) surface. TRAP reaction counterstained with hematoxylin. *D* dentin, *PL* periodontal ligament (bar, 100 lm). In (**b**), outlined area of (**a**), TRAP-positive osteoclasts (*arrows*) are adjacent to the bone surface. AB, alveolar process (bar, 50 lm). (**c**) Shows a layer of two to three elongated cells (*EP*) between the perforation in the floor of the pulp chamber (*P*) and the periodontal ligament (*PL*). In the PL, some bundles of collagen fibers (*CF*) penetrate into the root surfaces (*arrows*). D, dentin; AB, alveolar process. Masson's trichrome (bar, 100 lm). In (**d**), acidophilic and irregular material (*NF*) fills partially the perforation of the floor of the pulp chamber and is surrounded by numerous mononuclear cells and blood vessels (*BV*). Collagen fibers and fibroblasts (*arrows*) seem to be surrounding the material "NF." PL, peridontal ligament; D, dentin; AB, alveolar process. H&E (bar, 100 lm). In (**e**), outlined area of (**d**), homogeneous material "NF" contains lacunae (L) and, sometimes, cells inside them (*arrows*). Elongated and rounded cells (*arrowheads*) are in close juxtaposition to the irregular surface of "NF." BV, blood vessels. H&E (bar, 50 lm). In (**f**), some inflammatory cells (*IC*) are adjacent to the root surface. In the furcation region, fibroblasts (*arrows*) and bundles of collagen fibers (*CF*); some of them penetrate into the alveolar bone (*AB*) and cementum (*C*). D, dentin. H&E (bar, 100 lm) (Reprinted with permission from da Silva et al. [51] © 2010 *International Endodontic Journal*)

days and compared to DiaRoot BioAggregate. The materials were inserted into Teflon tubes and implanted subcutaneously. Blood samples were taken to investigate changes of kidney and liver functions. MTA induced side effects on the liver and kidney that were significantly more severe than BioAggregate (Verio Dental Co. Ltd., Vancouver, Canada) but with no permanent damage [97].

Clinical research on MTA is presented as specific case reports or randomized clinical trials. The case reports present a very low level of evidence due to lack of standardization as opposed to randomized clinical trials. From 1995 to date there have been 50 clinical trials on MTA. Most of the clinical trials were performed on treatment of primary teeth with a total of 27 reports (Table 3.1), 26 out of which MTA was used for pulpotomies and one report for MTA used as a direct pulp capping agent [186]. The clinical trials and outcome of clinical reports assessing the success rate of MTA used for the treatment of primary teeth are shown in Table 3.1. The assessment period ranged from 3 months to 84 months. Dentin bridge formation and absence of clinical and radiographic symptoms were used to assess the success rates. MTA was shown to exhibit same outcome as of other materials tested in 17 from the 26 cases reviewed. Two studies did not use a control material but assessed MTA only; thus, no comparisons could be made [110, 118]. Calcium hydroxide and MTA may be suitable materials for the treatment of the immature teeth. However, more studies evaluating the factors influencing success and failure in teeth should be conducted [46].

There have been five reports on the use of MTA for direct pulp capping [1, 67, 69, 84, 93] and two for indirect pulp capping [103, 136]; four for apexification [52, 64, 158, 163] and six for apexogenesis [14, 16, 64, 78, 125, 138]; and five studies for use as a root-end filler [47, 48, 104, 165, 191] and one for perforation repair [77]. Taking into consideration the randomized clinical trials with specific MTA use, it can be concluded that MTA was shown to be a successful root-end filling material [156] and was comparable to IRM and super EBA cement [47, 104, 165]. Furthermore, the type of tooth treated did not affect the outcome of treatment. MTA was shown to be better than Retroplast as a root-end filling material [191]. High success rates were reported, and the need to use a root-end filling material as opposed to resection and burnishing gutta-percha was highlighted [48].

Pulp capping with MTA is recommended for teeth with carious pulp exposures especially immature teeth with high potential for healing [70]. When used as a pulp capping agent, MTA exhibited comparable clinical and radiographic success rates to calcium hydroxide [103, 136], while in other clinical studies, MTA was shown to have better clinical success rates than calcium hydroxide [67, 84]. Both ProRoot MTA and MTA Angelus exhibited similar success rates [1]. No statistically significant differences were found for superficial and deep inflammatory cell response, presence of a dentin bridge, and pulp vitality between MTA and calcium hydroxide. A statistically significant difference was found for the diameter of exposure. Only a minimal association between clinical and histological findings could be established for either material [93].

For treatment of immature permanent teeth, cases treated with MTA exhibited complete root formation earlier. A good success and an effective option for apexification with the advantage of reduced treatment time, good sealing ability, and biocompatibility providing a barrier for immediate obturation were demonstrated from MTA [52]. One-visit apexification procedures are possible with MTA [163]. Although MTA was more successful, it is more expensive, and dentin bridges developed over canal orifices, complicating future root canal therapy [78]. MTA was comparable to calcium hydroxide [16, 65, 138] and calcium-enriched mixture in treatment of immature permanent molars by pulpotomy [14, 125].

Table 3.1 Clinical trials evaluating the success rates of MTA used in treatment of primary teeth

Year	Author	Assessment period (months)	Control material	Outcome
2013	Mehrdad et al. [114]	24	CEM	Same; calcific bridge formation
2012	Sushynski et al. [171]	6–24	FC	Gray MTA better than formocresol
	Fernández et al. [72]	24	FC, FS, NaOCl	Same
	Odabaş et al. [127]	12	FS	Same
	Airen et al. [4]	6, 12, 24	FC	MTA better
2011	Liu et al. [105]	/	$Ca(OH)_2$	MTA better; crown discoloration noted
	Malekafzali et al. [108]	12, 24	CEM	Same
	Srinivasan and Jayanthi [167]	3, 6, 9, 12	FC	MTA better
	Erdem et al. [66]	6, 12, 24	FC, FS, ZnO	Same. MTA better than ZnO
	Cardoso Silva et al. [39]	84	GMTA, WMTA	Same, gray better
2010	Zealand et al. [196]	6	FC	Same; MTA 22 % dentin bridge formation
	Ansari and Ranjpour [11]	6, 12, 24	FC	Same
	Doyle et al. [60]	24	FS (±eugenol)	MTA better; outcome worse with eugenol free FS
2009	Subramaniam et al. [170]	24	FC	MTA better
	Sakai et al. [154]	6, 12, 18, 24	Portland cement	Same; Portland cement caused more pulp obliteration
2008	Sonmez et al. [166]	24	FC, FS, $Ca(OH)_2$	Same; $Ca(OH)_2$ was the least appropriate
	Moretti et al. [117]	3, 6, 12, 18, 24	FC, $Ca(OH)_2$	MTA same as FC; better than $Ca(OH)_2$
	Noorollahian [124]	6, 12, 24	FC	Same
	Tuna and Olmez [186]	1–24	$Ca(OH)_2$	Same
2007	Aeinehchi et al. [2]	3, 6	FC	Same
2006	Percinoto et al. [135]	3, 6, 12	$Ca(OH)_2$	Same
2005	Farsi et al. [70]	24	FC	Clinical outcome same; MTA better radiographically
	Maroto et al. [110]	6	/	Dentin bridge formation; crown discoloration
	Holan et al. [86]	38	FC	Same
	Naik and Hegde [118]	6	/	Successful
2004	Agami et al. [3]	12	FC	Gray better than white; MTA better than FC
2001	Eidelman et al. [62]	6–30	FC	Same

CEM calcium-enriched mixture, *FC* formocresol, *FS* ferric sulfate

Conclusions

Although there are no standards for root-end filling materials or materials based on Portland cement to which MTA can conform, MTA was shown to exhibit adequate physical, chemical, antimicrobial, and biological properties which are comparable to other dental materials used for the same purpose. The clinical studies on MTA demonstrate similar data to the in vitro studies.

References

1. Accorinte ML, Loguercio AD, Reis A, Bauer JR, Grande RH, Murata SS, Souza V, Holland R. Evaluation of two mineral trioxide aggregate compounds as pulp-capping agents in human teeth. Int Endod J. 2009;42(2):122–8.
2. Aeinehchi M, Dadvand S, Fayazi S, Bayat-Movahed S. Randomized controlled trial of mineral trioxide aggregate and formocresol for pulpotomy in primary molar teeth. Int Endod J. 2007;40(4):261–7.
3. Agamy HA, Bakry NS, Mounir MM, Avery DR. Comparison of mineral trioxide aggregate and formocresol as pulp-capping agents in pulpotomized primary teeth. Pediatr Dent. 2004;26(4):302–9.
4. Airen P, Shigli A, Airen B. Comparative evaluation of formocresol and mineral trioxide aggregate in pulpotomized primary molars – 2 year follow up. J Clin Pediatr Dent. 2012;37(2):143–7.
5. Akbari M, Rouhani A, Samiee S, Jafarzadeh H. Effect of dentin bonding agent on the prevention of tooth discoloration produced by mineral trioxide aggregate. Int J Dent. 2012;2012:563203.
6. Alanezi AZ, Zhu Q, Wang YH, Safavi KE, Jiang J. Effect of selected accelerants on setting time and biocompatibility of mineral trioxide aggregate (MTA). Oral Surg Oral Med Oral Pathol Oral Radiol Endod. 2011;111(1):122–7.
7. Al-Hezaimi K, Al-Shalan TA, Naghshbandi J, Oglesby S, Simon JH, Rotstein I. Antibacterial effect of two mineral trioxide aggregate (MTA) preparations against Enterococcus faecalis and Streptococcus sanguis in vitro. J Endod. 2006;32(11):1053–6.
8. Al-Hezaimi K, Al-Shalan TA, Naghshbandi J, Simon JH, Rotstein I. MTA preparations from different origins may vary in their antimicrobial activity. Oral Surg Oral Med Oral Pathol Oral Radiol Endod. 2009;107(5):e85–8.
9. Al-Nazhan S, Al-Judai A. Evaluation of antifungal activity of mineral trioxide aggregate. J Endod. 2003;29(12):826–7.
10. Andreasen JO, Munksgaard EC, Bakland LK. Comparison of fracture resistance in root canals of immature sheep teeth after filling with calcium hydroxide or MTA. Dent Traumatol. 2006;22:154–6.
11. Ansari G, Ranjpour M. Mineral trioxide aggregate and formocresol pulpotomy of primary teeth: a 2-year follow-up. Int Endod J. 2010;43(5):413–8.
12. Antunes Bortoluzzi E, Jua´rez Broon N, Antonio Hungaro Duarte M, de Oliveira Demarchi AC, Monteiro Bramante C. The use of a setting accelerator and its effect on pH and calcium ion release of mineral trioxide aggregate and white Portland cement. J Endod. 2006;32:1194–7.
13. Arruda RA, Cunha RS, Miguita KB, Silveira CF, De Martin AS, Pinheiro SL, Rocha DG, Bueno CE. Sealing ability of mineral trioxide aggregate (MTA) combined with distilled water, chlorhexidine, and doxycycline. J Oral Sci. 2012;54(3):233–9.
14. Asgary S, Eghbal MJ. Treatment outcomes of pulpotomy in permanent molars with irreversible pulpitis using biomaterials: a multi-center randomized controlled trial. Acta Odontol Scand. 2013;71(1):130–6.
15. Balto HA. Attachment and morphological behavior of human periodontal ligament fibroblasts to mineral trioxide aggregate: a scanning electron microscope study. J Endod. 2004;30(1):25–9.
16. Barrieshi-Nusair KM, Qudeimat MA. A prospective clinical study of mineral trioxide aggregate for partial pulpotomy in cariously exposed permanent teeth. J Endod. 2006;32(8):731–5.
17. Bates CF, Carnes DL, del Rio CE. Longitudinal sealing ability of mineral trioxide aggregate as a root-end filling material. J Endod. 1996;22(11):575–8.
18. Belı´o-Reyes IA, Bucio L, Cruz-Chavez E. Phase composition of ProRoot mineral trioxide aggregate by X-ray powder diffraction. J Endod. 2009;35:875–8.
19. Belobrov I, Parashos P. Treatment of tooth discoloration after the use of white mineral trioxide aggregate. J Endod. 2011;37(7):1017–20.
20. Bernabé PF, Gomes-Filho JE, Bernabé DG, Nery MJ, Otoboni-Filho JA, Dezan-Jr E, Cintra LT. Sealing ability of MTA used as a root end filling material: effect of the sonic and ultrasonic condensation. Braz Dent J. 2013;24(2):107–10.
21. Bidar M, Naderinasab M, Talati A, Ghazvini K, Asgari S, Hadizadeh B, Gharechahi M, Mashadi NA. The effects of different concentrations of chlorhexidine gluconate on the antimicrobial properties of mineral trioxide aggregate and calcium enrich mixture. Dent Res J (Isfahan). 2012;9(4):466–71.
22. Bortoluzzi EA, Araújo GS, Guerreiro Tanomaru JM, Tanomaru-Filho M. Marginal gingiva discoloration by gray MTA: a case report. J Endod. 2007;33(3):325–7.
23. Bortoluzzi EA, Souza EM, Reis JM, Esberard RM, Tanomaru-Filho M. Fracture strength of bovine incisors after intra-radicular treatment with MTA in an experimental immature tooth model. Int Endod J. 2007;40(9):684–91.
24. Bramante CM, Kato MM, Assis GF, Duarte MA, Bernardineli N, Moraes IG, Garcia RB, Ordinola-Zapata R, Bramante AS. Biocompatibility and setting time of CPM-MTA and white Portland cement clinker with or without calcium sulfate. J Appl Oral Sci. 2013;21(1):32–6.
25. Bueno CE, Zeferino EG, Manhães Jr LR, Rocha DG, Cunha RS, De Martin AS. Study of the bismuth oxide concentration required to provide Portland cement with adequate radiopacity for endodontic use. Oral Surg Oral Med Oral Pathol Oral Radiol Endod. 2009;107(1):e65–9.
26. Camargo CH, Fonseca MB, Carvalho AS, Camargo SE, Cardoso FG, Valera MC. Microhardness and sealing ability of materials used for root canal perforations. Gen Dent. 2012;60(6):e393–7.
27. Camilleri J. Hydration mechanisms of mineral trioxide aggregate. Int Endod J. 2007;40:462–70.

28. Camilleri J. Characterization of hydration products of mineral trioxide aggregate. Int Endod J. 2008;41:408–17.
29. Camilleri J. Evaluation of the physical properties of an endodontic Portland cement incorporating alternative radiopacifiers used as root-end filling material. Int Endod J. 2010;43:231–40.
30. Camilleri J. Evaluation of the effect of intrinsic material properties and ambient conditions on the dimensional stability of white mineral trioxide aggregate and Portland cement. J Endod. 2011;37(2):239–45.
31. Camilleri J. The color stability of white mineral trioxide aggregate in contact with hypochlorite solution. J Endod. 2014;40(3):436–40.
32. Camilleri J, Gandolfi MG. Evaluation of the radiopacity of calcium silicate cements containing different radiopacifiers. Int Endod J. 2010;43(1):21–30.
33. Camilleri J, Kralj P, Veber M, Sinagra E. Characterization and analyses of acid-extractable and leached trace elements in dental cements. Int Endod J. 2012;45(8):737–43.
34. Camilleri J, Montesin FE, Brady K, Sweeney R, Curtis RV, Ford TR. The constitution of mineral trioxide aggregate. Dent Mater. 2005;21:297–303.
35. Camilleri J, Montesin FE, Di Silvio L, Pitt Ford TR. The chemical constitution and biocompatibility of accelerated Portland cement for endodontic use. Int Endod J. 2005;38(11):834–42.
36. Camilleri J, Montesin FE, Papaioannou S, McDonald F, Pitt Ford TR. Biocompatibility of two commercial forms of mineral trioxide aggregate. Int Endod J. 2004;37(10):699–704.
37. Camilleri J, Pitt Ford TR. Mineral trioxide aggregate: a review of the constituents and biological properties of the material. Int Endod J. 2006;39(10):747–54.
38. Camilleri J, Sorrentino F, Damidot D. Investigation of the hydration and bioactivity of radiopacified tricalcium silicate cement, Biodentine and MTA Angelus. Dent Mater. 2013;29(5):580–93.
39. Cardoso-Silva C, Barbería E, Maroto M, García-Godoy F. Clinical study of Mineral Trioxide Aggregate in primary molars. Comparison between Grey and White MTA-a long term follow-up (84 months). J Dent. 2011;39(2):187–93.
40. Cauwels RG, Pieters IY, Martens LC, Verbeeck RM. Fracture resistance and reinforcement of immature roots with gutta percha, mineral trioxide aggregate and calcium phosphate bone cement: a standardized in vitro model. Dent Traumatol. 2010;26(2):137–42.
41. Cavenago BC, Pereira TC, Duarte MA, Ordinola-Zapata R, Marciano MA, Bramante CM, Bernardineli N. Influence of powder-to-water ratio on radiopacity, setting time, pH, calcium ion release and a micro-CT volumetric solubility of white mineral trioxide aggregate. Int Endod J. 2014;47(2):120–6. doi:10.1111/iej.12120.
42. Chang SW, Baek SH, Yang HC, Seo DG, Hong ST, Han SH, Lee Y, Gu Y, Kwon HB, Lee W, Bae KS, Kum KY. Heavy metal analysis of ortho MTA and ProRoot MTA. J Endod. 2011;37(12):1673–6.
43. Chang SW, Shon WJ, Lee W, Kum KY, Baek SH, Bae KS. Analysis of heavy metal contents in gray and white MTA and 2 kinds of Portland cement: a preliminary study. Oral Surg Oral Med Oral Pathol Oral Radiol Endod. 2010;109(4):642–6.
44. Charland T, Hartwell GR, Hirschberg C, Patel R. An evaluation of setting time of mineral trioxide aggregate and EndoSequence root repair material in the presence of human blood and minimal essential media. J Endod. 2013;39(8):1071–2.
45. Chng HK, Islam I, Yap AU, Tong YW, Koh ET. Properties of a new root-end filling material. J Endod. 2005;31:665–8.
46. Chong BS. MTA or calcium hydroxide treatment for immature permanent teeth? Evid Based Dent. 2012; 13(1):11.
47. Chong BS, Pitt Ford TR, Hudson MB. A prospective clinical study of mineral trioxide aggregate and IRM when used as root-end filling materials in endodontic surgery. Int Endod J. 2003;36(8):520–6.
48. Christiansen R, Kirkevang LL, Hørsted-Bindslev P, Wenzel A. Randomized clinical trial of root-end resection followed by root-end filling with mineral trioxide aggregate or smoothing of the orthograde gutta-percha root filling–1-year follow-up. Int Endod J. 2009;42(2):105–14.
49. Coomaraswamy KS, Lumley PJ, Hofmann MP. Effect of bismuth oxide radioopacifier content on the material properties of an endodontic Portland cement-based (MTA-like) system. J Endod. 2007;33:295–8.
50. Coutinho-Filho T, De-Deus G, Klein L, Manera G, Peixoto C, Gurgel-Filho ED. Radiopacity and histological assessment of Portland cement plus bismuth oxide. Oral Surg Oral Med Oral Pathol Oral Radiol Endod. 2008;106(6):e69–77.
51. da Silva GF, Guerreiro-Tanomaru JM, Sasso-Cerri E, Tanomaru-Filho M, Cerri PS. Histological and histomorphometrical evaluation of furcation perforations filled with MTA, CPM and ZOE. Int Endod J. 2011;44(2):100–10.
52. Damle SG, Bhattal H, Loomba A. Apexification of anterior teeth: a comparative evaluation of mineral trioxide aggregate and calcium hydroxide paste. J Clin Pediatr Dent. 2012;36(3):263–8.
53. Dammaschke T, Gerth HU, Züchner H, Schäfer E E. Chemical and physical surface and bulk material characterization of white ProRoot MTA and two Portland cements. Dent Mater. 2005;21:731–8.
54. Danesh G, Dammaschke T, Gerth HU, Zandbiglari T, Schäfer E. A comparative study of selected properties of ProRoot mineral trioxide aggregate and two Portland cements. Int Endod J. 2006;39:213–9.
55. Danesh F, Tootian Z, Jahanbani J, Rabiee M, Fazelipour S, Taghva O, Shabaninia S. Biocompatibility and mineralization activity of fresh or set white mineral trioxide aggregate, biomimetic carbonated apatite, and synthetic hydroxyapatite. J Endod. 2010;36(6):1036–41.
56. De Bruyne MA, De Bruyne RJ, Rosiers L, De Moor RJ. Longitudinal study on microleakage of three

root-end filling materials by the fluid transport method and by capillary flow porometry. Int Endod J. 2005;38(2):129–36.
57. de Tenório de Franca TR, da Silva RJ, Sedycias de Queiroz M, Aguiar CM. Arsenic content in Portland cement: a literature review. Indian J Dent Res. 2010;21(4)):591–5.
58. De-Deus G, Audi C, Murad C, Fidel S, Fidel R. Similar expression of through-and-through fluid movement along orthograde apical plugs of MTA Bio and white Portland cement. Int Endod J. 2008;41(12):1047–53.
59. De-Deus G, de Souza MC, Sergio Fidel RA, Fidel SR, de Campos RC, Luna AS. Negligible expression of arsenic in some commercially available brands of Portland cement and mineral trioxide aggregate. J Endod. 2009;35(6):887–90.
60. Doyle TL, Casas MJ, Kenny DJ, Judd PL. Mineral trioxide aggregate produces superior outcomes in vital primary molar pulpotomy. Pediatr Dent. 2010;32(1):41–7.
61. Duarte MA, De Oliveira Demarchi AC, Yamashita JC, Kuga MC, De Campos Fraga S. Arsenic release provided by MTA and Portland cement. Oral Surg Oral Med Oral Pathol Oral Radiol Endod. 2005; 99(5):648–50.
62. Eidelman E, Holan G, Fuks AB. Mineral trioxide aggregate vs. formocresol in pulpotomized primary molars: a preliminary report. Pediatr Dent. 2001; 23(1):15–8.
63. Eldeniz AU, Hadimli HH, Ataoglu H, Orstavik D. Antibacterial effect of selected root-end filling materials. J Endod. 2006;32(4):345–9.
64. El-Meligy OA, Avery DR. Comparison of apexification with mineral trioxide aggregate and calcium hydroxide. Pediatr Dent. 2006;28(3):248–53.
65. El-Meligy OA, Avery DR. Comparison of mineral trioxide aggregate and calcium hydroxide as pulpotomy agents in young permanent teeth (apexogenesis). Pediatr Dent. 2006;28(5):399–404.
66. Erdem AP, Guven Y, Balli B, Ilhan B, Sepet E, Ulukapi I, Aktoren O. Success rates of mineral trioxide aggregate, ferric sulfate, and formocresol pulpotomies: a 24-month study. Pediatr Dent. 2011;33(2):165–70.
67. Eskandarizadeh A, Shahpasandzadeh MH, Shahpasandzadeh M, Torabi M, Parirokh M. A comparative study on dental pulp response to calcium hydroxide, white and grey mineral trioxide aggregate as pulp capping agents. J Conserv Dent. 2011;14(4): 351–5.
68. Estrela C, Bammann LL, Estrela CR, Silva RS, Pécora JD. Antimicrobial and chemical study of MTA, Portland cement, calcium hydroxide paste, Sealapex and Dycal. Braz Dent J. 2000;11(1):3–9.
69. Farsi N, Alamoudi N, Balto K, Al Mushayt A. Clinical assessment of mineral trioxide aggregate (MTA) as direct pulp capping in young permanent teeth. J Clin Pediatr Dent. 2006;31(2):72–6.
70. Farsi N, Alamoudi N, Balto K, Mushayt A. Success of mineral trioxide aggregate in pulpotomized primary molars. J Clin Pediatr Dent. 2005;29(4):307–11.
71. Felman D, Parashos P. Coronal tooth discoloration and white mineral trioxide aggregate. J Endod. 2013;39(4):484–7.
72. Fernández CC, Martínez SS, Jimeno FG, Lorente Rodríguez AI, Mercadé M. Clinical and radiographic outcomes of the use of four dressing materials in pulpotomized primary molars: a randomized clinical trial with 2-year follow-up. Int J Paediatr Dent. 2013;23(6):400–7.
73. Ford TR, Torabinejad M, McKendry DJ, Hong CU, Kariyawasam SP. Use of mineral trioxide aggregate for repair of furcal perforations. Oral Surg Oral Med Oral Pathol Oral Radiol Endod. 1995;79(6): 756–63.
74. Fridland M, Rosado R. Mineral trioxide aggregate (MTA) solubility and porosity with different water-to-powder ratios. J Endod. 2003;29(12):814–7.
75. Fridland M, Rosado R. MTA solubility: a long term study. J Endod. 2005;31:376–9.
76. Gancedo-Caravia L, Garcia-Barbero E. Influence of humidity and setting time on the push-out strength of mineral trioxide aggregate obturations. J Endod. 2006;32(9):894–6.
77. Ghoddusi J, Sanaan A, Shahrami F. Clinical and radiographic evaluation of root perforation repair using MTA. N Y State Dent J. 2007;73(3):46–9.
78. Ghoddusi J, Shahrami F, Alizadeh M, Kianoush K, Forghani M. Clinical and radiographic evaluation of vital pulp therapy in open apex teeth with MTA and ZOE. N Y State Dent J. 2012;78(3):34–8.
79. Giuliani V, Nieri M, Pace R, Pagavino G. Effects of pH on surface hardness and microstructure of mineral trioxide aggregate and Aureoseal: an in vitro study. J Endod. 2010;36(11):1883–6.
80. Gonçalves JL, Viapiana R, Miranda CE, Borges AH, Cruz Filho AM. Evaluation of physico-chemical properties of Portland cements and MTA. Braz Oral Res. 2010;24(3):277–83. PubMed PMID: 20877963.
81. Haglund R, He J, Jarvis J, Safavi KE, Spångberg LS, Zhu Q. Effects of root-end filling materials on fibroblasts and macrophages in vitro. Oral Surg Oral Med Oral Pathol Oral Radiol Endod. 2003;95(6): 739–45.
82. Hasan Zarrabi M, Javidi M, Naderinasab M, Gharechahi M. Comparative evaluation of antimicrobial activity of three cements: new endodontic cement (NEC), mineral trioxide aggregate (MTA) and Portland. J Oral Sci. 2009;51(3):437–42.
83. Hatibovic´-Kofman S, Raimundo L, Zheng L, Chong L, Friedman M, Andreasen JO. Fracture resistance and histological findings of immature teeth treated with mineral trioxide aggregate. Dent Traumatol. 2008;24:272–6.
84. Hilton TJ, Ferracane JL, Mancl L. Comparison of CaOH with MTA for direct pulp capping: a PBRN randomized clinical trial. J Dent Res. 2013;92(7 Suppl):16S–22.
85. Hirschberg CS, Patel NS, Patel LM, Kadouri DE, Hartwell GR. Comparison of sealing ability of MTA

and EndoSequence Bioceramic Root Repair Material: a bacterial leakage study. Quintessence Int. 2013;44(5):e157–62.
86. Holan G, Eidelman E, Fuks AB. Long-term evaluation of pulpotomy in primary molars using mineral trioxide aggregate or formocresol. Pediatr Dent. 2005;27(2):129–36.
87. Holland R, Bisco Ferreira L, de Souza V, Otoboni Filho JA, Murata SS, Dezan Jr E. Reaction of the lateral periodontium of dogs' teeth to contaminated and noncontaminated perforations filled with mineral trioxide aggregate. J Endod. 2007;33(10):1192–7.
88. Holland R, Filho JA, de Souza V, Nery MJ, Bernabé PF, Junior ED. Mineral trioxide aggregate repair of lateral root perforations. J Endod. 2001;27(4):281–4.
89. Holt DM, Watts JD, Beeson TJ, Kirkpatrick TC, Rutledge RE. The anti-microbial effect against Enterococcus faecalis and the compressive strength of two types of mineral trioxide aggregate mixed with sterile water or 2 % chlorhexidine liquid. J Endod. 2007;33(7):844–7.
90. International Standards Organization. ISO 9917-1. Dentistry-water-based cements. Part 1: powder/liquid acid–base cements. Geneva: International Standards Organization; 2007.
91. Islam I, Chng HK, Yap AU. X-ray diffraction analysis of mineral trioxide aggregate and Portland cement. Int Endod J. 2006;39:220–5.
92. Islam I, Chng HK, Yap AU. Comparison of the physical and mechanical properties of MTA and Portland cement. J Endod. 2006;32:193–7.
93. Iwamoto CE, Adachi E, Pameijer CH, Barnes D, Romberg EE, Jefferies S. Clinical and histological evaluation of white ProRoot MTA in direct pulp capping. Am J Dent. 2006;19(2):85–90.
94. Kang JY, Lee BN, Son HJ, Koh JT, Kang SS, Son HH, Chang HS, Hwang IN, Hwang YC, Oh WM. Biocompatibility of mineral trioxide aggregate mixed with hydration accelerators. J Endod. 2013;39(4):497–500.
95. Katsamakis S, Slot DE, Van der Sluis LW, Van der Weijden F. Histological responses of the periodontium to MTA: a systematic review. J Clin Periodontol. 2013;40(4):334–44.
96. Kayahan MB, Nekoofar MH, Kazandağ M, Canpolat C, Malkondu O, Kaptan F, Dummer PM. Effect of acid-etching procedure on selected physical properties of mineral trioxide aggregate. Int Endod J. 2009;42(11):1004–14.
97. Khalil WA, Eid NF. Biocompatibility of BioAggregate and mineral trioxide aggregate on the liver and kidney. Int Endod J. 2013;46(8):730–7.
98. Koçak MM, Koçak S, Aktuna S, Görücü J, Yaman SD. Sealing ability of retrofilling materials following various root-end cavity preparation techniques. Lasers Med Sci. 2011;26(4):427–31.
99. Krastl G, Allgayer N, Lenherr P, Filippi A, Taneja P, Weiger R. Tooth discoloration induced by endodontic materials: a literature review. Dent Traumatol. 2013;29(1):2–7.
100. Kurita LM, Cavalcante RB, Gurgel-Filho ED, De-Deus GA, Ximenes AB, Da Silva EJ. Response of mice connective tissue to three different endodontic materials. Microsc Res Tech. 2013;76(3):311–5.
101. Lee YL, Lee BS, Lin FH, Yun Lin A, Lan WH, Lin CP. Effects of physiological environments on the hydration behavior of mineral trioxide aggregate. Biomaterials. 2004;25(5):787–93.
102. Lenherr P, Allgayer N, Weiger R, Filippi A, Attin T, Krastl G. Tooth discoloration induced by endodontic materials: a laboratory study. Int Endod J. 2012;45(10):942–9.
103. Leye Benoist F, Gaye Ndiaye F, Kane AW, Benoist HM, Farge P. Evaluation of mineral trioxide aggregate (MTA) versus calcium hydroxide cement (Dycal®) in the formation of a dentine bridge: a randomised controlled trial. Int Dent J. 2012;62(1):33–9.
104. Lindeboom JA, Frenken JW, Kroon FH, van den Akker HP. A comparative prospective randomized clinical study of MTA and IRM as root-end filling materials in single-rooted teeth in endodontic surgery. Oral Surg Oral Med Oral Pathol Oral Radiol Endod. 2005;100(4):495–500.
105. Liu H, Zhou Q, Qin M. Mineral trioxide aggregate versus calcium hydroxide for pulpotomy in primary molars. Chin J Dent Res. 2011;14(2):121–5.
106. Lodiene G, Kleivmyr M, Bruzell E, Ørstavik D. Sealing ability of mineral trioxide aggregate, glass ionomer cement and composite resin when repairing large furcal perforations. Br Dent J. 2011;210(5):216–7.
107. Loxley EC, Liewehr FR, Buxton TB, McPherson 3rd JC. The effect of various intracanal oxidizing agents on the push-out strength of various perforation repair materials. Oral Surg Oral Med Oral Pathol Oral Radiol Endod. 2003;95(4):490–4.
108. Malekafzali B, Shekarchi F, Asgary S. Treatment outcomes of pulpotomy in primary molars using two endodontic biomaterials. A 2-year randomised clinical trial. Eur J Paediatr Dent. 2011;12(3):189–93.
109. Maltezos C, Glickman GN, Ezzo P, He J. Comparison of the scaling of Resilon, Pro Root MTA, and Super-EBA as root-end filling materials: a bacterial leakage study. J Endod. 2006;32(4):324–7.
110. Maroto M, Barbería E, Planells P, García GF. Dentin bridge formation after mineral trioxide aggregate (MTA) pulpotomies in primary teeth. Am J Dent. 2005;18(3):151–4.
111. Matsunaga T, Tsujimoto M, Kawashima T, Tsujimoto Y, Fujiwara M, Ookubo A, Hayashi Y. Analysis of arsenic in gray and white mineral trioxide aggregates by using atomic absorption spectrometry. J Endod. 2010;36(12):1988–90.
112. Matt GD, Thorpe JR, Strother JM, McClanahan SB. Comparative study of white and gray mineral trioxide aggregate (MTA) simulating a one- or two-step apical barrier technique. J Endod. 2004;30:876–9.
113. McNamara RP, Henry MA, Schindler WG, Hargreaves KM. Biocompatibility of accelerated

mineral trioxide aggregate in a rat model. J Endod. 2010;36(11):1851–5.
114. Mehrdad L, Malekafzali B, Shekarchi F, Safi Y, Asgary S. Histological and CBCT evaluation of a pulpotomised primary molar using calcium enriched mixture cement. Eur Arch Paediatr Dent. 2013;14(3):191–4.
115. Miyagak DC, de Carvalho EM, Robazza CR, Chavasco JK, Levorato GL. In vitro evaluation of the antimicrobial activity of endodontic sealers. Braz Oral Res. 2006;20(4):303–6.
116. Monteiro Bramante C, Demarchi AC, de Moraes IG, Bernadineli N, Garcia RB, Spångberg LS, Duarte MA. Presence of arsenic in different types of MTA and white and gray Portland cement. Oral Surg Oral Med Oral Pathol Oral Radiol Endod. 2008;106(6): 909–13.
117. Moretti AB, Sakai VT, Oliveira TM, Fornetti AP, Santos CF, Machado MA, Abdo RC. The effectiveness of mineral trioxide aggregate, calcium hydroxide and formocresol for pulpotomies in primary teeth. Int Endod J. 2008;41(7):547–55.
118. Naik S, Hegde AH. Mineral trioxide aggregate as a pulpotomy agent in primary molars: an in vivo study. J Indian Soc Pedod Prev Dent. 2005;23(1):13–6.
119. Nair U, Ghattas S, Saber M, Natera M, Walker C, Pileggi R. A comparative evaluation of the sealing ability of 2 root-end filling materials: an in vitro leakage study using Enterococcus faecalis. Oral Surg Oral Med Oral Pathol Oral Radiol Endod. 2011;112(2):e74–7.
120. Namazikhah MS, Nekoofar MH, Sheykhrezae MS, Salariyeh S, Hayes SJ, Bryant ST, Mohammadi MM, Dummer PM. The effect of pH on surface hardness and microstructure of mineral trioxide aggregate. Int Endod J. 2008;41(2):108–16.
121. Nekoofar MH, Adusei G, Sheykhrezae MS, Hayes SJ, Bryant ST, Dummer PM. The effect of condensation pressure on selected physical properties of mineral trioxide aggregate. Int Endod J. 2007;40(6):453–61.
122. Nekoofar MH, Aseeley Z, Dummer PM. The effect of various mixing techniques on the surface microhardness of mineral trioxide aggregate. Int Endod J. 2010;43(4):312–20.
123. Nekoofar MH, Oloomi K, Sheykhrezae MS, Tabor R, Stone DF, Dummer PM. An evaluation of the effect of blood and human serum on the surface microhardness and surface microstructure of mineral trioxide aggregate. Int Endod J. 2010;43(10): 849–58.
124. Noorollahian H. Comparison of mineral trioxide aggregate and formocresol as pulp medicaments for pulpotomies in primary molars. Br Dent J. 2008;204(11):E20.
125. Nosrat A, Seifi A, Asgary S. Pulpotomy in caries-exposed immature permanent molars using calcium-enriched mixture cement or mineral trioxide aggregate: a randomized clinical trial. Int J Paediatr Dent. 2013;23(1):56–63.
126. Odaba° ME, Cinar C, Akça G, Araz I, Ulusu T, Yücel H. Short-term antimicrobial properties of mineral trioxide aggregate with incorporated silver-zeolite. Dent Traumatol. 2011;27(3):189–94.
127. Odabaş ME, Alaçam A, Sillelioğlu H, Deveci C. Clinical and radiographic success rates of mineral trioxide aggregate and ferric sulphate pulpotomies performed by dental students. Eur J Paediatr Dent. 2012;13(2):118–22.
128. Oliveira MG, Xavier CB, Demarco FF, Pinheiro AL, Costa AT, Pozza DH. Comparative chemical study of MTA and Portland cements. Braz Dent J. 2007;18:3–7.
129. Oraie E, Ghassemi AR, Eliasifar G, Sadeghi M, Shahravan A. Apical sealing ability of MTA in different liquid to powder ratios and packing methods. Iran Endod J. 2012;7(1):5–9.
130. Osorio RM, Hefti A, Vertucci FJ, Shawley AL. Cytotoxicity of endodontic materials. J Endod. 1998;24(2):91–6.
131. Ozdemir HO, elik B, Karabucak B, Cehreli ZC. Calcium ion diffusion from mineral trioxide aggregate through simulated root resorption defects. Dent Traumatol. 2008;24:70–3.
132. Paranjpe A, Zhang H, Johnson JD. Effects of mineral trioxide aggregate on human dental pulp cells after pulp-capping procedures. J Endod. 2010;36(6): 1042–7.
133. Parirokh M, Torabinejad M. Mineral trioxide aggregate: a comprehensive literature review – part I: chemical, physical, and antibacterial properties. J Endod. 2010;36(1):16–27.
134. Parirokh M, Torabinejad M. Mineral trioxide aggregate: a comprehensive literature review – part III: clinical applications, drawbacks, and mechanism of action. J Endod. 2010;36(3):400–13.
135. Percinoto C, de Castro AM, Pinto LM. Clinical and radiographic evaluation of pulpotomies employing calcium hydroxide and trioxide mineral aggregate. Gen Dent. 2006;54(4):258–61.
136. Petrou MA, Alhamoui FA, Welk A, Altarabulsi MB, Alkilzy M, H Splieth C. A randomized clinical trial on the use of medical Portland cement, MTA and calcium hydroxide in indirect pulp treatment. Clin Oral Investig. 2013. doi 10.1007/s00784-013-1107-z.
137. Post LK, Lima FG, Xavier CB, Demarco FF, Gerhardt-Oliveira M. Sealing ability of MTA and amalgam in different root-end preparations and resection bevel angles: an in vitro evaluation using marginal dye leakage. Braz Dent J. 2010;21(5): 416–9.
138. Qudeimat MA, Barrieshi-Nusair KM, Owais AI. Calcium hydroxide vs mineral trioxide aggregates for partial pulpotomy of permanent molars with deep caries. Eur Arch Paediatr Dent. 2007;8(2): 99–104.
139. Reyes-Carmona JF, Felippe MS, Felippe WT. The biomineralization ability of mineral trioxide aggregate and Portland cement on dentin enhances the push-out strength. J Endod. 2010;36(2):286–91.
140. Ribeiro DA, Duarte MA, Matsumoto MA, Marques ME, Salvadori DM. Biocompatibility in vitro tests of

mineral trioxide aggregate and regular and white Portland cements. J Endod. 2005;31(8):605–7.
141. Ribeiro CS, Kuteken FA, Hirata Júnior R, Scelza MF. Comparative evaluation of antimicrobial action of MTA, calcium hydroxide and Portland cement. J Appl Oral Sci. 2006;14(5):330–3.
142. Ribeiro DA, Matsumoto MA, Duarte MA, Marques ME, Salvadori DM. Ex vivo biocompatibility tests of regular and white forms of mineral trioxide aggregate. Int Endod J. 2006;39(1):26–30.
143. Ribeiro CS, Scelza MF, Hirata Júnior R, Buarque de Oliveira LM. The antimicrobial activity of gray-colored mineral trioxide aggregate (GMTA) and white-colored MTA (WMTA) under aerobic and anaerobic conditions. Oral Surg Oral Med Oral Pathol Oral Radiol Endod. 2010;109(6):e109–12.
144. Roberts HW, Toth JM, Berzins DW, Charlton DG. Mineral trioxide aggregate material use in endodontic treatment: a review of the literature. Dent Mater. 2008;24(2):149–64.
145. Saatchi M, Hosseini HS, Farhad AR, Narimany T. The effect of various concentrations of iodine potassium iodide on the antimicrobial properties of mineral trioxide aggregate – a pilot study. Dent Traumatol. 2012;28(6):474–7.
146. Saghiri MA, Asgar K, Lotfi M, Garcia-Godoy F. Nanomodification of mineral trioxide aggregate for enhanced physiochemical properties. Int Endod J. 2012;45(11):979–88.
147. Saghiri MA, Asgar K, Lotfi M, Karamifar K, Neelakantan P, Ricci JL. Application of mercury intrusion porosimetry for studying the porosity of mineral trioxide aggregate at two different pH. Acta Odontol Scand. 2012;70(1):78–82.
148. Saghiri MA, Asgar K, Lotfi M, Nazari A, Karamifar K, Neelakantan P, Gutmann JL. Effect of storage temperature on sealing ability and solubility of white mineral trioxide aggregate. Acta Odontol Scand. 2012;70(6):536–40.
149. Saghiri MA, Garcia-Godoy F, Gutmann JL, Lotfi M, Asatourian A, Ahmadi H. Push-out bond strength of a nano-modified mineral trioxide aggregate. Dent Traumatol. 2013;29(4):323–7.
150. Saghiri MA, Garcia-Godoy F, Lotfi M, Ahmadi H, Asatourian A. Effects of diode laser and MTAD on the push-out bond strength of mineral trioxide aggregate-dentin interface. Photomed Laser Surg. 2012;30(10):587–91.
151. Saghiri MA, Lotfi M, Joupari MD, Aeinehchi M, Saghiri AM. Effects of storage temperature on surface hardness, microstructure, and phase formation of white mineral trioxide aggregate. J Endod. 2010;36(8):1414–8.
152. Saghiri MA, Shokouhinejad N, Lotfi M, Aminsobhani M, Saghiri AM. Push-out bond strength of mineral trioxide aggregate in the presence of alkaline pH. J Endod. 2010;36(11):1856–9.
153. Saidon J, He J, Zhu Q, Safavi K, Spångberg LS. Cell and tissue reactions to mineral trioxide aggregate and Portland cement. Oral Surg Oral Med Oral Pathol Oral Radiol Endod. 2003;95(4):483–9.
154. Sakai VT, Moretti AB, Oliveira TM, Fornetti AP, Santos CF, Machado MA, Abdo RC. Pulpotomy of human primary molars with MTA and Portland cement: a randomized controlled trial. Br Dent J. 2009;207(3):E5; discussion 128–9.
155. Saliba E, Abbassi-Ghadi S, Vowles R, Camilleri J, Hooper S, Camilleri J. Evaluation of the strength and radiopacity of Portland cement with varying additions of bismuth oxide. Int Endod J. 2009; 42(4):322–8.
156. Saunders WP. A prospective clinical study of periradicular surgery using mineral trioxide aggregate as a root-end filling. J Endod. 2008;34(6):660–5.
157. Schembri M, Peplow G, Camilleri J. Analyses of heavy metals in mineral trioxide aggregate and Portland cement. J Endod. 2010;36(7):1210–5.
158. Shah N, Logani A, Bhaskar U, Aggarwal V. Efficacy of revascularization to induce apexification/apexogensis in infected, nonvital, immature teeth: a pilot clinical study. J Endod. 2008;34(8):919–25; discussion 1157.
159. Shahi S, Rahimi S, Lotfi M, Yavari H, Gaderian A. A comparative study of the biocompatibility of three root-end filling materials in rat connective tissue. J Endod. 2006;32(8):776–80.
160. Shahi S, Yavari HR, Rahimi S, Eskandarinezhad M, Shakouei S, Unchi M. Comparison of the sealing ability of mineral trioxide aggregate and Portland cement used as root-end filling materials. J Oral Sci. 2011;53(4):517–22.
161. Shie MY, Huang TH, Kao CT, Huang CH, Ding SJ. The effect of a physiologic solution pH on properties of white mineral trioxide aggregate. J Endod. 2009;35:98–101.
162. Shokouhinejad N, Nekoofar MH, Iravani A, Kharrazifard MJ, Dummer PM. Effect of acidic environment on the push-out bond strength of mineral trioxide aggregate. J Endod. 2010;36(5):871–4.
163. Simon S, Rilliard F, Berdal A, Machtou P. The use of mineral trioxide aggregate in one-visit apexification treatment: a prospective study. Int Endod J. 2007;40(3):186–97.
164. Sluyk SR, Moon PC, Hartwell GR. Evaluation of setting properties and retention characteristics of mineral trioxide aggregate when used as a furcation perforation repair material. J Endod. 1998; 24:768–71.
165. Song M, Kim E. A prospective randomized controlled study of mineral trioxide aggregate and super ethoxy-benzoic acid as root-end filling materials in endodontic microsurgery. J Endod. 2012;38(7): 875–9.
166. Sonmez D, Sari S, Cetinbaş T. A comparison of four pulpotomy techniques in primary molars: a long-term follow-up. J Endod. 2008;34(8):950–5.
167. Srinivasan D, Jayanthi M. Comparative evaluation of formocresol and mineral trioxide aggregate as pulpotomy agents in deciduous teeth. Indian J Dent Res. 2011;22(3):385–90.
168. Storm B, Eichmiller FC, Tordik PA, Goodell GG. Setting expansion of gray and white mineral trioxide

aggregate and Portland cement. J Endod. 2008;34:80–2.
169. Stowe TJ, Sedgley CM, Stowe B, Fenno JC. The effects of chlorhexidine gluconate (0.12 %) on the antimicrobial properties of tooth-colored ProRoot mineral trioxide aggregate. J Endod. 2004;30(6): 429–31.
170. Subramaniam P, Konde S, Mathew S, Sugnani S. Mineral trioxide aggregate as pulp capping agent for primary teeth pulpotomy: 2 year follow up study. J Clin Pediatr Dent. 2009;33(4):311–4.
171. Sushynski JM, Zealand CM, Botero TM, Boynton JR, Majewski RF, Shelburne CE, Hu JC. Comparison of gray mineral trioxide aggregate and diluted formocresol in pulpotomized primary molars: a 6- to 24-month observation. Pediatr Dent. 2012;34(5): 120–8.
172. Tanomaru-Filho M, Faleiros FB, Silva GF, Bosso R, Guerreiro-Tanomaru JM. Sealing ability of retrograde obturation materials containing calcium hydroxide or MTA. Acta Odontol Latinoam. 2011; 24(1):110–4.
173. Tanomaru-Filho M, Luis MR, Leonardo MR, Tanomaru JM, Silva LA. Evaluation of periapical repair following retrograde filling with different root-end filling materials in dog teeth with periapical lesions. Oral Surg Oral Med Oral Pathol Oral Radiol Endod. 2006;102(1):127–32.
174. Tanomaru-Filho M, Tanomaru JM, Barros DB, Watanabe E, Ito IY. In vitro antimicrobial activity of endodontic sealers, MTA-based cements and Portland cement. J Oral Sci. 2007;49(1):41–5.
175. Torabinejad M, Higa RK, McKendry DJ, Pitt Ford TR. Dye leakage of four root end filling materials: effects of blood contamination. J Endod. 1994; 20(4):159–63.
176. Torabinejad M, Hong CU, Lee SJ, Monsef M, Pitt Ford TR. Investigation of mineral trioxide aggregate for root-end filling in dogs. J Endod. 1995;21(12): 603–8.
177. Torabinejad M, Hong CU, McDonald F, Pitt Ford TR. Physical and chemical properties of a new root-end filling material. J Endod. 1995;21:349–53.
178. Torabinejad M, Hong CU, Pitt Ford TR, Kaiyawasam SP. Tissue reaction to implanted super-EBA and mineral trioxide aggregate in the mandible of guinea pigs: a preliminary report. J Endod. 1995;21(11): 569–71.
179. Torabinejad M, Hong CU, Pitt Ford TR, Kettering JD. Antibacterial effects of some root end filling materials. J Endod. 1995;21(8):403–6.
180. Torabinejad M, Parirokh M. Mineral trioxide aggregate: a comprehensive literature review – part II: leakage and biocompatibility investigations. J Endod. 2010;36(2):190–202.
181. Torabinejad M, Pitt Ford TR, McKendry DJ, Abedi HR, Miller DA, Kariyawasam SP. Histologic assessment of mineral trioxide aggregate as a root-end filling in monkeys. J Endod. 1997;23(4):225–8.
182. Torabinejad M, Rastegar AF, Kettering JD, Pitt Ford TR. Bacterial leakage of mineral trioxide aggregate as a root-end filling material. J Endod. 1995;21(3): 109–12.
183. Torabinejad M, Smith PW, Kettering JD, Pitt Ford TR. Comparative investigation of marginal adaptation of mineral trioxide aggregate and other commonly used root-end filling materials. J Endod. 1995;21(6):295–9.
184. Torabinejad M, Watson TF, Pitt Ford TR. Sealing ability of a mineral trioxide aggregate when used as a root end filling material. J Endod. 1993;19:591–5.
185. Torabinejad M, White DJ, inventors; Loma Linda University, assignee. Tooth filling material and use. United States Patent Number 5,769,638. 16 May 1995.
186. Tuna D, Olmez A. Clinical long-term evaluation of MTA as a direct pulp capping material in primary teeth. Int Endod J. 2008;41(4):273–8.
187. Uyanik MO, Nagas E, Sahin C, Dagli F, Cehreli ZC. Effects of different irrigation regimens on the sealing properties of repaired furcal perforations. Oral Surg Oral Med Oral Pathol Oral Radiol Endod. 2009;107(3):e91–5.
188. Vallés M, Mercadé M, Duran-Sindreu F, Bourdelande JL, Roig M. Color stability of white mineral trioxide aggregate. Clin Oral Investig. 2013;17(4):1155–9.
189. Vallés M, Mercadé M, Duran-Sindreu F, Bourdelande JL, Roig M. Influence of light and oxygen on the color stability of five calcium silicate-based materials. J Endod. 2013;39(4):525–8.
190. Vivan RR, Ordinola-Zapata R, Bramante CM, Bernardineli N, Garcia RB, Hungaro Duarte MA, de Moraes IG. Evaluation of the radiopacity of some commercial and experimental root-end filling materials. Oral Surg Oral Med Oral Pathol Oral Radiol Endod. 2009;108(6):e35–8.
191. von Arx T, Hänni S, Jensen SS. Clinical results with two different methods of root-end preparation and filling in apical surgery: mineral trioxide aggregate and adhesive resin composite. J Endod. 2010;36(7):1122–9.
192. Wälivaara DÅ, Abrahamsson P, Isaksson S, Salata LA, Sennerby L, Dahlin C. Periapical tissue response after use of intermediate restorative material, gutta-percha, reinforced zinc oxide cement, and mineral trioxide aggregate as retrograde root-end filling materials: a histologic study in dogs. J Oral Maxillofac Surg. 2012;70(9):2041–7.
193. Yasuda Y, Kamaguchi A, Saito T. In vitro evaluation of the antimicrobial activity of a new resin-based endodontic sealer against endodontic pathogens. J Oral Sci. 2008;50(3):309–13.
194. Yildirim T, Er K, Taşdemir T, Tahan E, Buruk K, Serper A. Effect of smear layer and root-end cavity thickness on apical sealing ability of MTA as a root-end filling material: a bacterial leakage study. Oral Surg Oral Med Oral Pathol Oral Radiol Endod. 2010;109(1):e67–72.

195. Yildirim T, Oruçoğlu H, Cobankara FK. Long-term evaluation of the influence of smear layer on the apical sealing ability of MTA. J Endod. 2008;34(12):1537–40.
196. Zealand CM, Briskie DM, Botero TM, Boynton JR, Hu JC. Comparing gray mineral trioxide aggregate and diluted formocresol in pulpotomized human primary molars. Pediatr Dent. 2010;32(5):393–9.
197. Zhu Q, Haglund R, Safavi KE, Spangberg LS. Adhesion of human osteoblasts on root-end filling materials. J Endod. 2000;26(7):404–6.

4 Bioactivity of Mineral Trioxide Aggregate and Mechanism of Action

Franklin R. Tay

4.1 Introduction

In the grand scheme of things, a bioactive material may be broadly defined as 'one which has been designed to induce specific biological activity' [162]. Based on this generic definition, biologically active materials may include those that promote tissue regeneration by adhesion to soft and hard tissues of the human body and those that possess cell-instructive and molecular-signalling properties via functionalised ligands or incorporating growth factors for regulating cell proliferation, migration, differentiation, protein expression and mineralisation processes. Other bioactive materials include those that are designed for biosensing or biological recognition via physicochemical interactions, those that contain recognition sites for cleavage of enzymes involved in cell functions and those that possess antimicrobial or immunoregulatory activities by incorporating antimicrobial agents or molecules that mimic natural host-defence peptides [4, 21, 26, 82, 103]. Along the same line of thought, bioactive materials may also include those that incorporate bioactive peptides with antithrombotic, antihypertensive, opioid or antioxidative properties for controlled release [140].

F.R. Tay, BDSc (Hons), PhD
Department of Endodontics, Georgia Regents University College of Dental Medicine, Rm 2270, 1430 John Wesley Gilbert Drive, Augusta 30912, GA, USA
e-mail: tayfranklin7@gmail.com

Prior to the adoption of this contemporary interpretation of bioactivity, scientists in the field of tissue regeneration have been using a more focused definition of 'bioactivity' to describe the resistance of a calcium phosphosilicate glass to be removed from the host hard and soft tissues, after it was experimentally implanted in rat femurs and muscles [78]. The phenomenon of interfacial bonding between the implant and living tissues has subsequently been observed in other synthetic calcium phosphate ceramics and silicate-based, borate-based and phosphate-based glasses [79, 115], which form the foundation of the field of biomaterials science known as 'bioactive glass-ceramics'. A bioactive material, as defined by Hench and coworkers, is one that elicits a specific biological response at the interface of the material, which results in the formation of a bond between living tissues and the material [125]. A feature commonly identified from these materials is a time-dependent kinetic modification of the material's surface via the formation of a carbonated apatite surface layer following its implantation in vivo [40, 77].

The tissue regeneration definition of bioactivity has undergone a subtle paradigm drift, after the feature of in vivo carbonated apatite formation over an apatite/wollastonite glass-ceramic [86], being one of the stages that contributes to the bone-bonding ability of a bioactive material to living tissues, was found to be reproducible in vitro by immersing the material in a simulated body fluid designed to mimic human blood plasma [89]. Thus, according to Kokubo and Takadama, a bioactive material is one on which bone-like

J. Camilleri (ed.), *Mineral Trioxide Aggregate in Dentistry*,
DOI 10.1007/978-3-642-55157-4_4, © Springer-Verlag Berlin Heidelberg 2014

carbonated apatite will form selectively after it is immersed in a serum-like solution [90]. Over the years, the scientific community at large has intuitively accepted this paradigm drift, with the assumption that demonstrating this so-called in vitro bioactivity is the indirect equivalent of affirming a material's bone-bonding potential. Although in vitro bioactivity evaluation is appealing because of its simplicity and rapidity in data generation, a recent review cautioned the lack of adequate scientific evidence to support the assumption that a material that initiates the deposition of calcium phosphate salts on its surface after immersion in simulated body fluid will bond directly to bone following placement of the material in a surgical site [12]. For example, a host of sol–gel reaction-derived metallic oxides, including SiO_2, TiO_2, ZrO_2, Nb_2O5 and Ta_2O_5, were found to possess in vitro bioactivity after immersing in simulated body fluid [33, 109, 110, 123, 157]; however, the ability of these metallic oxide gels to bond to bone in vivo has not been demonstrated.

The introduction of hydraulic calcium (alumino)silicate cements has provided clinicians with alternative biomaterials for dentine replacement, pulp capping, pulpotomy, creation of apical barriers in teeth with open apices, repair of root perforation and resorptive defects, as well as orthograde or retrograde root canal fillings [39, 120, 121, 131]. Amongst their many desirable properties, hydraulic calcium silicate cements have been described as possessing bioactive properties that influence their surrounding environments [120]. A discussion of the bioactivity of hydraulic calcium silicate cements based on its generic definition is beyond the scope of this chapter; issues such as their cell-instructive and antimicrobial activities are addressed in depth in Chap. 3. Rather, the bioactivity of hydraulic calcium silicate cements will be discussed from a tissue regeneration perspective.

4.2 Biologically Inactive Versus Bioactive Inorganic Materials

When a biomaterial is implanted in the human body, the host tissue reacts towards the implant in different ways depending on the tissue response along the implant surface. Accordingly, a biomaterial may be classified into four types based on their tissue responses: nearly inert, porous, resorbable or bioactive [74]. As hydraulic calcium silicate cements are non-resorbable and do not possess pores that are large enough for ingrowth of bone or blood vessels, only the tissue responses of nearly inert and bioactive materials will be discussed.

No material implanted in living tissues is completely inert. Thus, the term 'bioinert' is designated to any material which, when implanted into the human body, elicits minimal interaction with its surrounding tissues. Examples of these materials are stainless steel, titanium, alumina, partially stabilised zirconia and ultrahigh molecular weight polyethylene. Following implantation of a foreign material into the body, the material's surface is immediately coated with proteins derived from blood and interstitial fluids. It is through this layer of adsorbed proteins that the cells sense foreign surfaces [163]. In response, the body's defence mechanism will stimulate the formation of a non-adherent fibrous capsule around the implant in an attempt to isolate it from the surrounding tissue. The thickness of this protective fibrous capsule depends on the chemical reactivity of the implanted material and on the motion and fit of the material at the interface [27]. Because the interface is not chemically or biologically bonded, micro-movement of the implant will result in progressive thickening of the non-adherent fibrous capsule and eventually leads to functional deterioration of the implanted material.

By contrast, a bioactive material creates an environment compatible with osteogenesis, and in some cases, compatible with soft tissues [165], by developing a natural bonding interface between living and nonliving materials. With the exception of calcite (calcium carbonate) and β-tricalcium phosphate, which are examples of resorbable bioceramics that bond directly to living bone [114], interfacial bonding of other bioactive materials with bone is initiated via ion-exchange reactions between the bioactive implant and surrounding body fluids. This results in the formation of a biologically active carbonated apatite layer on the implant surface that is chemically and crystallographically equivalent to the mineral phase in bone [66]. Human plasma is supersaturated with respect to calcium and phosphate ions. The presence of certain functional groups, such as silanol (Si–OH), on the material surface induces nucleation of carbonated apatite crystallites from the amorphous calcium phosphate that is deposited over the initially formed silica gel layer. For bone, interfacial bonding occurs because of the rapid turnover of bone, as well as the biological equivalence of the carbonated apatite deposits with the inorganic portion of bone, which enables a collagen matrix to be deposited by osteoblasts over the carbonated apatite layer. Subsequent mineralisation of the collagen fibrils results in bonding of the living tissues to the implanted material [74]. For bonding to soft tissues, collagen fibrils are chemisorbed on the porous silica gel layer via electrostatic, ionic and/or hydrogen bonding [107, 174].

The first bioactive glass-ceramic invented and the most extensively studied was the SiO_2–Na_2O–CaO–P_2O_5 melt-derived quaternary glass system invented by Dr. Hench [75], commonly known as 45S5 Bioglass® (US Biomaterials Corp., Alachua, FL, USA). Based on this formulation and subsequently developed bioactive glass formulations, the ability of these materials to bond to bone tissue was thought to occur in 11 stages (Table 4.1). These stages represent the combined results of the surface chemical reactivity of bioactive glasses in physiological media (stages 1–5), and the body's healing and regenerative responses (stages 6–11) [74]. Reaction stages 1–5 in bioactive glasses lead to rapid release of soluble ionic species and formation of a porous hydrated silica gel and polycrystalline carbonated apatite bilayer on the glass surface. These reaction layers enhance the adsorption of proteins and growth factors (stage 6), influence the length of time macrophages are required to clear the surgical site of debris for tissue repair (stage 7) and promote attachment (stage 8), proliferation and differentiation of osteoblasts from mesenchymal stem cells (stage 9). Deposition of an extracellular collagen matrix (stage 10) and subsequent mineralisation of the collagen matrix deposited by osteoblasts (stage 11) follow, ultimately resulting in mature osteocytes encased in a collagen-carbonated apatite matrix.

It has been shown that fibroblasts do not spread and proliferate on bioactive glass surfaces, contrary to what occurs on the surface of bioinert materials [139]. The exact mechanism is not clear, but may be due to the selective adsorption of serum proteins on the surface of bioactive materials. Bioactive glass containing a calcium phosphate-rich layer was found to preferentially adsorb fibronectin, which contains the integrin-binding arginine-glycine-aspartic acid (RGD) amino acid sequence for enhanced osteoblast adhesion [59]. Other researchers observed that the configuration of fibronectin adsorbed was different depending on the type of surface exposed by the biomaterial. A specific fibronectin conformation present on bioactive glasses that have reacted with simulated body fluid to form a surface Ca/P amorphous layer was found to induce very strong osteoblast adhesion [46]. This is important, since mesenchymal stem cells take time to migrate from their niches to a surgical site and arrive later than fibroblasts after a bioactive material is implanted. Thus, if fibroblasts proliferate, a non-adherent fibrous capsule forms, which inhibits interfacial bonding between the implanted material and the host tissue. When fibroblasts remain 'quiescent' along the surface of bioactive glass, new bone tissue can be produced upon differentiation of the mesenchymal stem cells and endothelial progenitor cells into osteoblasts and endothelial cells of the blood vessel wall, respectively.

A Bioactivity Index (IB) was introduced to rank the level of bioactivity of a specific material [73]. This index is defined as the time taken for more than 50 % of the interface to bond to bone ($t_{0.5}$) and is represented by $IB = 100/t_{0.5bb}$. Materials exhibiting an IB value greater than eight (e.g. 45S5 Bioglass®) will bond to both soft and hard tissues. Materials with an IB value less than 8 but greater than 0 (e.g. synthetic hydroxyapatite) will bond only to hard tissue [74]. The presence of silica was found to be crucial for a material to exhibit bioactivity. This is due to the partial dissolution of the material in an alkaline environment, which releases Si^{4+} ions to form the silica gel surface layer in stages 2 and 3 and creates

Table 4.1 Reaction stages in 45S5 Bioglass® with increasing time

Stage	Reaction event	Response
1	Sodium and calcium hydrogen ion exchange on glass surface	Chemical
2	Dissolution of surface silica and formation of surface silanol	
3	Condensation and repolymerisation of silanol to form SiO_2-rich surface layer	Occurs in vitro or in vivo
4	Precipitation of amorphous calcium phosphate on the silica gel surface layer	
5	Nucleation and crystallisation of amorphous calcium phosphate to carbonated apatite	
6	Protein adsorption (growth factors, etc.) to the surface carbonated apatite layer	Biological
7	Action of macrophages to remove debris from surgical site	
8	Attachment of mesenchymal stem cells on bioactive surface	
9	Differentiation of stem cells to form bone-growing cells, osteoblasts	Occurs only in vivo
10	Generation of extracellular matrix by osteoblasts to form bone	
11	Mineralisation of extracellular matrix to enclose bone cells, osteocytes	

silanol groups to act as sites for the nucleation of carbonated apatite from the amorphous calcium phosphate deposited over the silica gel layer in stage 5 (Table 4.1). Nevertheless, incorporation of increasing concentrations of silica in the glass resulted in a diminished rate of bioactivity. Increasing the silica content of the glasses decreases their dissolution rates by reducing the release of modifier ions such as Ca^{2+} and HPO_4^- ions, which inhibits the development of the silica gel layer on the glass surface. Complete loss of bone-bonding ability occurred with further increases in SiO_2 concentration, the exact concentration of which was dependent upon whether the glasses were melt-derived (>60 mol%) [76] or sol–gel reaction-derived (>90 mol%) [96]. The presence of P_2O_5 and Na_2O was initially thought to be essential for glass-ceramics to be bioactive. However, sol–gel-derived CaO–SiO_2 binary calcium silicate gel glasses were also found to bond firmly to bone tissues after intraosseous implantation [135, 136]. The information suggests that the absence of phosphate from most hydraulic calcium silicate cements does not preclude these cements from exhibiting bioactive behaviour. Conversely, partial substitution of CaO with Al_2O_3 in the binary CaO–SiO_2 glass composition to produce ternary CaO–Al_2O_3–SiO_2 glasses resulted in an Al_2O_3 concentration-dependent reduction/inhibition of the ability to form a calcium phosphate surface layer after exposure of these ternary glass formulations to simulated body fluid [16]. Addition of as little as three mass% Al_2O_3 completely inhibited the bone-bonding ability of bioactive glass [67]. The inhibitory effect of Al^{3+} on bone bonding was attributed to an increased resistance of the bioactive glass to ion-exchange surface reactions, to the precipitation of the multivalent ions as oxides, hydroxides or carbonates and to the shift of isoelectric point of the surface from negative to positive at physiological pH [173]. As tricalcium aluminate is a component of most hydraulic calcium silicate cements, the potential effect of aluminium on the bioactivity of these cements will be discussed in subsequent sections.

A functional bioactivity classification has been used to rate biomaterials designed for use as orthopaedic implants [164]. Class A materials demonstrate *osteoproduction*, which means that they can actively recruit cellular elements involved in bone formation (mesenchymal stem cells and endothelial progenitor cells) after implantation in a surgical site. These materials have IB values of 12. Class B materials show only *osteoconduction* [1]. These materials have IB values of 3–6 and function only as passive structural scaffolds for inward migration of cellular elements involved in bone formation. The term *osteoproduction* is similar to the contemporary terminology *osteoinduction*, meaning that primitive, undifferentiated and pluripotent cells are stimulated to differentiate into bone-forming and blood vessel-forming cell lineages [1]. *Osteoproduction* was used in the bioactive glass literature to describe bone proliferation resulting from the combined properties (i.e. osteoinduction, osteoconduction and/or osteogenic properties) of a grafting material. Based on this classification, a material is considered *osteoproductive* if it elicits both intracellular and extracellular responses at its interface (e.g. 45S5 Bioglass®) and *osteoconductive* if it triggers only an extracellular response (e.g. synthetic hydroxyapatite).

Release of inorganic ions by class A biomaterials may trigger intracellular responses [81]. Of the elements released by bioactive glasses, Si is known to be an essential element for metabolic processes associated with calcification of bone tissues [28] and induction of the apatite precipitation [38]. Dietary intake of Si has been shown to increase bone mineral density [84]. Orthosilicic acid stimulates type I collagen synthesis and osteoblast differentiation in human osteoblast-like cells in vitro [14, 127, 143]. Inorganic monomeric and polymeric silica/silicate have been shown to increase the expression of osteoprotegerin in osteogenic cells and modulate the crosstalk between osteoblasts and osteoclasts. Osteoprotegerin is a decoy receptor for the receptor activator of nuclear factor kappa B ligand (RANKL). Osteoprotegerin binding to RANKL on osteoblast/stromal cells blocks the RANKL–RANK ligand interaction between osteoblast/stromal cells and osteoclast precursors. This has the effect of inhibiting the differentiation of osteoclast precursors into mature osteoclasts. Thus, inorganic silica/silicate has the potential to stimulate osteogenesis in vivo by inhibiting osteoclast growth and differentiation [138]. Release of calcium ions favours osteoblast proliferation, differentiation and extracellular matrix mineralisation [98], activates Ca-sensing receptors in osteoblasts and increases expression of growth factors such as insulin-like growth factor-I (IGF-I) or IGF-II [104, 158]. Additional extracellular responses may be produced by adsorption of bone growth factor proteins, such as plasma-derived transforming growth factor-β1, by the surface silica gel layer. Bioactive glasses have also been shown to promote angiogenesis by stimulating the secretion of vascular endothelial growth factor by human fibroblasts [60, 61, 64, 95].

The information in this section represents only the tip of the iceberg of the humongous amount of research published on the bioactivity of glass and glass-ceramics. Nevertheless, the information provides the background for evaluating the bioactivity of hydraulic calcium silicate cements.

4.3 In Vitro Bioactivity of MTA

4.3.1 Direct Demonstration of In Vitro Bioactivity

Mineral trioxide aggregate (MTA) is the most well known and most thoroughly investigated of all the hydraulic calcium cements available to date. It is a clinker-derived Portland cement composed of different phases, including tricalcium silicate, dicalcium silicate, tricalcium aluminate, tetracalcium aluminoferrite and calcium sulphate. MTA is the first hydraulic calcium silicate cement patented for endodontic applications [155], which contains all the aforementioned mineral phases as well as bismuth oxide as a radiopacifier [24]. The aluminoferrite phase in the grey version of MTA is absent from the white version of MTA [124]. The compositions of other commercially available hydraulic calcium silicate cements designed for use as endodontic cements and sealers are covered in Chaps. 7 and 8.

Although bioactivity is not as esteemed property for industrial applications of Portland cements, in vitro bioactivity of white Portland cement has been reported after it was immersed in simulated body fluid for 7 days [36]. Using a combination of X-ray diffraction (XRD) and Fourier transform-infrared spectroscopy (FT-IR), the authors reported the formation of a layer of hydroxyapatite on the surface of white Portland cement after immersion of the set cement in simulated body fluid. Dissolution of portlandite (calcium hydroxide) and formation of calcite (calcium carbonate; reaction product of calcium hydroxide with atmospheric carbon dioxide) were also observed on contact of set white Portland cement with simulated body fluid. In another study, set white Portland cement was immersed in phosphate-containing fluid and the resultant calcium phosphate phase examined using XRD and FT-IR, in combination with scanning electron microscopy, transmission electron microscopy and electron diffraction [149]. The authors reported that the initial calcium phosphate phase formed was amorphous calcium phosphate. This precursor phase was subsequently transformed into calcium-deficient, poorly crystalline, B-type apatite (i.e. the PO_4^{3-} groups in apatite being substituted by CO_3^-). The authors concluded that the in vitro bioactivity of MTA materials is likely to be attributed to their Portland cement component. Identification of the amorphous calcium phosphate phase is of biological significance because the latter is the key intermediate calcium phosphate precursor phase that precedes biological apatite formation in in vivo osteogenesis [99–101]. As will be discussed below, identification of amorphous calcium phosphate precursors bridges the missing link in the sequence of stages that contribute to the in vitro bioactivity of hydraulic calcium silicate cements. In addition, by using the contemporary principles of biomineralisation, strategies have been developed with the use of polyanionic acid analogues of noncollagenous proteins for stabilising the amorphous calcium phosphate precursor phase to prevent its premature transformation into carbonated apatite. The resultant polyanionic acid-stabilised amorphous calcium phosphate precursors have been used experimentally for biomimetic intrafibrillar mineralisation of collagen fibrils in demineralised dentine [116]. Such a technology has potential applications in remineralisation of hybrid layers created by dentine adhesives to prevent their degradation by matrix metalloproteinases and cysteine capthepsins, as well as in the remineralisation of dentinal caries.

The two major components of Portland cements, tricalcium silicate and dicalcium silicate, have been produced separately using sol–gel reactions to create experimental, pure tricalcium silicate [160, 172] and dicalcium silicate [65] cements. These pure calcium silicate cements also demonstrated in vitro bioactivity by the precipitation of apatite crystallites on the cement surface after immersion in simulated body fluid. These results have led to the preparation of experiment bioactive tricalcium silicate [30, 48] and dicalcium silicate [25] cements for endodontic applications. The use of these experimental calcium silicate cements should alleviate potential concerns regarding aluminium-induced neurotoxicity [69, 141, 171] that may arise with the clinical use of clinker-derived tricalcium aluminate-containing hydraulic calcium (alumino)silicate cements.

By and large, the in vitro bioactivity observed in Portland cements and pure calcium silicate cements is recapitulated in MTA and the MTA-like clan of commercially available or experimental hydraulic calcium silicate cements designed for restorative and endodontic uses [5, 10, 15, 20, 25, 49, 51–58, 70–72, 128, 137, 142, 146, 147, 151]. These calcium phosphate reaction products were observed after the cements were immersed in simulated body fluid based on Kokubo's formula or its modification [12, 89, 90], Dulbecco's phosphate-buffered saline, Hank's balanced salt solution or simply phosphate-containing fluid, with different degrees of reactivity. The ultimate reaction product formed on the surface of the set cements was, according to most of those publications, hydroxyapatite.

4.3.2 Mechanism of Action

The in vitro bioactivity of MTA and MTA-like materials is tissue independent and may proceed sequentially in stages that parallel those proposed for bioactive glasses. For comparative purposes, a similar sequence of events will be used in this discussion. These stages are schematically represented in Fig. 4.1.

Stage 1 – Hydrolysis and ion exchange. Ion exchange occurs following hydration of the calcium silicate particles, with rapid exchange of Ca^{2+} with H^+ or H_3O^+ ions from the aqueous mixing solution to form a solid–liquid interface [57]. Reaction of Ca^{2+} ions with OH^- ions derived from water results in the formation of calcium hydroxide (portlandite) [22] that creates a highly alkaline environment. Although these reactions occur almost immediately after cement hydration, continuous release of

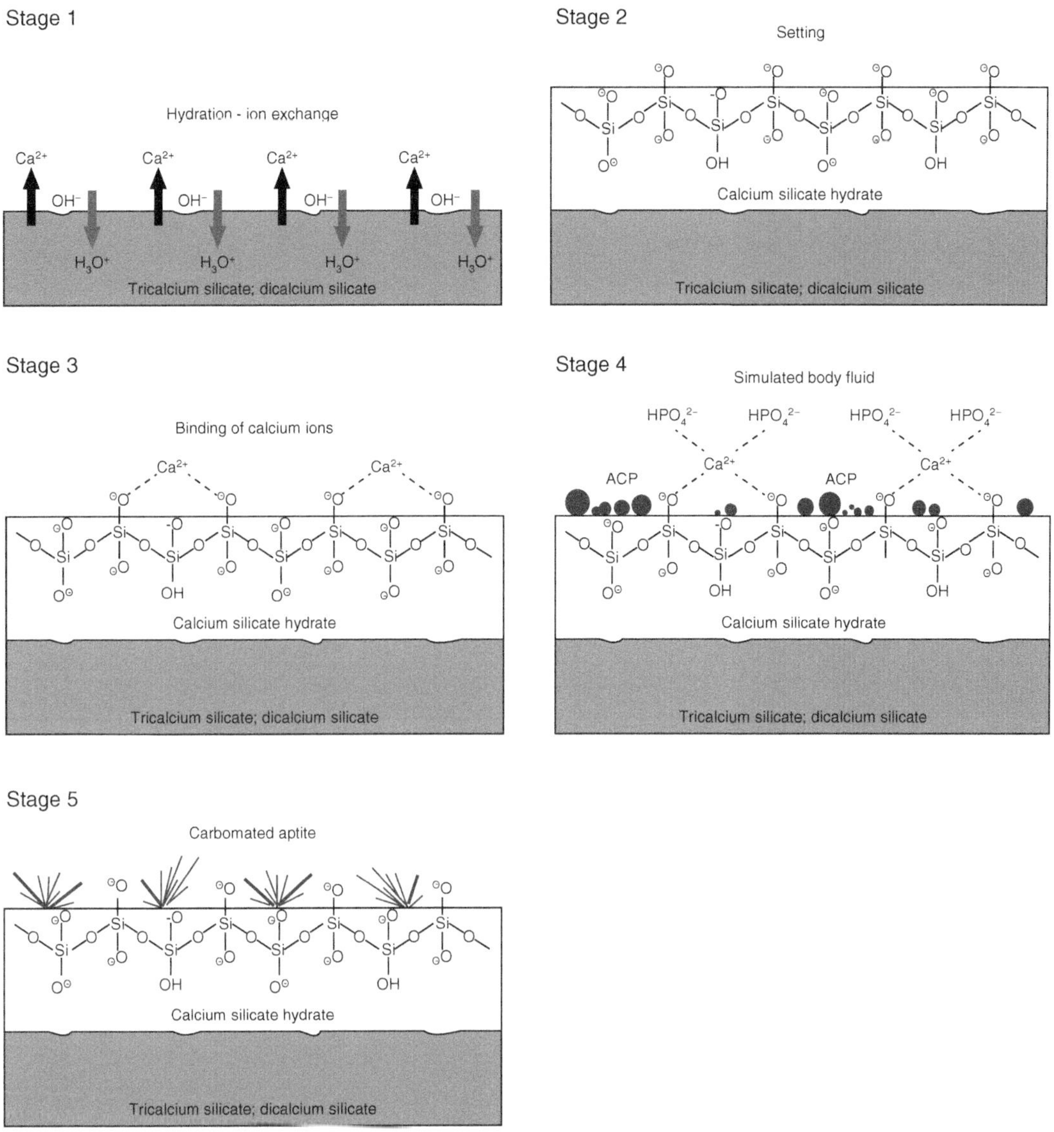

Fig. 4.1 A schematic of the five sequential stages of events that contribute to the manifestation of in vitro bioactivity of hydraulic calcium silicate cements after the latter is immersed in simulated body fluid (not to scale). *ACP* amorphous calcium phosphate

Ca^{2+} and Si^{4-} after initial setting, together with the release of minor amounts of Al^{3+}, Fe^{3+} and $SO4^{2-}$, depending on the type of material, result in the formation of other inorganic mineral phases (Chap. 2).

Stage 2 – Formation of calcium silicate hydrate. Cation exchange increases the hydroxyl concentration of the solution. The surfaces of the calcium silicate particles are attacked by OH^- ions in solution, resulting in hydrolysis of SiO^{4-} group in an alkaline environment. The result is the formation of an amorphous calcium silicate hydrate phase on the surface of the mineral particles (Fig. 4.2a). Calcium silicate hydrate is a non-stoichiometric, porous, water-containing silicate gel layer [129] containing silanol (Si–OH) groups that forms the main binding phase in a set cement matrix.

Stage 3 – Binding of calcium silicate hydrate with calcium ions. Deprotonation of silanol groups in the calcium silicate hydrate phase at alkaline pH produces a negatively charged surface with SiO^- functional groups [91, 97]:

$$\equiv SiOH + H_2O \leftrightarrow \equiv SiO^- + H_3O^+ \quad (4.1)$$

This negatively charged surface attracts cations released into solution, such as Ca^{2+}, via electrostatic interaction to decrease the total energy of the system, resulting in an increase of cations on the set cement surface:

$$\equiv SiO^- + Ca^{2+} \rightarrow \equiv SiO^- \ldots Ca^{2+} \quad (4.2)$$

This region, consisting of a charged surface and an equal but opposite charge in the solution, is called an electric double layer on which other substances may deposit under suitable conditions.

Stage 4 – Precipitation of amorphous calcium phosphate. When the set calcium silicate cement is immersed in a phosphate-containing solution, which contains hydrolysed HPO_4^{2-} ions, electrostatic interaction occurs between the $HPO4^{2-}$ ions with the Ca^{2+}-rich CSH surface:

$$H_2O + PO_4^{3-} \leftrightarrow HPO_4^{2-} + OH^- \equiv SiO^- \ldots Ca^{2+}$$
$$+HPO_4^{2-} \rightarrow \equiv SiO^- \ldots Ca^{2+} \ldots HPO_4^{2-} \quad (4.3)$$

Continued release of calcium ions from the set cement into the phosphate-containing solution leads to supersaturation of Ca^{2+} and $HPO4^{2-}$ ions in the solution, which in turn results in the formation of an amorphous calcium phosphate precursor phase in the solution. These initially formed subnanometre-sized amorphous calcium phosphate precursors are known as prenucleation clusters and have an average diameter of 0.87 ± 0.2 nm [41]. They remain relatively stable in the phosphate-containing solution in the absence of a nucleation-inducing surface. In the presence of a nucleation-inducing surface, aggregation of the prenucleation clusters leads to their densification near the cement surface, producing a 'dense liquid' CaP-rich phase [43]. Coalescence of the densified prenucleation clusters subsequently results in the deposition of globular amorphous calcium phosphate on the set cement surface (Fig. 4.2b), with the general formula $Ca_9(PO_4)_{6-x}(HPO_4)_x(OH)_x$ [37]. Apart from the observation of amorphous calcium phosphate formation in Portland cement [149], amorphous calcium phosphate in the form of aggregated spherulites was also reported after ProRoot MTA (Dentsply Tulsa Dental Specialties, Tulsa, OK, USA), MTA Angelus (Angelus Soluções Odontológicas, Londrina, PR, Brazil), MTA Branco (Angelus) and MTA BIO (Angelus) were immersed in phosphate-buffered saline or Hank's balanced salt solution [52, 128].

Stage 5 – Nucleation and transformation of amorphous calcium phosphate into carbonated apatite. In the presence of a nucleation-inducing CSH surface ($\equiv SiO^- \ldots Ca^{2+} \ldots HPO_4^{2-}$), the amorphous calcium phosphate undergoes phase transformation over time into carbonated apatite [44, 117] (Fig. 4.3a, b). This transformation occurs via an octacalcium phosphate intermediate phase ($Ca_8H_2(PO_4)_6 \cdot 5H_2O$) [11, 45, 93, 156]. Whilst it is indisputable that apatite represents the endpoint of this phase transformation, the morphology of the calcium phosphate phases presented in the endodontic literature on in vitro bioactivity of hydraulic calcium silicate cements is highly variable, ranging from acicular, lathlike, petal-like, platelike, globular structures to needle-shaped [5, 10, 15, 20, 25, 49, 51–58, 70–72, 128, 137, 142, 146, 147, 151], with different Ca/P molar ratios (ranging from 1.33 to 1.67) (Fig. 4.4). Although it is possible that some of these represent calcium-deficient apatite with variable degrees of lattice substitutions by cations such as Na^+ and Mg^{2+} and anions such as Cl^-, it is likely some of these crystalline morphologies represent the intermediate octacalcium phosphate (OCP) phase described in classic calcium phosphate characterisation studies. Formation of an intermediate OCP phase by MTA or MTA-like materials was sparsely discussed in the endodontic literature except in a couple of studies [52, 128]. Indiscriminate use

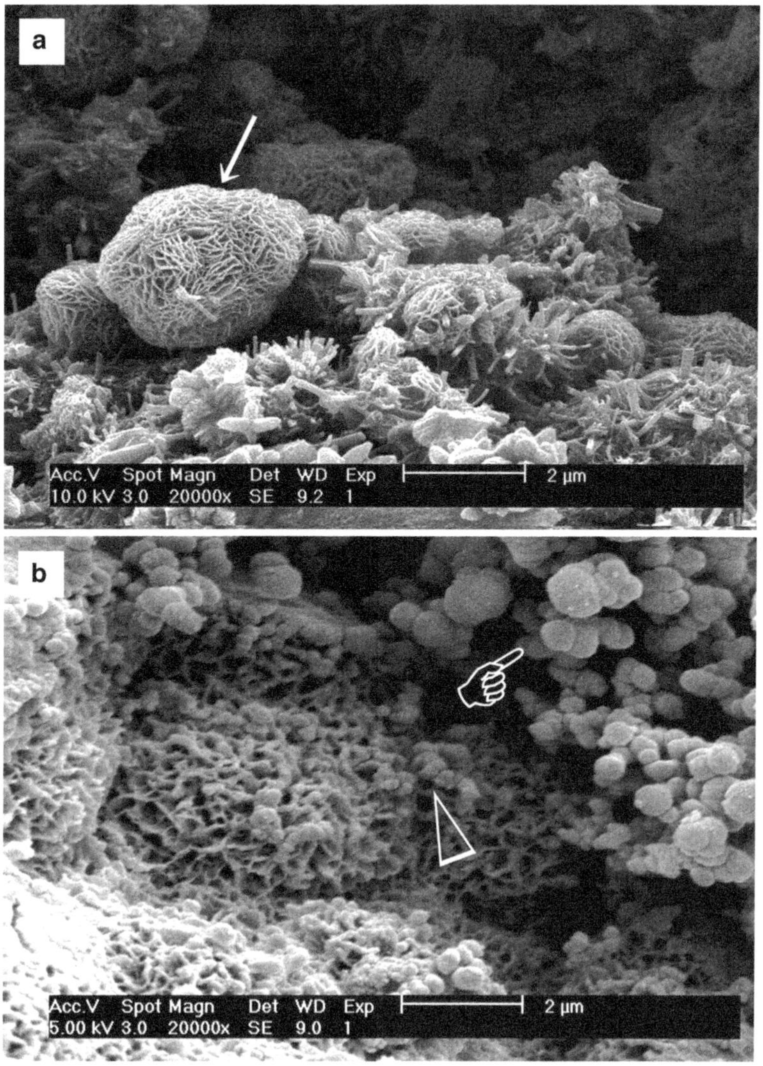

Fig. 4.2 (**a**) Scanning electron microscopy (SEM) image of the surface of set white MTA powder showing formation of a calcium silicate hydrate layer (*arrow*) over the surface of the mineral particles after hydration of the powder. (**b**) SEM image of the surface of set white MTA powder after immersion in phosphate-containing fluid for 8 h. Amorphous calcium phosphate is deposited over the surface of the calcium silicate hydrate reaction phase in the form of spherule clusters (*pointer*). Some of the smaller amorphous calcium phosphate spherules are dispersed within the calcium silicate hydrate phase (*open arrowhead*)

of the term 'hydroxyapatite' (HA) in most of these endodontic studies is reflected by the inadequate chemo-analytical techniques employed for characterising the calcium phosphate precipitates. The so-formed apatite is not stoichiometric HA but is carbonated apatite, which represents the biological apatite found in bone, cartilage enamel and dentine [32, 42]. Accurate characterisation of calcium phosphate phases requires the simultaneous use of XRD and FT-IR; the latter may be further complemented with micro-Raman spectroscopy [50, 92, 105]. It should be emphasised that CaP mineral phase information derived from XRD cannot be substituted by the peak designations derived from the combined use of FT-IR and micro-Raman spectroscopy. Even with the use of all these techniques, differentiation between octacalcium phosphate and apatite is extremely difficult [18, 19, 148] and often required high-resolution transmission electron microscopy of the crystalline lattice planes to determine the length of the unit cell axes and their crystallographic orientation [166]. The crystal structure of octacalcium phosphate has been described as an alternative stacking of apatite layers and hydrated layers along its [142] direction [18, 106]. The

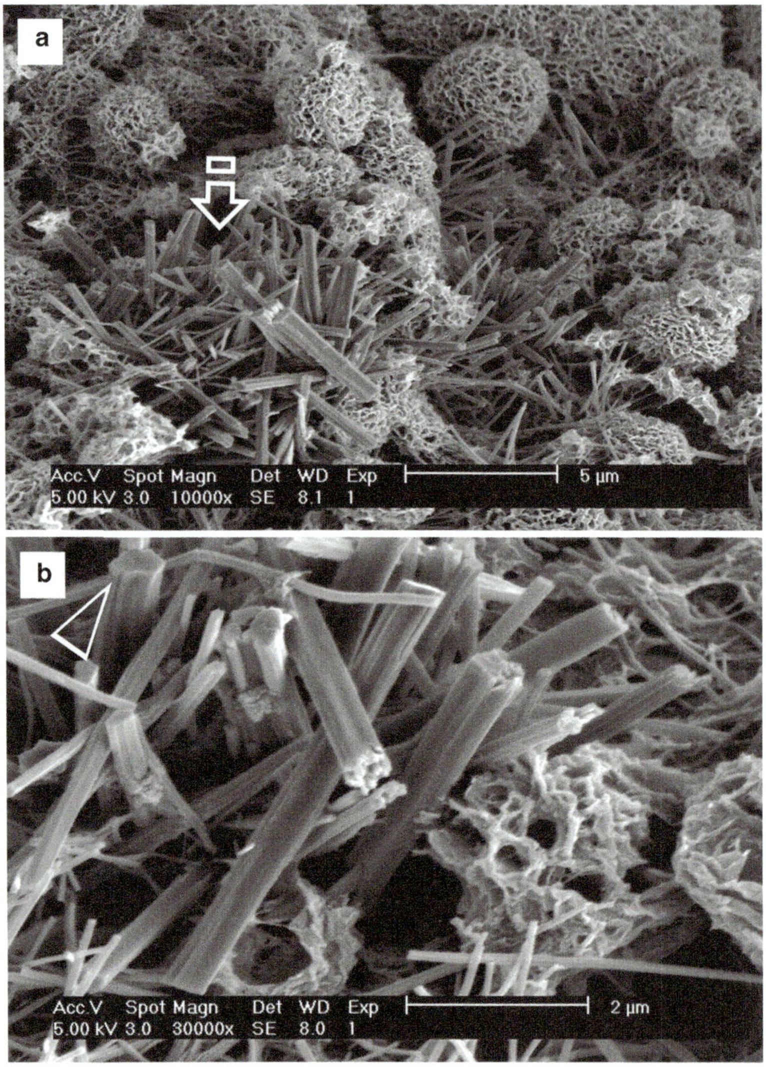

Fig. 4.3 (**a**) SEM image of the surface of hydrated white MTA powder after immersion in phosphate-containing fluid for 168 h. A crystalline calcium phosphate mineral phase (*open arrow*) is scattered around the calcium silicate hydrate-coated MTA mineral particles (energy dispersive X-ray analysis data not shown). Amorphous calcium phosphate spherules can no longer be observed. (**b**) High-magnification image of the calcium phosphate mineral phase in (a). These crystallites have short a-axis and b-axis but long c-axis, forming needle-shaped crystallites with hexagonal cross sections (*open arrowhead*)

similarity of the apatite layer in OCP and the structure in HA provide geometrically favourable conditions for phase transformation from octacalcium phosphate to carbonated apatite. In a model of OCP–HA transformation, it has been suggested that transformation of OCP to HA occurs through epitaxial growth of HA on the OCP surface along the OCP[100]/HA[100] and OCP [001]/HA[100] crystalline planes [19]. Transformation of OCP to HA may be accomplished in solution through dissolution–precipitation or occur by solid-state transformation via one of the two processes [47]:

$$5Ca_8H_2(PO_4)_6 \cdot 5H_2O \rightarrow 4Ca_{10}(PO_4)_6(OH)_2 + 6H_3PO_4 + 17H_2O$$
$$Ca_8H_2(PO_4)_6\ 5H_2O + 2Ca^{2+} \rightarrow Ca_{10}(PO_4)_6(OH)_2 + 3H_2O + 4H^+ \quad (4.4)$$

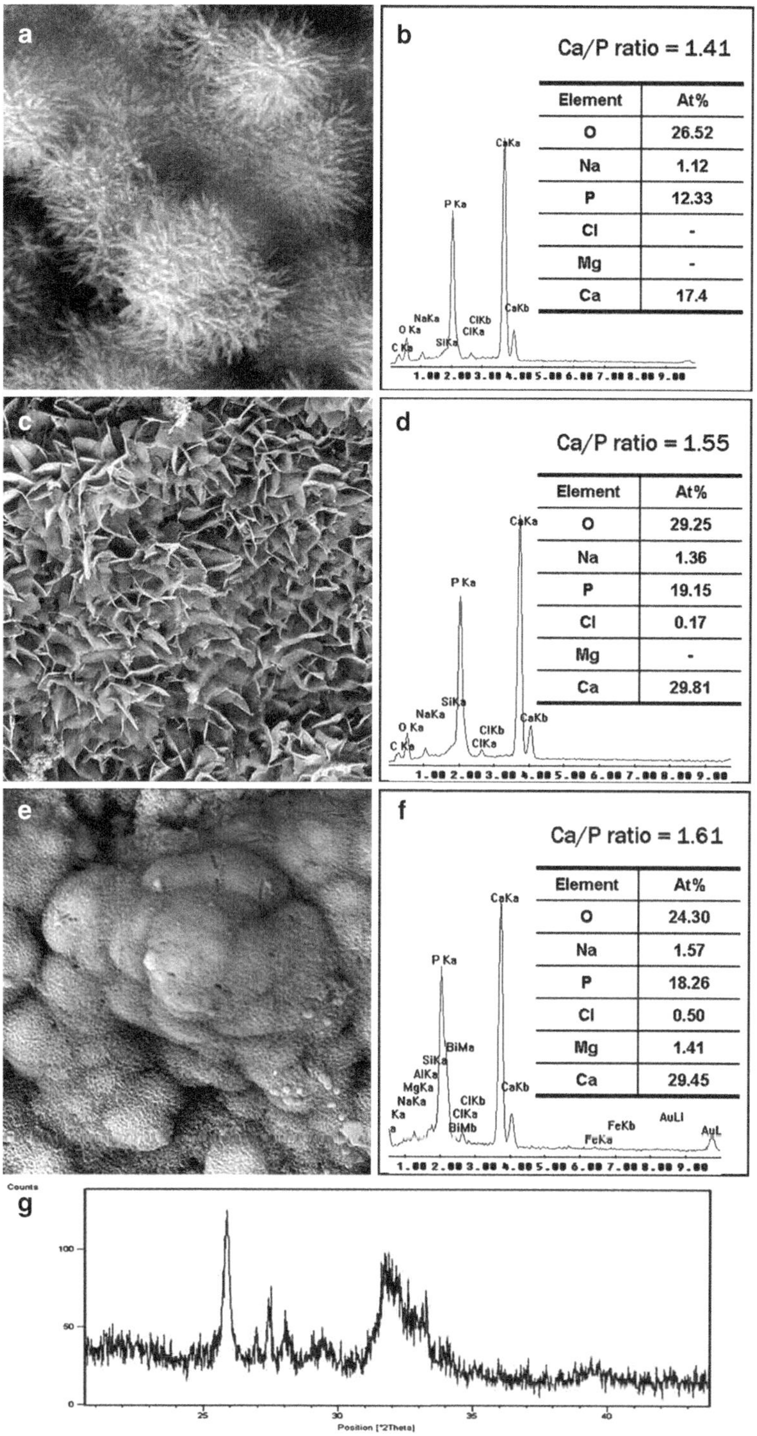

Fig. 4.4 Characterisation of precipitates formed by MTA BIO after 2 months of immersion in phosphate-buffered saline. (**a**) SEM image showing the acicular nature of spherules (original magnification, 8,000×). (**b**) Energy dispersive X-ray (EDAX) spectrum for precipitates in (a) and semi-quantitative chemical composition showing their Ca/P molar ratio. (**c**) SEM image showing petal-like precipitates (original magnification, 1,000×). (**d**) EDAX spectrum for precipitates in (c) revealed a greater Ca/P molar ratio and lattice substitution of Na and Cl. (**e**) SEM image of compact lathlike precipitates (original magnification, 1,000×). (**f**) Semi-quantitative analysis of the EDAX data derived from (e) indicates that the precipitates have a Ca/P molar ratio of 1.61 with lattice substitution of Na, Cl and Mg. (**g**) X-ray diffraction pattern of the calcium phosphate precipitates obtained after 2 months of immersion in phosphate-buffered saline, revealing the presence of poorly crystalline apatite (Reprinted from Reyes-Carmona et al. [128], copyright 2009, with permission from Elsevier)

The first reaction represents solid-state transformation and may occur in experiments that examined desiccated calcium silicate cements after they are immersed in phosphate-containing fluids. The second reaction requires an additional supply of calcium ions and is more likely to occur in solutions containing calcium. Such a scenario may be found when there is continuous leaching of calcium ions from the set hydraulic calcium silicate cements after they are immersed in phosphate-containing fluids or serum.

Taken together, evidence is abundant in the literature showing that hydraulic calcium silicate cements exhibit in vitro activity. However, these studies were not performed as rigorously as those examining bioactive glasses. Although there have been attempts to compare the in vitro bioactivity of different commercially available or experimental hydraulic calcium silicate cements, most of the works were qualitative in nature. In particular, there was no adoption of a matrix such as the use of an in vitro version of the Bioactive Index, in systematically quantifying the percentage of the cement surface covered by calcium phosphate salts or the variation in thickness of the apatite or apatite-like mineral layer over time.

4.3.3 Indirect Evidence of In Vitro Bioactivity

Interestingly, in vitro bioactivity of hydraulic calcium phosphate cements was demonstrated in dentine instead of bone. Sarkar et al. [137] were the first to show the formation of an apatite-rich interfacial layer along the cement–dentine interface when grey MTA was placed on top of dentine and immersed in phosphate-containing fluid for 2 months in vitro. According to the authors, this interfacial layer was firmly attached to the dentinal walls with no observable gap between the interfacial layer and dentine. Subsequently, Reyes-Carmona et al. [128] reported the formation of a similar interfacial layer along the cement–dentine interface after ProRoot MTA, MTA Branco and MTA BIO were immersed in phosphate-buffered saline for 2 months in vitro. Apatite-rich tags were also demonstrated in the dentinal tubules and their lateral branches. Han and Okiji [70] demonstrated similar interfacial layers and taglike structures within dentinal tubules after white ProRoot MTA (Dentsply Tulsa Dental Specialties) and Biodentine (Septodont, Saint-Maur-des-Fossés, France) were placed in instrumented root canals of bovine incisors that were irrigated with ethylenediaminetetraacetic acid and sodium hypochlorite and followed by immersion in Ca- and Mg-free phosphate-buffered saline for up to 3 months.

The mechanism involved in formation of an interfacial cement–dentine layer with the use of hydraulic calcium silicate cements is different from what occurs in dentine bonding or with the use of glass ionomer cements. In the absence of adjunctive chemical treatment, it is not possible for an inorganic layer to bond chemically or even interlock mechanically with the surface of highly mineralised dentine, which consists predominantly of mineralised type I collagen. In dentine bonding, for example, bonding of adhesive resin monomers to dentine is achieved by demineralisation of the dentine surface with acid or acidic resin monomers to create a partially demineralised collagen matrix. Hydrophilic adhesive resin monomers infiltrate this collagen matrix and polymerise in situ to create a hybrid layer that bonds the pure resin layer above to the mineralised dentine below [122, 159]. In glass ionomer cements and resin-modified glass ionomer cements, chemical bonding occurs after treatment of the dentine with polyalkenoic acid. An interfacial zone or intermediate layer is created between the glass ionomer cement and dentine, which represents the summation of the infiltration of polyalkenoic acid and subsequent deposition of ion-exchange reaction products into the partially demineralised collagen matrix [150, 170].

In the case of calcium silicate cements, a new type of interfacial interaction known as the 'mineral infiltration zone' has recently been reported [6]. In this interaction, the highly caustic (alkaline) calcium silicate cement hydration products are responsible for the degradation of the collagenous component of intertubular dentine. A porous intertubular dentine layer is produced in which the collagen fibrils are depleted, leaving behind porous 'mineral ghosts' [102] that enable the permeation of high concentrations of calcium, hydroxyl and carbonate ions to form a hypermineralised layer [6]. Such a process has been termed 'alkaline etching' [6], to distinguish it from the 'acid etching' process associated with the use of dentine adhesives and glass ionomer cements. Prior to this report (Atmeh et al.) [6], a similar hypermineralised layer was observed on the of the resin-dentine interface (i.e. hybrid layer) when set white Portland cement was used to remineralise hybrid layers created in severely compromised bonded dentine [102]. Whilst this 'mineral infiltration zone' enables a calcium silicate cement to 'bond' to dentine, it is likely to be highly brittle because type I collagen, which is responsible for the toughness of biological mineralised tissues [8, 94], is destroyed by the alkalinity of the calcium silicate cements. It has been shown that hypermineralisation of cortical bone produces localised regions with reduction in fracture toughness that are prone to subcritical crack formation within the hypermineralised region [9]. These cracks provide sites for crack initiation following an impact. Similarly, dentine with high mineral/collagen ratios exhibits reduction in flexural strength and energy to fracture [132], which may contribute to increase in brittleness and decrease in fracture toughness of human dentine with age [83, 113]. To date, the long-term effect of taking advantage of the in vitro bioactivity of calcium silicate cements to bond to dentine is unknown, particularly for dental restorative procedures that involve placement of a fast-setting calcium silicate cement in dentinal cavities as a dentine replacement material [23].

4.4 In Vivo Bioactivity of Hydraulic Calcium Silicate Cements

As discussed in the introductory section, scientific evidence is lacking to support the assumption that a biomaterial that initiates the deposition of calcium phosphate salts on its surface after immersion in simulated body fluid will bond directly to bone following placement of the material in a surgical site [12]. Thus, it is appropriate to review the in vivo bioactive potential of hydraulic calcium silicate cements following their surgical implantation in appropriate animal models. Understandably, hydraulic calcium silicate cements employed in dentistry are not designed for complete filling of a surgical wound. However, it is important to see if the in vitro bioactivity reported for Portland cement and other hydraulic calcium silicate cements marketed for clinical use can be reproduced in vivo. Specifically, it is pertinent to identify if these materials can bond directly to bone without encasement by a fibrous connective tissue, the latter being the property of a bioinert material.

Because biocompatibility is not the subject of discussion in this chapter, studies that involved subcutaneous implantation of set calcium silicate cements will be excluded from the discussion. Likewise, histological studies that involved testing of calcium silicate cements as a root-end filling material will be excluded, as the tissue response involves migration of fibroblasts from the adjacent periodontal ligament to produce a layer of cementum over the material. Thus, only quantitative histological studies that involved the placement of calcium silicate cements as intraosseous implants will be examined. Of those studies, four studies [34, 35, 62, 63] that involved placement of calcium silicate cement-loaded polyethylene tubes into extraction sockets in a rat model were also excluded, as those implants were perceived to fit rather loosely within the surgical site. The results from the six studies selected based on these inclusion and exclusion criteria are summarised in Table 4.2.

Although in vitro bioactivity has been reported for most of the calcium silicate cements available for clinical use, evaluation of the bone-bonding potential of these cements was almost exclusive focused on grey MTA (ProRoot MTA, Dentsply Tulsa Dental Specialties) [111, 126, 133, 144, 153, 154]. Although a Bioactivity Index similar to that utilised in in vivo bioactive glass research has not been employed to quantify the time required for more than 50 % of the calcium silicate cement interface to bond to bone, there were

Table 4.2 Studies on in vivo bioactivity (bone-bonding responses) of hydraulic calcium silicate cements following intraosseous implantation

Reference	Material investigated	Animal model	Surgical site	Number of intraosseous implants	Time period (days)	Delivery method	Results: New bone apposition in direct contact with material Number (%)	Results: New bone separated from material by fibrous connective tissue Number (%)	Results: Mixed (incomplete direct bone contact) Number (%)
[154]	Grey MTA	Guinea pig	Mandible	5	60	Teflon cup	1 (20 %)	4 (80 %)	NA
[153]	Grey MTA	Guinea pig	Mandible	10	70	Teflon cup	1 (10 %)	9 (90 %)	0 (0 %)
			Tibia	11	80		5 (45.45 %)	5 (45.45 %)	1 (9.1 %)
[111]	Grey MTA	Rat	Parietal bone	20	15	Freshly mixed; direct placement	0 (0 %)[a]	20 (100 %)[b]	0 (0 %)[c]
				18	30		0 (0 %)[a]	14 (77.8 %)[b]	4 (22.2 %)[c]
				18	60		2 (11.2 %)[a]	8 (44.4 %)[b]	8 (44.4 %)[c]
[133]	Grey MTA	Guinea pig	Mandible	13	14	Teflon cup	8 (81.5 %)	5 (38.5 %)	NA
				13	84		7 (53.8 %)	6 (46.2 %)	
	Portland cement			13	14		7 (53.8 %)	6 (46.2 %)	
				13	84		10 (76.9 %)	3 (23.1 %)	
[144]	Grey MTA	Guinea pig	Mandible	10	28	Teflon cup	Unspecified specimen numbers – fibrous capsule (absent/slight), new bone in close contact with material (extensive) for both time periods. Negative control (empty Teflon cup) – thin fibrous capsule for both time periods		
				12	84				
[126][d]	Grey MTA	Rat	Femur	15	7	Freshly mixed; direct placement		15 (100 %)[b]	
				15	28				15 (100 %)[c]
				15	56		15 (100 %)[a]		

[a]Defined as extensive (complete coverage or 'bridging' of the material surface with bone)
[b]Defined as slight (occasional islands of osteogenesis over the material surface; less than 25 % of the material surface covered with bone)
[c]Defined as moderate (at least 50 % of the material surface partially covered with bone)
[d]Results questionable – negative control groups (no material placement in implant cavity) for each time period exhibited the same results as the experimental groups

attempts in some studies to classify the bone apposition responses in terms of the percentage of exposed cement surface area that is in direct contact with new bone [111, 126] or the temporal changes in bone apposition responses prior to the sacrifice of the animals [111, 126, 133, 144].

With the exception of one study in which the results are questionable due to the similar bioactivity responses elicited by grey MTA and the negative control (no material placement in intraosseous site) [126], the rest of the studies were unanimous in demonstrating direct apposition of bone to grey MTA is possible without the new bone being separated from the material by a fibrous capsule. However, such a hallmark of in vivo bioactivity could not be predictably achieved in all the five studies [111, 133, 144, 153, 154]. For example, in a guinea pig model employed by a group of authors [153], 90 % of the grey MTA specimens that were implanted in the mandible were incapable of direct bonding to bone, with the histological manifestation of fibrous connective tissue between the newly formed bone and the set cement. In the same study, 45.45 % of the specimens implanted in the tibia were incapable of direct bonding to bone, whilst 9.1 % of the specimens demonstrated incomplete direct bone contact with intervening fibrous tissues. These unfavourable results could not have been attributed to the displacement of the implanted cup containing the tested material into the surrounding tissues, as those specimens could not be sectioned satisfactorily and would not have been reported [153]. Likewise, these unfavourable results could not be accounted for by implanting grey MTA in a bioinert Teflon cup, as similar results were achieved when freshly mixed grey MTA was directly placed into the intraosseous site [111]. In any scientific discipline that involves hypothesis testing, a hypothesis can seldom be accepted if 90 % or even 50 % of the results are contrary to what is proposed. Yet, in a subsequent comprehensive review by those authors, MTA was described as bioactive based on its ability to form an apatite layer on its surface when it comes in contact with physiological fluids in vivo or with simulated body fluids in vitro [121]. In the age of evidence-based endodontics [152], it is worth pondering the question raised by Bohner and Lemaitre in a leading opinion biomaterials paper: ‘can bioactivity be tested in vitro with simulated body fluid solution?’ [12].

Similar results were achieved in another study that compared the in vivo bone-bonding ability of grey MTA versus Portland cement in a guinea pig model [133]. The study concluded that there is no statistical significance between a clinical-grade and an industrial-grade hydraulic calcium silicate cement in terms of their ability to bond to bone. In that study, the authors used grooved Teflon cups for filling the calcium silicate cements to prevent dislodgement of the implants from the intraosseous sites. They also examined the biological responses after two time periods, 14 and 84 days. For both Portland cement and grey MTA, both direct contact of the cement with new bone (Fig. 4.5a) and the presence of a thin layer of fibrous connective tissue between the cement and new bone (Fig. 4.5b) were observed. Although not explicitly mentioned in that paper, an important result was obtained after reanalysis of the data presented by comparing the responses of each material over the two time periods. That is, there is no statistically significant increase in specimens exhibiting direct bone–cement contact with time, for either grey MTA or Portland cement (Fisher exact tests, $p>0.05$).

Since direct bone apposition occurs in grey MTA and Portland cement intraosseous implants, it is envisaged that the in vivo stages of bioactivity (i.e. stages 6–11; Table 4.1) that were described for bioactive glasses should be recapitulated in these calcium silicate cements, as these stages represent the body's physiological healing and regeneration processes. Adsorption of proteins on the apatite-coated cement surface (stage 6) should enable the mesenchymal stem cells that migrate into the bony defect to ‘see’ a bone-like surface complete with organic components, and not a foreign material. There is only one study in the endodontic literature that attempted to analyse the surfaces of grey MTA and white MTA when these cements were allowed to set in the presence of fetal bovine serum [151]. This would have been the perfect opportunity to analyse the type of proteins/

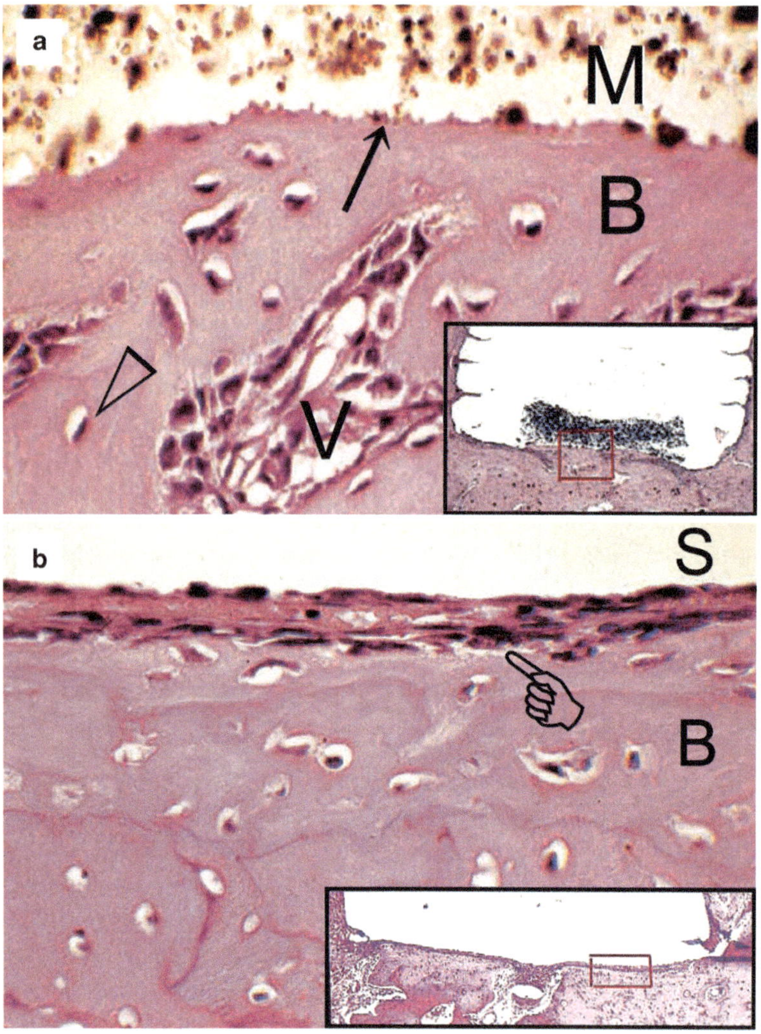

Fig. 4.5 (**a**) Light microscopy image of the tissue response following implantation of grey MTA (ProRoot MTA) in an intraosseous site for 2 weeks. The material–hard tissue interface (*arrow*) shows new bone (*B*) apposition in direct contact with the material (*M*). *Open arrowhead*: osteocyte; *V*, capillary blood vessel. *Inset*: grey MTA-filled Teflon tube (removed, space left behind) and adjacent tissues showing remnants of grey MTA and the location (*red box*) from which the high-magnification image is derived (haematoxylin–eosin-stained section; original magnification, 250×). (**b**) Light microscopy image of the tissue response following implantation of grey MTA in another intraosseous site for 2 weeks. The grey MTA was lost during histological preparation (*S*). The bone tissue (*B*) has healed well, but a thin layer of fibrous connective tissue (*pointer*) separates the newly formed bone from direct contact with the implanted grey MTA. *Inset*: grey MTA-filled Teflon tube (dislodged) and adjacent tissues showing the location (*red box*) from which the high-magnification image is derived (haematoxylin–eosin-stained section; original magnification, 250×) (Images courtesy of Dr. Kamran Safavi)

growth factors that preferentially attached to the set cement surfaces. Unfortunately, the study only analysed the surface inorganic chemical composition of the set cement and nothing was performed to characterise the protein components. The effect of macrophages on clearing the debris around the implanted material for tissue repair (stage 7), being part of the host inflammatory response, has been shown in many studies [34, 35, 133].

Inasmuch as the in vivo bone-bonding potential of grey MTA was unpredictably achieved, there was no explanation in the studies involved with regard to why this is so. Thus, it is logical to ask why a non-adherent fibrous capsule is sometimes formed that prevents direct contact of the newly formed bone with the set cement. One of the reasons is probably due to the initial high alkalinity [150] of the intraosseous site following implantation of the grey MTA. Although part of the calcium hydroxide formed in the initiate hydrolysis of tricalcium silicate and late hydrolysis of dicalcium silicate is deposited as crystalline portlandite, saturated aqueous calcium hydroxide is also present as 'pore solution' within the bulk of the set hydrated cement [17, 29]. Leaching of this 'pore solution' results in coagulation necrosis of the tissues in contact with the material and causes an initial mild to moderate inflammatory response that may result in the formation of granulation tissue by fibroblasts on resolution of the inflammation [35]. Nevertheless, no study has attempted to correlate the extent of inflammation around the intraosseous implants with the subsequent ability of the grey MTA to bond directly to bone.

The major cations that leach from set grey MTA were reported to be (in parts per million) Ca 176.7±3.3, Si 13.4±0.6, Bi 6.1±0.5, Fe 2.5±0.4, Al 2.3±0.2 and Mg 1.0±0.1 [137]. The beneficial effects of Ca and Si ions on osteogenesis have already been described in the section on bioactive glasses. It is envisaged that leaching of these cations from set grey MTA and Portland cement will exert similar beneficial effects on osteogenesis and contribute to the in vivo bioactivity of these calcium silicate cements. It was also mentioned in the section on bioactive glasses that addition of as little as three mass% Al_2O_3 completely inhibited the in vivo bone-bonding ability of bioactive glass [67]. Portland cement contains 4.7 mass% Al_2O_3, with the calculated constitution of tricalcium aluminate and tetracalcium aluminoferrite being 7.9 and 8.1 mass%, respectively [39]. Although some of the leached Al ions may be incorporated into the calcium silicate hydrate phase of set calcium silicate cements [3, 118, 130], part of the leach ions may still exist in solution, which may have an adverse effect on the in vivo bioactivity of grey MTA and Portland cement. To date, no information is available on the in vivo bioactivity of other commercially available calcium silicate cements. To test whether aluminium has a detrimental effect on the in vivo bioactivity of calcium silicate cements, it is necessary to compare the bone-bonding potential of white MTA with the corresponding grey versions of the cement, because tricalcium aluminate is negligible, and tetracalcium aluminoferrite is virtually absent from white MTA [24, 124]. Future studies should also examine the in vivo bioactivity of aluminium-free, sol–gel reaction-derived calcium silicate cements and compare the results with aluminium-containing, clinker-derived calcium silicate cements.

For the other cations released by grey MTA, magnesium has been shown to stimulate adhesion of osteoblastic cells to implant surfaces by interacting with integrins of osteoblast cells which are responsible for cell adhesion [168, 176]. By contrast, iron has an inhibitory effect on bone morphogenetic protein 2-induced osteoblastogenesis [169]. Addition of 20 mass% Bi_2O_3 to a dicalcium silicate cement resulted in lower cell proliferation, differentiation and formation of calcium deposits by MG63 human osteosarcoma cells in cell culture experiments [31]. Of the minor inorganic phases formed on the cement surface following hydration, the potential effects of ettringite and calcium monosulphate aluminate hydrate on osteogenesis is unknown. Calcite, which is frequently formed on the cement surface, has been shown to bond directly to bone without the formation of a carbonated apatite surface layer [114].

It has been mentioned in the section on bioactive glasses that fibroblasts do not spread and proliferate on bioactive glass surfaces, contrary to what occurs on the surface of bioinert materials [139]. Although set MTA provides an excellent surface for the attachment of bone-forming cells or osteoblast-like cells [2, 87, 88, 108, 112, 175], mesenchymal stem cells take 24–72 h to migrate from their stem cell niches to the surgical site before they can attach to the surface of the intraosseous implant (stage 8). Unlike bioactive glass, MTA surfaces also provide a highly favourable environment for fibroblasts to attach and proliferate [7, 13, 68, 134]. Thus, at least, theoretically, there is a competition between fibroblasts and osteogenic cells for attachment to the protein-coated calcium silicate cement surface in vivo. In a more recent study on the attachment and proliferation of fibroblasts and osteoblasts on calcium silicate cements, it was found that human periodontal ligament fibroblasts and human osteoblasts attach and proliferate well on MTA-based materials. However, the osteoblasts exhibited lower proliferation rates compared with fibroblasts [161]. Because the two cell lines require different growth media in cell culture environments to support osteogenic differentiation of the osteoblasts, experiments on the fibroblasts and osteoblasts were performed separately. The study should be repeated by culturing both cell lines in the same medium and without stimulating osteogenic differentiation of the osteoblasts. Quantitating the cell type that preferentially attaches to the surface of MTA-based materials should provide an in-depth appreciation of whether competition between fibroblasts and osteoblasts for attachment is responsible for unpredictable bone bonding following intraosseous implantation of hydraulic calcium silicate cements. That said, it does not mean that demonstration of a fibrous capsule over the set calcium silicate cement surface is an indication of the suboptimal clinical effectiveness of these cements. Rather, attachment of periodontal ligament fibroblasts to the cement surface provides a means for regenerating the periodontal ligament and deposition of cementum, as discussed in detail in a recent systematic review [85]. Formation of cementum provides the justification for the clinical superiority in using hydraulic calcium silicate cements as clinical root-end filling materials.

In terms of the osteoconductivity and osteoinductivity of calcium silicate cements, the literature is dichotomous with respective to how these cements should be classified. For example, Moretton et al. compared tissue reactions after subcutaneous and intraosseous implantation of grey MTA in a rat model [111]. The authors concluded that grey MTA is not osteoinductive because osteogenesis was not observed in subcutaneous implants. Nevertheless, the authors concluded that grey MTA is osteoconductive because osteogenesis occurred erratically with intraosseous implants. Conversely, using subcutaneous implants of MTA materials in rat models, other studies reported dystrophic calcifications within the fibrous capsule formed around the cement surface [80, 119, 145, 167]. Those authors opined that production of calcific structures in subcutaneous implants is a sign of osteoinductivity of the MTA materials.

Conclusion

MTA has been reported and promoted as bioactive materials based on its ability to produce apatite after interacting with phosphate ions derived from physiological or simulated body fluids. As this attribute was first observed in a SiO_2–Na_2O–CaO–P_2O_5 quaternary bioactive glass, the same definitions employed for establishing in vitro bioactivity and in vivo bioactivity in glass or glass-ceramic systems and the proposed mechanisms involved in these phenomena are used as blueprints for reviewing whether these activities are identifiable in MTA and other calcium silicate cements. As far as in vitro bioactivity is concerned, all papers published on this phenomenon clearly demonstrated that some forms of calcium phosphate deposition on the surface of calcium silicate cements after these materials were immersed in simulated body fluids or phosphate-containing fluids. It is likely that these calcium phosphate deposits represent the amorphous or crystalline precursors of carbonated apatite, or carbonated apatite per se, depending on the condition and timing upon which the specimens were examined and the techniques employed for analysing these inorganic precipitations. In this regard, the phenomenon of in vitro bioactivity of calcium silicate cements is indisputable. However, studies performed on calcium silicate cements lack the robustness that was demonstrated in similar studies performed on bioactive glasses, in terms of quantifying the spatiotemporal events associated with the activity. Based on these studies, the mechanisms that are responsible for the in vitro bioactivity of calcium silicate cements may be generally described in stages that are analogous to those exhibited by bioactive glass or glass-ceramics.

Based on the same definition adopted for bioactive glass and glass-ceramics, in vivo bioactivity has been demonstrated for at least grey MTA and Portland cement. However, a fibrous connective tissue layer is frequently observed along the newly formed bone–cement interface that is reminiscent of the responses observed in bioinert materials. The composition, constitutional phases and hydration characteristics of a clinker-derived calcium silicate cement are much more complex compared to a quaternary or even a ternary melt-derived bioactive glass system. The contribution of early and late hydration of different constitutional phases in clinker-derived calcium silicate cements to the rate and extent of carbonated apatite formation has not been established. Data is also lacking on the potential in vivo bioactivity of other calcium silicate cements such as white MTA and MTA-like materials, as well as and single-phase calcium silicate cements. In matters of style, it is tempting to swim with the current by endorsing that hydraulic calcium silicate cements exhibit predictable in vivo bioactive behaviour akin to those observed in 45S5 bioactive glass. In matters of principle, however, one has to acknowledge that there is presently insufficient scientific evidence to support this assumption. More importantly, the parameters responsible for this uncertainty have not been recognised. Even though this assumption may be valid, the current methods generally employed by the endodontic community for validating this assumption leave room for improvement in terms of understanding how the composition (including types of opacifier), hydration phases and alkalinity of different calcium silicate cements may influence the predictability of their in vivo bone-bonding responses. In addition, universally acceptable criteria are lacking for objective appraisal of the relative in vivo bioactivity of different hydraulic calcium silicate cements. As such, the term 'bioactivity' is used rather ambiguously and loosely defined in studies on these cements. Appraisal criteria should be developed by reputable organisations such as the International Organization for Standardization (ISO) or the American Society for Testing and Materials (ASTM), to guide manufacturers, or scientists who are interested in patenting their own inventions, in more accurately defining the bioactivity profiles of novel calcium silicate cements that are introduced for restorative and endodontic applications.

References

1. Albrektsson T, Johansson C. Osteoinduction, osteoconduction and osseointegration. Eur Spine J. 2001;10 Suppl 2:S96–101.
2. Al-Rabeab E, Perinpanayagam H, MacFarland D. Human alveolar bone cells interact with ProRoot and tooth-colored MTA. J Endod. 2006;32:872–5.
3. Andersen MD, Jakobsen HJ, Skibsted J. Incorporation of aluminum in the calcium silicate hydrate (C-S-H) of hydrated Portland cements: a high-field 27Al and 29Si MAS NMR investigation. Inorg Chem. 2003; 42:2280–7.
4. Asefa T, Duncan CT, Sharma KK. Recent advances in nanostructured chemosensors and biosensors. Analyst. 2009;134:1980–90.
5. Asgary S, Eghbal MJ, Parirokh M, Ghoddusi J. Effect of two storage solutions on surface topography of two root-end fillings. Aust Endod J. 2009;35:147–52.
6. Atmeh AR, Chong EZ, Richard G, Festy F, Watson TF. Dentin-cement interfacial interaction: calcium silicates and polyalkenoates. J Dent Res. 2012;91: 454–9.
7. Balto HA. Attachment and morphological behavior of human periodontal ligament fibroblasts to mineral trioxide aggregate: a scanning electron microscope study. J Endod. 2004;30:25–9.
8. Beniash E. Biominerals-hierarchical nanocomposites: the example of bone. Wiley Interdiscip Rev Nanomed Nanobiotechnol. 2011;3:47–69.
9. Bertassoni LE, Orgel JP, Antipova O, Swain MV. The dentin organic matrix – limitations of restorative dentistry hidden on the nanometer scale. Acta Biomater. 2012;8:2419–33.
10. Bird DC, Komabayashi T, Guo L, Opperman LA, Spears R. In vitro evaluation of dentinal tubule penetration and biomineralization ability of a new root-end filling material. J Endod. 2012;38:1093–6.
11. Bodier-Houllé P, Steuer P, Voegel JC, Cuisinier FJ. First experimental evidence for human dentine crystal formation involving conversion of octacalcium phosphate to hydroxyapatite. Acta Crystallogr D Biol Crystallogr. 1998;54(Pt 6 Pt 2):1377–81.

12. Bohner M, Lemaitre J. Can bioactivity be tested in vitro with SBF solution? Biomaterials. 2009;30:2175–9.
13. Bonson S, Jeansonne BG, Lallier TE. Root-end filling materials alter fibroblast differentiation. J Dent Res. 2004;83:408–13.
14. Bosetti M, Zanardi L, Hench L, Cannas M. Type I collagen production by osteoblast-like cells cultured in contact with different bioactive glasses. J Biomed Mater Res A. 2003;64:189–95.
15. Bozeman TB, Lemon RR, Eleazer PD. Elemental analysis of crystal precipitate from gray and white MTA. J Endod. 2006;32:425–8.
16. Branda F, Arcobello-Varlese F, Costantini A, Luciani G. Effect of the substitution of M2O3 (M = La, Y, In, Ga, Al) for CaO on the bioactivity of 2.5CaO x 2SiO2 glass. Biomaterials. 2002;23:711–6.
17. Brouwers HJH, van Eijk RJ. Alkali concentrations of pore solution in hydrating OPC. Cement Concrete Res. 2003;33:191–6.
18. Brown WE. Octacalcium phosphate and hydroxyapatite: crystal structure of octacalcium phosphate. Nature. 1962;196:1048–50.
19. Brown WE, Smith JP, Lehr JR, Frazier AW. Octacalcium phosphate and hydroxyapatite: crystallographic and chemical relations between octacalcium phosphate and hydroxyapatite. Nature. 1962;196:1050–5.
20. Budiraharjo R, Neoh KG, Kang ET, Kishen A. Bioactivity of novel carboxymethyl chitosan scaffold incorporating MTA in a tooth model. Int Endod J. 2010;43:930–9.
21. Cado G, Aslam R, Séon L, Garnier T, Fabre R, Parat A, Chassepot A, Voegel J-C, Senger B, Schneider F, Frère Y, Jierry L, Schaaf P, Kerdjoudj H, Metz-Boutique M-H, Boulmedais F. Self-defensive biomaterial coating against bacteria and yeasts: polysaccharide multilayer film with embedded antimicrobial peptide. Adv Funct Mater. 2013. doi:10.1002/adfm.201300416.
22. Camilleri J. Hydration mechanisms of mineral trioxide aggregate. Int Endod J. 2007;40:462–70.
23. Camilleri J. Investigation of Biodentine as dentine replacement material. J Dent. 2013;41:600–10.
24. Camilleri J, Montesin FE, Brady K, Sweeney R, Curtis R, Pitt Ford TR. The constitution of mineral trioxide aggregate. Dent Mater. 2005;21:297–303.
25. Camilleri J, Sorrentino F, Damidot D. Investigation of the hydration and bioactivity of radiopacified tricalcium silicate cement, Biodentine and MTA Angelus. Dent Mater. 2013;29:580–93.
26. Campoccia D, Montanaro L, Arciola CR. A review of the biomaterials technologies for infection-resistant surfaces. Biomaterials. 2013;34:8533–54.
27. Cao W, Hench LL. Bioactive materials. Ceram Int. 1996;22:493–507.
28. Carlisle EM. Silicon: a possible factor in bone calcification. Science. 1970;167:279–80.
29. Chen W, Brouwers HJH. Alkali binding in hydrated Portland cement paste. Cement Concrete Res. 2010;40:716–22.
30. Chen CC, Ho CC, David Chen CH, Wang WC, Ding SJ. In vitro bioactivity and biocompatibility of dicalcium silicate cements for endodontic use. J Endod. 2009;35:1554–7.
31. Chiang TY, Wei CK, Ding SJ. Effects of bismuth oxide on physicochemical properties and osteogenic activity of dicalcium silicate cements. J Med Biol Eng. 2013. doi:10.5305/jmbe.1386.
32. Chickerur NS, Tung MS, Brown WE. A mechanism for incorporation of carbonate into apatite. Calcif Tissue Int. 1980;32:55–62.
33. Cho SB, Nakanishi K, Kokubo T, Soga N, Ohtsuki C, Nakamura T. Apatite formation on silica gel in simulated body fluid: its dependence on structures of silica gels prepared in different media. J Biomed Mater Res. 1996;33:145–51.
34. Cintra LT, Bernabé PF, de Moraes IG, Gomes-Filho JE, Okamoto T, Consolaro A, Pinheiro TN. Evaluation of subcutaneous and alveolar implantation surgical sites in the study of the biological properties of root-end filling endodontic materials. J Appl Oral Sci. 2010;18:75–82.
35. Cintra LT, de Moraes IG, Estrada BP, Gomes-Filho JE, Bramante CM, Garcia RB, Bernardinelli N. Evaluation of the tissue response to MTA and MBPC: microscopic analysis of implants in alveolar bone of rats. J Endod. 2006;32:556–9.
36. Coleman NJ, Nicholson JW, Awosanya K. A preliminary investigation of the in vitro bioactivity of white Portland cement. Cement Concrete Res. 2007;37:1518–23.
37. Combes C, Rey C. Amorphous calcium phosphates: synthesis, properties and uses in biomaterials. Acta Biomater. 2010;6:3362–78.
38. Damen JJM, Ten Cate JM. Silica-induced precipitation of calcium phosphate in the presence of inhibitors of hydroxyapatite formation. J Dent Res. 1992;71:453–7.
39. Darvell BW, Wu RC. "MTA"-an hydraulic silicate cement: review update and setting reaction. Dent Mater. 2011;27:407–22.
40. Davies JE, editor. The bone-biomaterial interface. Toronto: University of Toronto Press; 1993.
41. Dey A, Bomans PH, Müller FA, Will J, Frederik PM, de With G, Sommerdijk NA. The role of prenucleation clusters in surface-induced calcium phosphate crystallization. Nat Mater. 2010;9:1010–4.
42. Dorozhkin SV. Calcium orthophosphates: occurrence, properties, biomineralization, pathological calcification and biomimetic applications. Biomatter. 2011;1:121–64.
43. Dorvee JR, Veis A. Water in the formation of biogenic minerals: peeling away the hydration layers. J Struct Biol. 2013;183:278–303.
44. Eanes ED. Amorphous calcium phosphate. Monogr Oral Sci. 2001;18:130–47.
45. Eidelman N, Chow LC, Brown WE. Calcium phosphate phase transformations in serum. Calcif Tissue Int. 1987;41:18–26.
46. El-Ghannam A, Ducheyne P, Shapiro IM. Effect of serum proteins on osteoblast adhesion to surface-modified bioactive glass and hydroxyapatite. J Orthop Res. 1999;17:340–5.
47. Elliot JC. Studies in inorganic chemistry 18: structure and chemistry of the apatites and other calcium orthophosphates. Amsterdam: Elsevier; 1994.
48. Formosa LM, Mallia B, Bull T, Camilleri J. The microstructure and surface morphology of radiopaque

tricalcium silicate cement exposed to different curing conditions. Dent Mater. 2012;28:584–95.
49. Formosa LM, Mallia B, Camilleri J. The chemical properties of light- and chemical-curing composites with mineral trioxide aggregate filler. Dent Mater. 2013;29:e11–9.
50. Fowler BO, Marković M, Brown WE. Octacalcium phosphate. 3. Infrared and Raman vibrational spectra. Chem Mater. 1993;5:1417–23.
51. Gandolfi MG, Ciapetti G, Taddei P, Perut F, Tinti A, Cardoso MV, Van Meerbeek B, Prati C. Apatite formation on bioactive calcium-silicate cements for dentistry affects surface topography and human marrow stromal cells proliferation. Dent Mater. 2010;26:974–92.
52. Gandolfi MG, Taddei P, Modena E, Siboni F, Prati C. Biointeractivity-related versus chemi/physisorption-related apatite precursor-forming ability of current root end filling materials. J Biomed Mater Res B Appl Biomater. 2013. doi:10.1002/jbm.b.32920.
53. Gandolfi MG, Taddei P, Siboni F, Modena E, Ciapetti G, Prati C. Development of the foremost light-curable calcium-silicate MTA cement as root-end in oral surgery. Chemical-physical properties, bioactivity and biological behavior. Dent Mater. 2011;27:e134–57.
54. Gandolfi MG, Taddei P, Siboni F, Modena E, Ginebra MP, Prati C. Fluoride-containing nanoporous calcium-silicate MTA cements for endodontics and oral surgery: early fluorapatite formation in a phosphate-containing solution. Int Endod J. 2011;44:938–49.
55. Gandolfi MG, Taddei P, Tinti A, De Stefano DE, Prati C. Alpha-TCP improves the apatite-formation ability of calcium-silicate hydraulic cement soaked in phosphate solutions. Mater Sci Eng C. 2011;31:1412–22.
56. Gandolfi MG, Taddei P, Tinti A, De Stefano DE, Rossi PL, Prati C. Kinetics of apatite formation on a calcium-silicate cement for root-end filling during ageing in physiological-like phosphate solutions. Clin Oral Investig. 2010;14:659–68.
57. Gandolfi MG, Taddei P, Tinti A, Prati C. Apatite-forming ability (bioactivity) of ProRoot MTA. Int Endod J. 2010;43:917–29.
58. Gandolfi MG, Van Landuyt K, Taddei P, Modena E, Van Meerbeek B, Prati C. Environmental scanning electron microscopy connected with energy dispersive x-ray analysis and Raman techniques to study ProRoot mineral trioxide aggregate and calcium silicate cements in wet conditions and in real time. J Endod. 2010;36:851–7.
59. García AJ, Ducheyne P, Boettiger D. Effect of surface reaction stage on fibronectin-mediated adhesion of osteoblast-like cells to bioactive glass. J Biomed Mater Res. 1998;40:48–56.
60. Gerhardt LC, Widdows KL, Erol MM, Burch CW, Sanz-Herrera JA, Ochoa I, Stämpfli R, Roqan IS, Gabe S, Ansari T, Boccaccini AR. The pro-angiogenic properties of multi-functional bioactive glass composite scaffolds. Biomaterials. 2011;32:4096–108.
61. Gerhardt LC, Widdows KL, Erol MM, Nandakumar A, Roqan IS, Ansari T, Boccaccini AR. Neocellularization and neovascularization of nanosized bioactive glass-coated decellularized trabecular bone scaffolds. J Biomed Mater Res A. 2013;101:827–41.
62. Gomes-Filho JE, de Moraes Costa MM, Cintra LT, Duarte PC, Takamiya AS, Lodi CS, Bernabé PF. Evaluation of rat alveolar bone response to Angelus MTA or experimental light-cured mineral trioxide aggregate using fluorochromes. J Endod. 2011;37:250–4.
63. Gomes-Filho JE, de Moraes Costa MT, Cintra LT, Lodi CS, Duarte PC, Okamoto R, Bernabé PF, Nery MJ, Cannon M. Evaluation of alveolar socket response to Angelus MTA and experimental light-cure MTA. Oral Surg Oral Med Oral Pathol Oral Radiol Endod. 2010;110:e93–7.
64. Gorustovich AA, Roether JA, Boccaccini AR. Effect of bioactive glasses on angiogenesis: a review of in vitro and in vivo evidences. Tissue Eng Part B Rev. 2010;16:199–207.
65. Gou Z, Chang J, Zhai W, Wang J. Study on the self-setting property and the in vitro bioactivity of beta-Ca2SiO4. J Biomed Mater Res B Appl Biomater. 2005;73:244–51.
66. Greenspan DC. Bioactive glass: mechanism of bone bonding. Tandläkartidningen Årk 1999;91(8):1–32.
67. Greenspan DC, Hench LL. Chemical and mechanical behavior of bioglass-coated alumina. J Biomed Mater Res. 1976;10:503–9.
68. Hakki SS, Bozkurt SB, Ozcopur B, Purali N, Belli S. Periodontal ligament fibroblast response to root perforations restored with different materials: a laboratory study. Int Endod J. 2012;45:240–8.
69. Han S, Lemire J, Appanna VP, Auger C, Castonguay Z, Appanna VD. How aluminum, an intracellular ROS generator promotes hepatic and neurological diseases: the metabolic tale. Cell Biol Toxicol. 2013;29:75–84.
70. Han L, Okiji T. Uptake of calcium and silicon released from calcium silicate-based endodontic materials into root canal dentine. Int Endod J. 2011;44:1081–7.
71. Han L, Okiji T. Bioactivity evaluation of three calcium silicate-based endodontic materials. Int Endod J. 2013;46:808–14.
72. Han L, Okiji T, Okawa S. Morphological and chemical analysis of different precipitates on mineral trioxide aggregate immersed in different fluids. Dent Mater J. 2010;29:512–7.
73. Hench LL. Bioactive ceramics. In: Ducheyne P, Lemons JE, editors. Bioceramics: materials characteristics versus in vivo behavior, Annals of the New York Academy of Sciences, vol. 523. New York: New York Academy of Sciences; 1988. p. 54.
74. Hench LL. Bioceramics: from concept to clinic. J Am Ceram Soc. 1991;74:1487–510.
75. Hench LL. The story of Bioglass®. J Mater Sci Mater Med. 2006;17:967–78.
76. Hench LL, Anderson ÖH. Bioactive glasses. In: Hench LL, Wilson J, editors. An introduction of bioceramics. London: World Scientific; 1993. p. 41–62.
77. Hench LL, Ethridge EC. Biomaterials – an interfacial approach. New York: Academic; 1982.

78. Hench LL, Paschall HA. Histochemical responses at a biomaterial's interface. J Biomed Mater Res. 1974;8:49–64.
79. Hench LL, Splinter RJ, Allen WC, Greenlee TK. Bonding mechanisms at the interface of ceramic prosthetic materials. J Biomed Mater Res. 1971;5:117–41.
80. Holland R, De Souza R, Nery MJ, Filho JAO, Bernabe PF, Dezan E. Reaction of rat connective tissue to implanted dentin tubes filled with mineral trioxide aggregate or calcium hydroxide. J Endod. 1999;25:161–6.
81. Hoppe A, Güldal NS, Boccaccini AR. A review of the biological response to ionic dissolution products from bioactive glasses and glass-ceramics. Biomaterials. 2011;32:2757–74.
82. Hubbell JA. Bioactive biomaterials. Curr Opin Biotechnol. 1999;10:123–9.
83. Ivancik J, Majd H, Bajaj D, Romberg E, Arola D. Contributions of aging to the fatigue crack growth resistance of human dentin. Acta Biomater. 2012;8:2737–46.
84. Jugdaohsingh R, Tucker KL, Qiao N, Cupples LA, Kiel DP, Powell JJ. Dietary silicon intake is positively associated with bone mineral density in men and premenopausal women of the Framingham Offspring cohort. J Bone Miner Res. 2004;19:297–307.
85. Katsamakis S, Slot DE, Van der Sluis LWM, Van der Weijden F. Histological responses of the periodontium to MTA: a systematic review. J Clin Periodontol. 2013;40:334–44.
86. Kitsugi T, Nakamura T, Yamamuro T, Kokubo T, Shibuya T, Takagi M. SEM-EPMA observation of three types of apatite containing glass ceramics implanted in bone: the variance of a Ca, P-rich layer. J Biomed Mater Res. 1987;21:1255–71.
87. Koh ET, McDonald F, Pitt Ford TR, Torabinejad M. Cellular response to mineral trioxide aggregate. J Endod. 1998;24:543–7.
88. Koh ET, Torabinejad M, Pitt Ford TR, Brady K, McDonald F. Mineral trioxide aggregate stimulates a biological response in human osteoblasts. J Biomed Mater Res. 1997;37:432–9.
89. Kokubo T, Kushitani H, Sakka S, Kitsugi T, Yamamuro T. Solutions able to reproduce in vivo surface-structure change in bioactive glass-ceramic A–W. J Biomed Mater Res. 1990;24:721–34.
90. Kokubo T, Takadama H. How useful is SBF in predicting in vivo bone bioactivity? Biomaterials. 2006;27:2907–15.
91. Labbez C, Jönsson B, Pochard I, Nonat A, Cabane C. Surface charge density and electrokinetic potential of highly charged minerals: experiments and Monte Carlo simulations on calcium silicate hydrate. J Phys Chem B. 2006;110:9219–30.
92. LeGeros RZ. Calcium phosphate in oral biology and medicine. Basel: Karger; 1991.
93. LeGeros RZ. Biological and synthetic apatites. In: Brown PW, Constantz B, editors. Hydroxyapatite and related material. Boca Raton: CRC Press; 1994. p. 3–28.
94. Leiendecker AP, Qi YP, Sawyer AN, Niu LN, Agee KA, Loushine RJ, Weller RN, Pashley DH, Tay FR. Effects of calcium silicate-based materials on collagen matrix integrity of mineralized dentin. J Endod. 2012;38:829–33.
95. Leu A, Stieger SM, Dayton P, Ferrara KW, Leach JK. Angiogenic response to bioactive glass promotes bone healing in an irradiated calvarial defect. Tissue Eng Part A. 2009;15:877–85.
96. Li R, Clark AE, Hench LL. An investigation of bioactive glass powders by sol-gel processing. J Appl Biomater. 1991;2:231–9.
97. Liu X, Ding C, Chu PK. Mechanism of apatite formation on wollastonite coatings in simulated body fluids. Biomaterials. 2004;25:1755–61.
98. Maeno S, Niki Y, Matsumoto H, Morioka H, Yatabe T, Funayama A, Toyama Y, Taguchi T, Tanaka J. The effect of calcium ion concentration on osteoblast viability, proliferation and differentiation in monolayer and 3D culture. Biomaterials. 2005;26:4847–55.
99. Mahamid J, Addadi L, Weiner S. Crystallization pathways in bone. Cells Tissues Organs. 2011;194:92–7.
100. Mahamid J, Aichmayer B, Shimoni E, Ziblat R, Li C, Siegel S, Paris O, Fratzl P, Weiner S, Addadi L. Mapping amorphous calcium phosphate transformation into crystalline mineral from the cell to the bone in zebrafish fin rays. Proc Natl Acad Sci U S A. 2010;107:6316–21.
101. Mahamid J, Sharir A, Addadi L, Weiner S. Amorphous calcium phosphate is a major component of the forming fin bones of zebrafish: Indications for an amorphous precursor phase. Proc Natl Acad Sci U S A. 2008;105:12748–53.
102. Mai S, Kim YK, Kim J, Yiu CK, Ling J, Pashley DH, Tay FR. In vitro remineralization of severely compromised bonded dentin. J Dent Res. 2010;89:405–10.
103. Maia FR, Bidarra SJ, Granja PL, Barrias CC. Functionalization of biomaterials with small osteoinductive moieties. Acta Biomater. 2013;9(11):8773–89. pii: S1742-7061(13)00396-6.
104. Marie PJ. The calcium-sensing receptor in bone cells: a potential therapeutic target in osteoporosis. Bone. 2010;46:571–6.
105. Marković M, Fowler BO, Tung MS. Preparation and comprehensive characterization of a calcium hydroxyapatite reference material. Natl Inst Stan Technol. 2004;109:553–68.
106. Matthew M, Takagi S. Structure of biological minerals in dental research. J Res Natl Inst Stan Technol. 2001;106:1035–44.
107. Merwin GE, Atkins JS, Wilson J, Hench LL. Comparison of ossicular replacement materials in a mouse ear model. Otolaryngol Head Neck Surg. 1982;90:461–9.
108. Mitchell PJ, Pitt Ford TR, Torabinejad M, McDonald F. Osteoblast biocompatibility of mineral trioxide aggregate. Biomaterials. 1999;20:167–73.

109. Miyazaki T, Kim HM, Kokubo T, Kato H, Nakamura T. Induction and acceleration of bone-like apatite formation on tantalum oxide gel in simulated body fluid. J Sol Gel Sci Technol. 2001;21:83–8.
110. Miyazaki T, Kim HM, Kokubo T, Ohtsuki C, Kato H, Nakamura T. Apatite-forming ability of niobium oxide gels in a simulated body fluid. J Ceram Soc Japan. 2001;109:929–33.
111. Moretton TR, Brown Jr CE, Legan JJ, Kafrawy AH. Tissue reactions after subcutaneous and intraosseous implantation of mineral trioxide aggregate and ethoxybenzoic acid cement. J Biomed Mater Res. 2000;52:528–33.
112. Nakayama A, Ogiso B, Tanabe N, Takeichi O, Matsuzaka K, Inoue T. Behaviour of bone marrow osteoblast-like cells on mineral trioxide aggregate: morphology and expression of type I collagen and bone-related protein mRNAs. Int Endod J. 2005;38:203–10.
113. Nazari A, Bajaj D, Zhang D, Romberg E, Arola D. Aging and the reduction in fracture toughness of human dentin. J Mech Behav Biomed Mater. 2009;2:550–9.
114. Neo M, Kotani S, Fujita Y, Nakamura T, Yamamuro T, Bando Y, Ohtsuki C, Kokubo T. Differences in ceramic-bone interface between surface-active ceramics and resorbable ceramics: a study by scanning and transmission electron microscopy. J Biomed Mater Res. 1992;26:255–67.
115. Neo M, Nakamura T, Ohtsuki C, Kokubo T, Yamamuro T. Apatite formation on three kinds of bioactive material at an early stage in vivo: a comparative study by transmission electron microscopy. J Biomed Mater Res. 1993;27:999–1006.
116. Niu LN, Zhang W, Pashley DH, Breschi L, Mao J, Chen JH, Tay FR. Biomimetic remineralization of dentin. Dent Mater. 2013;30(1):77–96, pii: S0109-5641(13)00175-9.
117. Pan H, Liu XY, Tang R, Xu HY. Mystery of the transformation from amorphous calcium phosphate to hydroxyapatite. Chem Commun (Camb). 2010;46:7415–7.
118. Pardal X, Pochard I, Nonat A. Experimental study of Si–Al substitution in calcium-silicate-hydrate (C-S-H) prepared under equilibrium conditions. Cement Concrete Res. 2009;39:637–53.
119. Parirokh M, Mirsoltani B, Raoof M, Tabrizchi H, Haghdoost AA. Comparative study of subcutaneous tissue responses to a novel root-end filling material and white and grey mineral trioxide aggregate. Int Endod J. 2011;44:283–9.
120. Parirokh M, Torabinejad M. Mineral trioxide aggregate: a comprehensive literature review – part I: chemical, physical, and antibacterial properties. J Endod. 2010;36:16–27.
121. Parirokh M, Torabinejad M. Mineral trioxide aggregate: a comprehensive literature review – part III: clinical applications, drawbacks, and mechanism of action. J Endod. 2010;36:400–13.
122. Pashley DH, Tay FR, Breschi L, Tjäderhane L, Carvalho RM, Carrilho M, Tezvergil-Mutluay A. State of the art etch-and-rinse adhesives. Dent Mater. 2011;27:1–16.
123. Peltola T, Pätsi M, Rahiala H, Kangasniemi I, Yli-Urpo A. Calcium phosphate induction by sol-gel-derived titania coatings on titanium substrates in vitro. J Biomed Mater Res. 1998;41:504–10.
124. Primus CM, inventor: DENTSPLY International, Inc., assignee. Dental material. United States Patent 7,892,342. 22 Feb 2011.
125. Rahaman MN, Day DE, Bal BS, Fu Q, Jung SB, Bonewald LF, Tomsia AP. Bioactive glass in tissue engineering. Acta Biomater. 2011;7:2355–73.
126. Rahimi S, Mokhtari H, Shahi S, Kazemi A, Asgary S, Eghbal MJ, Mesgariabbasi M, Mohajeri D. Osseous reaction to implantation of two endodontic cements: mineral trioxide aggregate (MTA) and calcium enriched mixture (CEM). Med Oral Patol Oral Cir Bucal. 2012;17:e907–11.
127. Reffitt DM, Ogston N, Jugdaohsingh R, Cheung HFJ, Evans BAJ, Thompson RPH, Powell JJ, Hampson GN. Orthosilicic acid stimulates collagen type 1 synthesis and osteoblastic differentiation in human osteoblast-like cells in vitro. Bone. 2003;32: 127–35.
128. Reyes-Carmona JF, Felippe MS, Felippe WT. Biomineralization ability and interaction of mineral trioxide aggregate and white portland cement with dentin in a phosphate-containing fluid. J Endod. 2009;35:731–6.
129. Richardson G. The calcium silicate hydrates. Cement Concrete Res. 2008;38:137–58.
130. Richardson IG, Brough AR, Brydson R, Groves GW, Dobson CM. Location of aluminum in substituted calcium silicate hydrate (C-S-H) gels as determined by 29Si and 27Al NMR and EELS. J Am Ceram Soc. 1995;76:2285–8.
131. Roberts HW, Toth JM, Berzins DW, Charlton DG. Mineral trioxide aggregate material use in endodontic treatment: a review of the literature. Dent Mater. 2008;24:149–64.
132. Ryou H, Amin N, Ross A, Eidelman N, Wang DH, Romberg E, Arola D. Contributions of microstructure and chemical composition to the mechanical properties of dentin. J Mater Sci Mater Med. 2011;22:1127–35.
133. Saidon J, He J, Zhu Q, Safavi K, Spångberg LS. Cell and tissue reactions to mineral trioxide aggregate and Portland cement. Oral Surg Oral Med Oral Pathol Oral Radiol Endod. 2003;95:483–9.
134. Samara A, Sarri Y, Stravopodis D, Tzanetakis GN, Kontakiotis EG, Anastasiadou E. A comparative study of the effects of three root-end filling materials on proliferation and adherence of human periodontal ligament fibroblasts. J Endod. 2011;37: 865–70.
135. Saravanapavan P, Jones JR, Pryce RS, Hench LL. Bioactivity of gel-glass powders in the CaO-SiO2 system: a comparison with ternary (CaO-P2O5-

SiO2) and quaternary glasses (SiO2-CaO-P2O5-Na2O). J Biomed Mater Res A. 2003;66:110–9.
136. Saravanapavan P, Jones JR, Verrier S, Beilby R, Shirtliff VJ, Hench LL, Polak JM. Binary CaO-SiO2 gel-glasses for biomedical applications. Biomed Mater Eng. 2004;14:467–86.
137. Sarkar NK, Caicedo R, Ritwik P, Moiseyeva R, Kawashima I. Physicochemical basis of the biologic properties of mineral trioxide aggregate. J Endod. 2005;31:97–100.
138. Schröder HC, Wang XH, Wiens M, Diehl-Seifert B, Kropf K, Schloßmacher U, Müller WE. Silicate modulates the cross-talk between osteoblasts (SaOS-2) and osteoclasts (RAW 264.7 cells): inhibition of osteoclast growth and differentiation. J Cell Biochem. 2012;113:3197–206.
139. Seitz TL, Noonan KD, Hench LL, Noonan NE. Effect of fibronectin on the adhesion of an established cell line to a surface reactive biomaterial. J Biomed Mater Res. 1982;16:195–207.
140. Sharma S, Singh R, Rana S. Bioactive peptides: a review. Int J Bioautomation. 2011;15:223–50.
141. Shaw CA, Tomljenovic L. Aluminum in the central nervous system (CNS): toxicity in humans and animals, vaccine adjuvants, and autoimmunity. Immunol Res. 2013;56:304–16.
142. Shokouhinejad N, Nekoofar MH, Razmi H, Sajadi S, Davies TE, Saghiri MA, Gorjestani H, Dummer PM. Bioactivity of EndoSequence root repair material and bioaggregate. Int Endod J. 2012;45:1127–34.
143. Silver IA, Deas J, Erecińska M. Interactions of bioactive glasses with osteoblasts in vitro: effects of 45S5 Bioglass, and 58S and 77S bioactive glasses on metabolism, intracellular ion concentrations and cell viability. Biomaterials. 2001;22:175–85.
144. Sousa CJ, Loyola AM, Versiani MA, Biffi JC, Oliveira RP, Pascon EA. A comparative histological evaluation of the biocompatibility of materials used in apical surgery. Int Endod J. 2004;37:738–48.
145. Sumer M, Muglali M, Badrumlu E, Guvenc T. Reactions of connective tissue to amalgam, intermediate restorative material, mineral trioxide aggregate and mineral trioxide aggregate mixed with chlorhexidine. J Endod. 2006;32:1094–6.
146. Taddei P, Tinti A, Gandolfi MG, Rossi PL, Prati C. Ageing of calcium silicate cements for endodontic use in simulated body fluids: a micro-Raman study. J Raman Spectrosc. 2009;40:1858–66.
147. Taddei P, Tinti A, Gandolfi MG, Rossi PL, Prati C. Vibrational study on the bioactivity of portland cement-based materials for endodontic use. J Mol Struct. 2009;924–926:548–54.
148. Taves DR. Similarity of octacalcium phosphate and hydroxyapatite structures. Nature. 1963;200:1312–3.
149. Tay FR, Pashley DH, Rueggeberg FA, Loushine RJ, Weller RN. Calcium phosphate phase transformation produced by the interaction of the Portland cement component of white mineral trioxide aggregate with a phosphate-containing fluid. J Endod. 2007;33:1347–51.
150. Tay FR, Sidhu SK, Watson TF, Pashley DH. Water-dependent interfacial transition zone in resin-modified glass-ionomer cement/dentin interfaces. J Dent Res. 2004;83(8):644–9.
151. Tingey MC, Bush P, Levine MS. Analysis of mineral trioxide aggregate surface when set in the presence of fetal bovine serum. J Endod. 2008;34:45–9.
152. Torabinejad M, Bahjri K. Essential elements of evidenced-based endodontics: steps involved in conducting clinical research. J Endod. 2005;31:563–9.
153. Torabinejad M, Ford TR, Abedi HR, Kariyawasam SP, Tang HM. Tissue reaction to implanted root-end filling materials in the tibia and mandible of guinea pigs. J Endod. 1998;24:468–71.
154. Torabinejad M, Hong CU, Pitt Ford TR, Kaiyawasam SP. Tissue reaction to implanted super-EBA and mineral trioxide aggregate in the mandible of guinea pigs: a preliminary report. J Endod. 1995;21:569–71.
155. Torabinejad M, White DJ, inventors: Loma Linda University, assignee. Tooth filling material and method of use. United States Patent 5,415,547. 23 Apr 1993.
156. Tseng YH, Mou CY, Chan JC. Solid-state NMR study of the transformation of octacalcium phosphate to hydroxyapatite: a mechanistic model for central dark line formation. J Am Chem Soc. 2006;128:6909–18.
157. Uchida M, Kim HM, Kokubo T, Nakamura T. Bonelike apatite formation induced on zirconia gel in simulated body fluid and its modified solutions. J Am Ceram Soc. 2001;84:2041–4.
158. Valerio P, Pereira MM, Goes AM, Leite MF. Effects of extracellular calcium concentration on the glutamate release by bioactive glass (BG60S) preincubated osteoblasts. Biomed Mater. 2009;4:045011.
159. Van Meerbeek B, Yoshihara K, Yoshida Y, Mine A, De Munck J, Van Landuyt KL. State of the art of self-etch adhesives. Dent Mater. 2011;27:17–28.
160. Wan XH, Chang CK, Mao DL, Jiang L, Li M. Preparation and in vitro bioactivities of calcium silicate nanophase materials. Mater Sci Eng C. 2005;25:455–61.
161. Willershausen I, Wolf T, Kasaj A, Weyer V, Willershausen B, Marroquin BB. Influence of a bioceramic root end material and mineral trioxide aggregates on fibroblasts and osteoblasts. Arch Oral Biol. 2013;58:1232–7.
162. Williams DF, editor. Definitions in biomaterials. Amsterdam/Oxford/New York/Tokyo: Elsevier; 1987.
163. Wilson CJ, Clegg RE, Leavesley DI, Pearcy MJ. Mediation of biomaterial-cell interactions by adsorbed proteins: a review. Tissue Eng. 2005;11:1–18.
164. Wilson J, Low SJ. Bioactive ceramics for periodontal treatment: comparative studies in the Patus monkey. J Appl Biomater. 1992;3:123–9.
165. Wilson J, Noletti D. Bonding of soft tissues to Bioglass®. In: Yamamuro T, Hench LL, Wilson J, editors. Handbook of bioactive ceramics vol. 1: bioactive glasses and glass-ceramics. Boca Raton: CRC Press; 1990.

166. Xin R, Leng Y, Wang N. In situ TEM examinations of octacalcium phosphate to hydroxyapatite transformation. J Cryst Growth. 2006;289:339–44.
167. Yaltirik M, Ozbas H, Bilgic B, Issever H. Reactions of connective tissue to mineral trioxide aggregate and amalgam. J Endod. 2004;30:95–9.
168. Yamasaki Y, Yoshida Y, Okazaki M, Shimazu A, Uchida T, Kubo T, Akagawa Y, Hamada Y, Takahashi J, Matsuura N. Synthesis of functionally graded MgCO3 apatite accelerating osteoblast adhesion. J Biomed Mater Res. 2002;62:99–105.
169. Yang Q, Jian J, Abramson SB, Huang X. Inhibitory effects of iron on bone morphogenetic protein 2-induced osteoblastogenesis. J Bone Miner Res. 2011;26:1188–96.
170. Yip HK, Tay FR, Ngo HC, Smales RJ, Pashley DH. Bonding of contemporary glass ionomer cements to dentin. Dent Mater. 2001;17:456–70.
171. Zhang L, Jin C, Liu Q, Lu X, Wu S, Yang J, Du Y, Zheng L, Cai Y. Effects of subchronic aluminum exposure on spatial memory, ultrastructure and L-LTP of hippocampus in rats. J Toxicol Sci. 2013;38:255–68.
172. Zhao W, Wang J, Zhai W, Wang Z, Chang J. The self-setting properties and in vitro bioactivity of tricalcium silicate. Biomaterials. 2005;26:6113–21.
173. Zhong J, Latorre G, Greenspan D, Hench LL. Alumina inhibitory effect on the formation of hydroxyapatite. In: Wilson J, Greenspan D, Hench LL, editors. Bioceramics, vol. 8. Oxford/London: Elsevier Science; 1995. p. 489–92.
174. Zhong JP, LaTorre GP, Hench LL. The kinetics of bioactive ceramics part VII: binding of collagen to hydroxyapatite and bioactive glass. In: Andersson OH, Yli-Urpo A, editors. Bioceramics, vol. 7. Oxford: Pergamon; 1994. p. 61–6.
175. Zhu Q, Haglund R, Safavi KE, Spångberg LS. Adhesion of human osteoblasts on root-end filling materials. J Endod. 2000;26:404–6.
176. Zreiqat H, Howlett CR, Zannettino A, Evans P, Schulze-Tanzil G, Knabe C, Shakibaei M. Mechanisms of magnesium-stimulated adhesion of osteoblastic cells to commonly used orthopaedic implants. J Biomed Mater Res. 2002;62:175–84.

Reactivity and Environmental Factors

5

Josette Camilleri and Paul Dummer

5.1 Introduction

Hydrated mineral trioxide aggregate (MTA) is composed of un-hydrated cement particles, which acts as a core around which a reaction rim of hydration products is formed (Fig. 2.5). When mixed with water, the tricalcium and dicalcium silicate react forming calcium silicate hydrate (honeycomb appearance) and calcium hydroxide (hexagonal plates) (Fig. 2.6), which is leached in solution. The presence of calcium hydroxide has been verified by X-ray diffraction analysis as it produces a typical peak for portlandite at 18° 2θ (Fig. 2.9), whilst the leaching of calcium has been measured by inductively coupled plasma. The particular microstructure of MTA and the presence of calcium hydroxide in solution make the material susceptible to environmental factors. The use of MTA brings it into contact with other materials, tissues and fluids, and a number of changes occur within or on the surface of the material in various environmental conditions.

J. Camilleri, BChD, MPhil, PhD, FIMMM, FADM (✉)
Department of Restorative Dentistry, Faculty of Dental Surgery, Medical School, Mater Dei Hospital, University of Malta, Msida, MSD 2090, Malta
e-mail: josette.camilleri@um.edu.mt

P. Dummer, BDS, MScD, PhD, DDSc, FDSRCS(Ed)
School of Dentistry, College of Biomedical and Life Sciences, Cardiff University, Heath Park, Cardiff CF14 4XY, Wales, UK
e-mail: dummer@cardiff.ac.uk

5.2 Effect of Environmental Factors on the Set Material

MTA has a variety of applications mostly in Endodontics. These various uses have been discussed [60] and are outlined in Chap. 6.

5.2.1 Dental Materials

5.2.1.1 Glass Ionomer

Covering MTA with glass ionomer cement when it is used as a pulp capping agent results in physical changes to the materials at their interface (Fig. 5.1a). A sizable gap has been observed at the interface attributed to the movement of water out of MTA into the glass ionomer. This movement of water out of MTA can inhibit its hydration and increases its porosity [9]. There is no evidence that covering MTA with a glass ionomer has an effect on the glass ionomer cement itself with regard to setting time and setting reaction [5, 36]. However, migration of strontium from glass ionomer to MTA has been observed [9], although its effects are unknown.

5.2.1.2 Base Materials

Zinc oxide eugenol-based cements are used as temporary filling materials and come into contact with MTA when it is used for pulp capping. Zinc is a retarder of cement hydration [47], and zinc salts form calcium hydrozincate ($Ca(Zn(OH)_3H_2O)_2$), an insoluble hydroxide in alkaline solution that creates a coating on MTA particles. In addition, zinc

J. Camilleri (ed.), *Mineral Trioxide Aggregate in Dentistry*,
DOI 10.1007/978-3-642-55157-4_5,

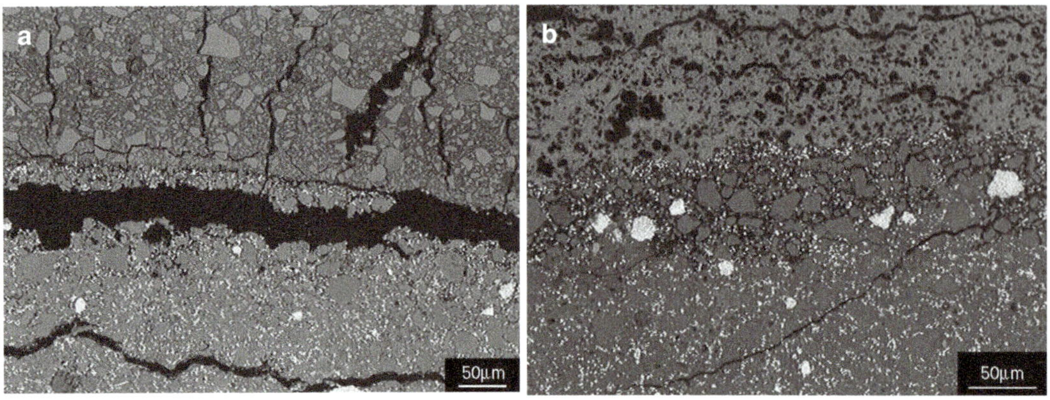

Fig. 5.1 (**a**) Interaction of glass ionomer cement with MTA leading to failure of glass ionomer and (**b**) layering of MTA with zinc oxide eugenol with a resultant retardation of setting of MTA (Reprinted from Camilleri [9], copyright 2011, with permission from Elsevier)

oxide retards the hydration of tricalcium silicate, although it does not interfere with the tricalcium aluminate/gypsum reaction. Zinc is incorporated into the calcium silicate hydrate gel phase [46], and the migration of zinc from zinc oxide cement into MTA has been reported. Furthermore, MTA in contact with intermediate restorative material (IRM) (Dentsply Caulk, Milford, DE, USA) exhibits a high degree of porosity resulting from incomplete hydration (Fig. 5.1b) [9].

5.2.1.3 Composite

The shear bond strengths of different composite adhesive systems to white MTA has been compared [6] with the conclusion that an etch-and-rinse adhesive system was preferred when placing compomer materials upon white MTA because it exhibited significantly higher shear bond strength values than self-etch adhesive systems. MTA used as pulp capping material necessitates the layering of MTA with composite for immediate restoration of the tooth. The use of bonding agent has been shown to reduce gaps at the material interface. Contact with both bonding agent and composite can reduce the micro-hardness of MTA in the early stages of its hydration [65].

5.2.2 Intra-canal Medicaments

When used inside the root canal for furcal repair and apexification procedures, MTA may come into contact with medicaments such as non-setting calcium hydroxide paste. No consensus has been reached on whether the calcium hydroxide in medicaments affects the sealing ability of MTA [20, 58]. However, calcium hydroxide does create an alkaline environment, which increases the porosity and un-hydrated microstructure of MTA [49], although no microstructural changes have been observed within MTA following contact with calcium hydroxide paste. On the other hand, migration of silicon and aluminium from MTA into calcium hydroxide medicaments has been observed [9].

5.2.3 Intra-canal Solutions

5.2.3.1 Bleaching Agents

MTA has been reported to be more easily displaced when in contact with sodium perborate mixed with saline, Superoxol (Sultan Healthcare, Hackensack, New Jersey, USA), and sodium perborate mixed with Superoxol, whereas IRM was not affected by the treatments used clinically for tooth bleaching [34]. Bleaching agents have also been shown to affect the elemental distribution of MTA [64]. A decrease in calcium and an increase in silicon were observed, and this tendency was especially pronounced when higher concentrations of hydrogen peroxide were used. The acidic conditions induced by bleaching agents also deteriorate the surface of

MTA. Overall, these findings suggest that MTA is not an effective barrier during tooth bleaching and should be protected by a more suitable material.

5.2.3.2 Chelators

Calcium chelators used as irrigating solutions affect the strength and microstructure of MTA. It has been reported that ethylenediaminetetraacetic acid (EDTA) significantly reduced the hardness and flexural strength of MTA compared with distilled water. Indeed, when in contact with EDTA, set MTA had a reduced Ca/Si molar ratio, a reduced calcium hydroxide production, lack of biocompatibility and reduced micro-hardness [31]. Therefore, after use of EDTA in the root canal system, a final flush with distilled water is advocated before placement of MTA [1]. EDTA and BioPure MTAD (Dentsply, Tulsa Dental Specialities, Tulsa, Oklahoma, USA) decreased the sealing efficacy of MTA 24 h after placement to suggest it may be beneficial to seal furcal repair sites where MTA has been used with a protective lining material before commencement of chemo-mechanical root canal preparation [66].

5.2.3.3 BioPure MTAD

BioPure MTAD-treated MTA surfaces exhibit greater surface roughness and more calcium loss when compared with EDTA treatment. Decomposition of the particle-binding hydration phases by acid erosion raises potential concern over the strength and sealing properties of MTA-repaired perforations following final irrigation using BioPure MTAD [57]. The seal of MTA used to repair root perforations has been reported to be negatively affected by irrigating solutions. Fluid conductance was affected by the type of irrigating regime used with mixtures of sodium hypochlorite and EDTA/MTAD resulting in increased leakage using the fluid filtration method to assess sealing ability of MTA [66].

5.2.3.4 Sodium Hypochlorite

NaOCl is used routinely as an irrigant in root canal treatment. Interestingly, its interaction with MTA has not been investigated extensively. However, NaOCl has been shown to enhance the push-out bond strength of MTA in the early stages of hydration [26]. MTA exhibits dark brown discoloration in contact with sodium hypochlorite solution [10], (Fig. 5.2). It is postulated that since sodium hypochlorite is reduced to sodium chloride, the oxygen present can destabilise the bismuth oxide in MTA rendering it reactive with the atmospheric carbon dioxide to be converted to bismuth carbonate, which is light sensitive and thus turns black when exposed to light. The sensitivity of MTA to different light sources has been demonstrated [67, 68].

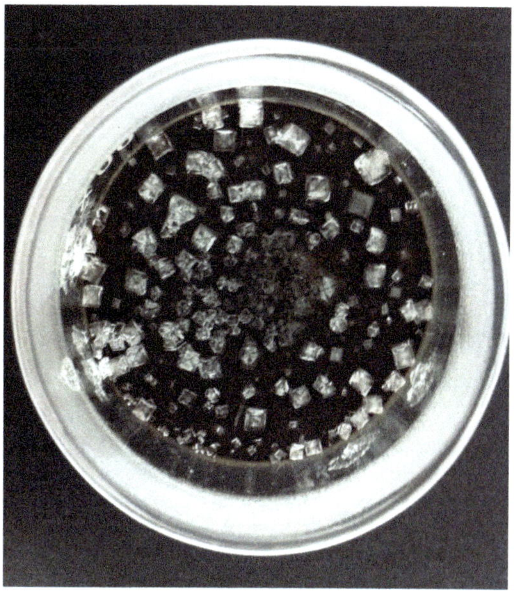

Fig. 5.2 Photograph of dried bismuth oxide powder after immersion for 24 h in sodium hypochlorite solution, showing surface crystalline deposits

5.2.4 Root Canal Sealers

MTA in contact with formaldehyde exhibits black discolouration Marciano MA, Hungaro Duarte MA University of Bauru (Personal Communication). Formaldehyde is released from resin-based sealers containing hexamethylenetetramine, such as AH 26, and Sealer 26 as a result of a chemical reaction between bisphenol A resin and hexamethylenetetramine.

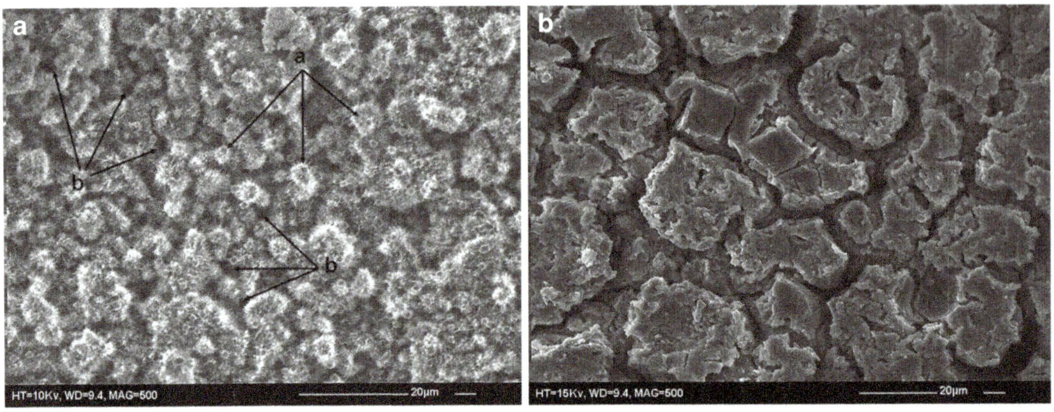

Fig. 5.3 (**a**) Intact surface of unetched mineral trioxide aggregate after 24 h. Irregular needlelike crystals that cover globular formulations (*a*) and cross sections of several micro-channels (*b*) can be seen (mag. 500×). (**b**) Etched enamel surface after 24 h. Selective loss of matrix from around the crystalline structures and relatively uniform honeycomb etched pattern with minimal loss of the cement can be seen. No needlelike crystals were observed (mag. 500×) (Reprinted with permission from Kayahan et al. [28]. © 2009 *International Endodontic Journal*)

5.2.5 Acid Etching

It is well known that exposure of MTA to a low pH environment will influence its physical and chemical properties [14, 70]. It is therefore not surprising that in the laboratory environment application of acid etch has adverse effects in the short term, on the push-out bond strength [56], porosity, micro-hardness [37] and compressive strength [28] of MTA, suggesting it would be better to postpone restorative procedures to allow more advanced hydration of the cement. Over longer time periods after placement, the application of etchants on some brands of MTA does not appear to affect its compressive strength [29]; however, other brands were more susceptible to etchant and have a reduced strength.

Following the laboratory evaluation of acid etchant on various materials [44], it was concluded that etching of MTA did not improve its shear bond strength to composite resin and that the surface etching of MTA was not necessary prior to composite placement using a total-etch adhesive resin. Furthermore, it is advised that when MTA is used in vital pulp therapies, it is better to cover the material with glass ionomer cement. However, it must be emphasised that these reports are based on laboratory investigations and that clinical trials have not been reported on the use and effects of acid etchant on MTA in a clinical setting.

The effects of exposing MTA to acid etching have been demonstrated by SEM analysis. In general, a selective loss of matrix from around the crystalline structures of MTA has been observed resulting in a relatively uniform 'honeycomb' pattern without penetrating deeply or removing substantial amounts of cement. In addition, etching has revealed crystalline structures such as plate-shaped and laminated crystals on the MTA surface; however, needlelike crystals have been reported to be missing (Fig. 5.3a, b) [28]. Further investigation on the material microstructure after exposure to acid etch in order to identify crystal morphology is necessary. The significance of these morphological changes is unclear.

5.2.6 Blood

The contamination of MTA by blood has been investigated in a number of laboratory studies in terms of the effect on its physical properties, leakage, displacement, marginal adaptation and colour. There is little doubt that blood contamination on the surface of MTA and, in particular, when incorporated into the material is detrimental

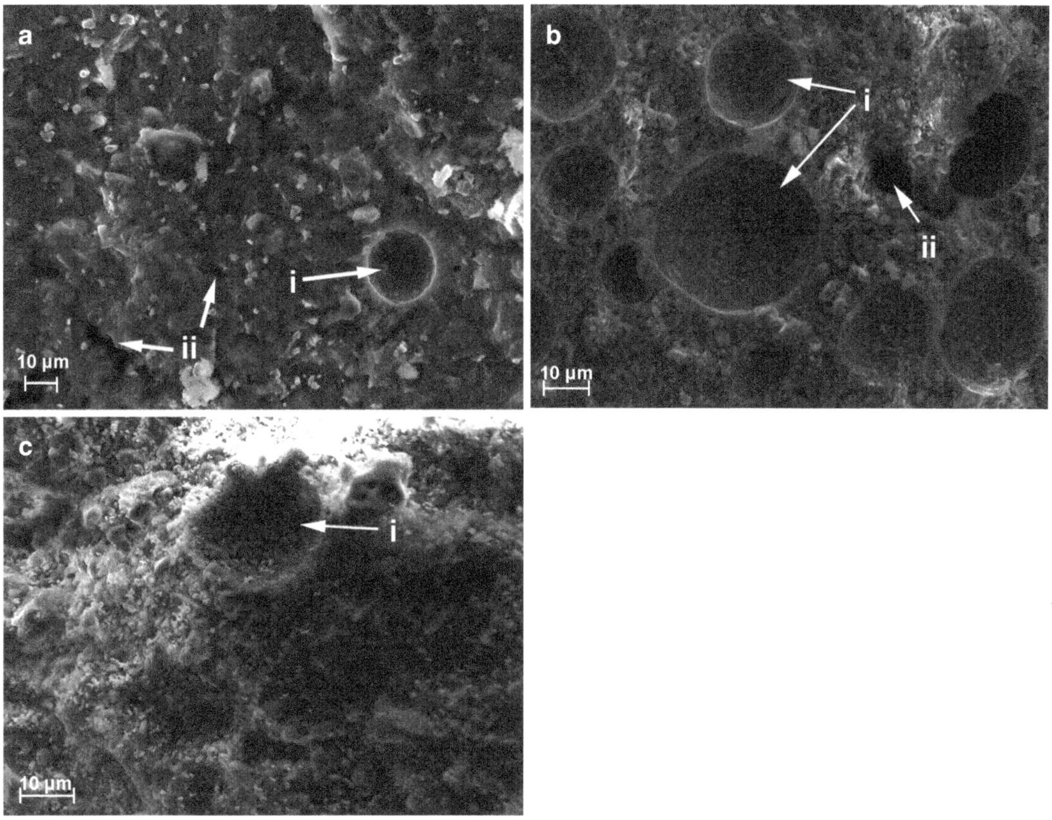

Fig. 5.4 Scanning electron microscopy images of mineral trioxide aggregate specimens mixed entirely with water (**a**), partially (**b**) and entirely (**c**) with whole, fresh human blood. Porosity (*i*) and presence of cross sections of micro-channels (*ii*) can be observed (Reprinted with permission from Nekoofar et al. [39]. © 2011 *International Endodontic Journal*)

to its hydration and thus its ultimate physical properties and performance. Unfortunately, MTA is often placed in contact with vital tissues that ooze blood/serum (pulp capping) or in situations where blood pools on its surface (root-end filling), and the impact of blood contamination is important and must be minimised.

5.2.6.1 Physical Properties

Mixing MTA with blood has a negative effect on its surface hardness, microstructure [41] and compressive strength [42]. Essentially, it has been reported that when blood becomes incorporated into MTA, its compressive strength is reduced with the result that in clinical situations in which blood becomes mixed with MTA, its physical properties are likely to be compromised [42], even when used with accelerators [43]. Similar effects have been reported when foetal bovine serum was used to contaminate the surface of MTA [30].

The hydration state of MTA mixed with blood has also been reported [39] with specimens partially mixed with blood being more completely hydrated than those mixed entirely with blood and less than specimens hydrated completely with water. Lack of formation of the crystalline calcium hydroxide in the early stage of the hydration process and the absent of acicular crystals, characteristic of ettringite crystals, in blood-contaminated specimens are common findings (Fig. 5.4).

5.2.6.2 Leakage

In laboratory studies, it has been reported that blood contamination of the surface of MTA increases leakage of root-end fillings when using tracer dyes [25]. An earlier study did not exhibit any leakage when root-end restorations were contaminated with blood and leakage was assessed using dyes [63].

5.2.6.3 Displacement

The push-out bond strength of MTA in the presence of blood contamination when used as a perforation repair material has been shown to be reduced [2, 69]. Conversely, other researchers reported increased values [45].

5.2.6.4 Marginal Adaptation

It has been reported that exposure to blood during setting has a negative effect on marginal adaptation of MTA [52].

5.2.6.5 Colour

Contamination of MTA with blood has been shown to have an adverse effect on tooth colour [33].

In summary, it is likely that the detrimental effects of blood on MTA will have a negative impact on its physical characteristics and thus on its performance in a variety of laboratory tests. From a clinical perspective it seems sensible to avoid blood contamination if possible.

5.2.7 Bone Grafting Materials

Demineralised and mineralised graft materials appear to have a differential effect on the microhardness of white MTA. White MTA microhardness values when in contact with Bio-Oss (Geistlich Pharma, Princeton, New Jersey, USA), MinerOss (BioHorizons, Markham, Ontario, Canada) and Puros (Zimmer Dental, Carlsbad, California, USA) have been reported to be lower than those for OraGraft (Salvin Dental Specialities, Charlotte, North Carolina, USA) and control groups regardless of incubation period [53].

5.2.8 Variable pH

A number of laboratory studies have evaluated the physical properties of MTA specimens following exposure to a range of acidic environments during hydration on the basis that in some situations the tissues or fluids that come into contact with MTA are acidic. The mean pH of pus from periapical abscesses was generally acidic, although some samples were neutral and some were alkaline [40]. It has been reported that surface hardness of MTA was reduced in an acidic environment [37] as is push-out strength [56]. Leakage of root-end fillings has also been reported to be affected by low pH [50]. The effect of acidic environment on the dislodgement resistance of MTA when used as a perforation repair material has been compared, and it was concluded that its dislodgment resistance was significantly reduced after exposure to acid [23]. Alkaline pH has also been reported to have a negative impact on push-out strength [51], surface hardness and porosity [49].

5.2.9 Saliva

Since MTA is known to have relatively poor physical properties in terms of strength and wear resistance, it has never been recommended for use when in contact with saliva. Thus, the contamination of MTA with saliva is unlikely in most situations, but may occur if the material is used to repair perforations that communicate with the mouth, i.e. in perforations occurring within periodontal pockets. Despite this, a number of laboratory studies have been conducted on salivary contamination of MTA with conflicting results. It has been reported that saliva reduces [24], increases [36] or has no effect [25] on leakage of MTA when used as a root-end filling material. The leakage of MTA when exposed to saliva and used as an orifice barrier [71] and an orthograde filling material [3] has also been evaluated with conflicting results. Overall, it must be remembered that the validity of leakage studies has been questioned and the conclusions of these and other similar studies are likely to be meaningless.

5.2.10 Tissue Fluid and Simulated Tissue Fluid

Mineral trioxide aggregate used as a root-end filling comes into contact with tissue fluid before complete hydration is achieved. When MTA is in contact with tissue fluid, the setting time is extended and in certain cases the material may not set at all [11, 19]. Immersion in tissue fluid has been reported to result in incomplete setting of MTA as the presence of phosphates in solution retards its hydration. The retardation is induced by the formation of insoluble hydroxides in the alkaline solution. The insoluble hydroxides form a coating over the cement particles. The adsorption of phosphate ions on the surface of the clinker phase or on the hydration product is thought to result in the precipitation of calcium phosphates [46]. Glucose, which is present in Hank's balanced salt solution, is also a known retarder of cement hydration [46].

The retardation of setting is apparent under the scanning electron microscope when the surface microstructure of MTA in contact with Hank's balanced salt solution was investigated. MTA in contact with simulated body fluid exhibits no evidence of hydration (Fig. 5.5). The cement in contact with simulated body fluid exhibits micro-cracking, which is caused by expansion of the cement [11].

When set MTA is stored in Hank's balanced salt solution, the pH of the storage solution becomes less alkaline. This could be due to the presence of buffers in simulated body fluids. These buffers are added to these solutions to maintain their pH. Regardless of the less alkaline pH, calcium ion release has been demonstrated in Hank's balanced salt solution. The leaching of calcium is higher in simulated body fluid than in distilled water both when tested after 1 day of immersion and at 28 days of material contact with the solution [8, 17].

The compressive strength of MTA stored in Hank's balanced salt solution is lower than when stored in a humid environment or immersed in water [18]. The dimensional stability of MTA in contact with different soaking solutions has been investigated and a net expansion has been reported when the materials were placed in contact with physiological solutions [8, 59]. MTA materials achieved approximately half of their final linear setting expansion by 300 min, with approximately 75 % of expansion occurring by 460 min and the final 25 % of total expansion occurring between 460 min and 24 h [59].

5.2.11 Effect on Dentine and Pulp

MTA releases calcium hydroxide as a by-product of hydration. The calcium hydroxide has a beneficial effect on the pulp, and dentine bridge formation has been reported. Random controlled clinical trials have shown that MTA is associated with the best clinical outcomes when used as a pulp capping material and for apexification/apexogenesis procedures (as discussed in Chap. 3; Table 3.1). The metallic ions released by set and setting MTA when placed clinically, may release dentine matrix components that potentially influence cellular events for dentine repair and regeneration [61].

When in contact with dentine, MTA altered the toughness more than the strength and stiffness of dentine after ageing in 100 % relative humidity. Dentine toughness is attributed to its collagen matrix; thus, MTA seems to affect the dentine collagen matrix [54]. Prolonged contact of mineralised dentine with MTA has an adverse effect on the integrity of the dentine collagen matrix. However, the amount of collagen extracted was limited to the contact surface. Clinicians are thus advised to use MTA with caution when it is applied to thin dentinal walls [32].

Along the material-dentine interface, MTA forms a taglike structure that is composed of either Ca- and P-rich crystalline deposits or the material itself. The width of a Ca- and Si-rich layer detected along the dentine layer of the material-dentine interface increases over time [21]. The selective diffusion of silicon, calcium and phosphorous across the cement-dentine interface has been demonstrated [16]. The movement of calcium is difficult to show using scanning electron microscopy and elemental mapping since calcium is present in both the material and dentine. However, elemental migration is clearly shown across the interface (Fig. 5.6). Together with calcium, silicon and phosphorus, migration of bismuth is also evident. Migration of bismuth into dentine can be problematic as bismuth oxide has been shown to react with collagen resulting in a change in colour of both MTA and the tooth [35] (Fig. 5.7).

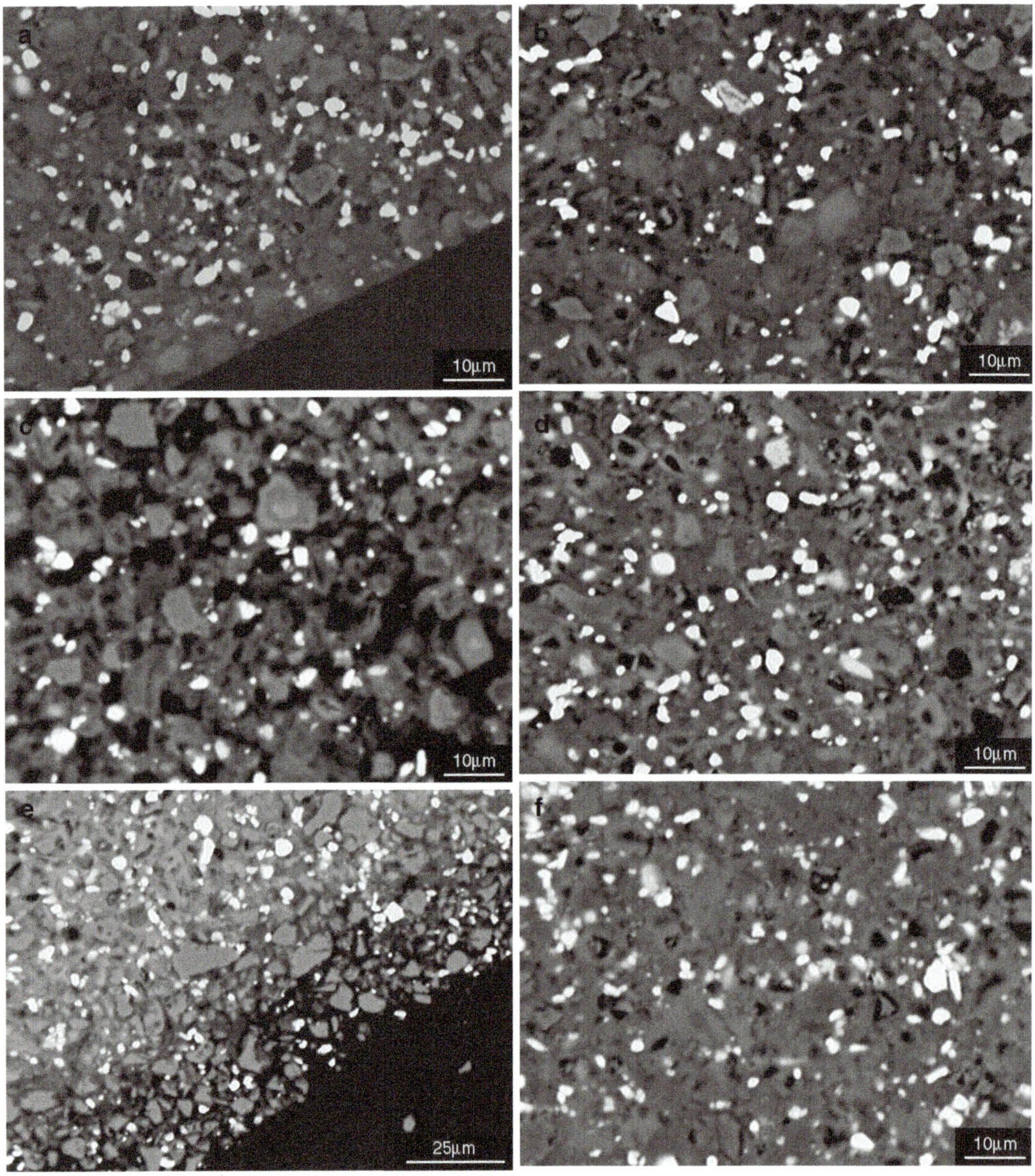

Fig. 5.5 Scanning electron micrographs of MTA stored in different environmental conditions (**a**, **b**) dry, (**c**, **d**) immersed in water (**e**, **f**) immersed in HBSS. (**a**, **c**, **e**) Depict the outer region whilst (**b**, **d**, **f**) the core region (Reprinted from Camilleri et al. [11]. © 2013 *International Endodontic Journal*. Published by John Wiley & Sons Ltd)

5.2.12 Chemical Reagents

Subjecting MTA to phosphate-buffered glutaraldehyde, a reagent used routinely for fixing cells in biocompatibility studies, results in the production of calcium phosphate crystals, which are deposited on the MTA surface [12]. The structure of set MTA is severely affected when subjected to acidic dyes such as rhodamine B used to test its sealing ability. The use of rhodamine B as a tracer increased the apparent leakage of MTA as the acidity affected the material and the dye preferentially passed into and

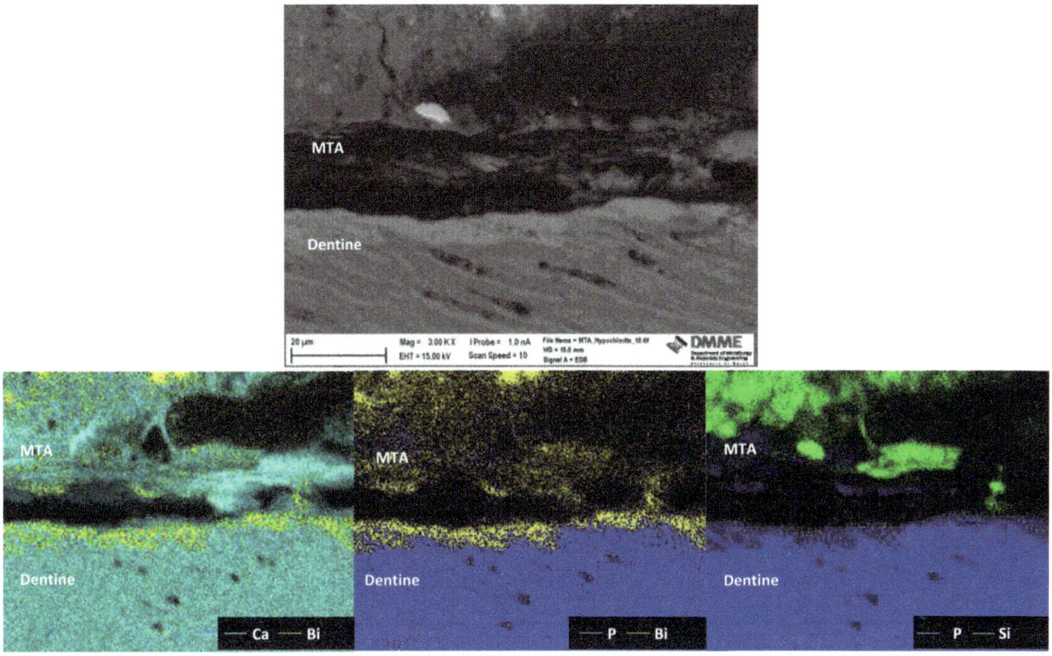

Fig. 5.6 Scanning electron micrograph of MTA to tooth interface and elemental maps for bismuth, calcium, silicon and phosphorus showing elemental migration from the MTA to the tooth at the interface

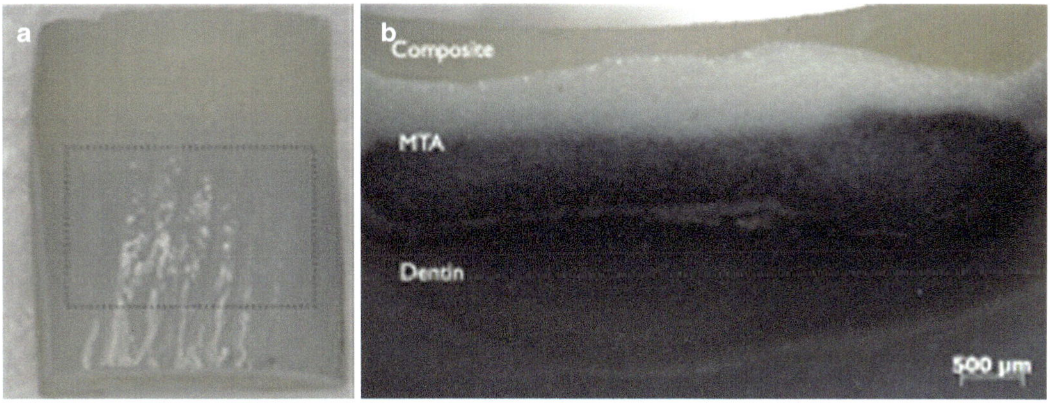

Fig. 5.7 (**a**) Labial surface of bovine tooth filled with MTA showing grey staining highlighted in the dotted rectangle; (**b**) section through tooth showing marked dentin staining. The dark discolouration was concentrated near dentin surface (Reprinted from Marciano et al. [35])

through it rather than along the tooth to material interface [14]. Furthermore, subjecting MTA to critical point drying, which is also a routine procedure used to dry cells for biocompatibility studies using osteoblasts, results in changes to the MTA surface. Critical point drying uses high temperatures, pressure and carbon dioxide to dry the material. This reacts with the calcium hydroxide depositing calcium carbonate over the MTA surface. Due to the low pressure, the calcium carbonate is deposited in various crystalline forms, namely, as calcite vaterite and aragonite [13]. Changes on the surface of set MTA have also been reported in the presence of foetal bovine serum with the material surface having a homogenous distribution of chemicals and a relatively smooth

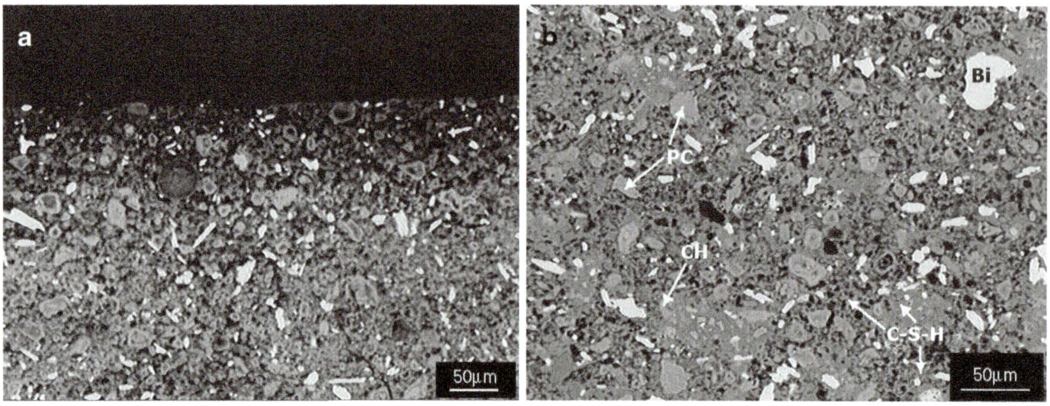

Fig. 5.8 Cross section through hydrated MTA showing (**a**) the surface area in contact with the fluid that was strongly leached with no calcium hydroxide present and the calcium silicate hydrate was strongly decalcified; (**b**) less leaching evident in the region approximately 200 μm from the surface. *PC*: cement particle; *CH*: calcium hydroxide; *C-S-H*: calcium silicate hydrate; *Bi*: bismuth oxide (Reprinted with permission from Camilleri [7]. © 2008 *International Endodontic Journal*)

globular appearance. The surface of the MTA/water was biphasic, containing large hexagonal crystalline plates composed of calcium embedded in a pool of globular crystals [60]. In addition, a recent study investigating the setting of MTA Angelus and ProRoot MTA in the presence of foetal bovine serum demonstrated a lack of hydration in contact with the solution [30]. The micro-hardness of MTA was adversely affected when the material was placed in contact with foetal bovine serum [27]. The glucose leakage model was shown to be inappropriate for use with MTA and related materials as MTA reacts with the glucose thus producing erroneous results for sealing ability [55].

5.2.13 Exposure to Air and Distilled Water

The calcium hydroxide produced as a by-product of hydration is susceptible to reaction when exposed to air and water or other liquids. When MTA is placed in water, it leaches calcium ions in solution [7] and the surface is modified. When viewed under the scanning electron microscope, MTA pastes show patterns of leaching, which are not uniform throughout the material surface. The surface area in contact with the fluid is strongly leached with no calcium hydroxide present and the calcium silicate hydrate is substantially decalcified (Fig. 5.8a). In the region approximately 200 μm from the surface, the leaching is less evident (Fig. 5.8b) [7]. Humidity significantly increased the push-out strength of MTA fillings [19].

MTA immersed in saline solution exhibits no crystalline deposits on its surface [4]. In distilled water, the material surface exhibits cubic crystals containing approximately 17 % calcium, 66 % oxygen and 17 % carbon. Phase analysis has revealed the presence of calcium hydroxide in the precipitate as well as calcium carbonate [22]. The surface carbonation of MTA exposed to air in humid conditions has not been well documented. This phenomenon is well known in the concrete industry where concrete structures undergo surface carbonation. Carbonation occurs on the surface of a Portland cement-based material when the carbon dioxide present in the air reacts with the calcium hydroxide produced by the cement with calcium carbonate being deposited over the surface (Fig. 5.9). Clinically, this would imply that the material surface is likely to be modified with less calcium hydroxide being available for reaction with tissue fluid. In summary, it is important to avoid surface carbonation of MTA.

5.2.14 Storage Temperature

Set MTA surface hardness is affected by storage temperature with lower temperatures leading to a decreased micro-hardness value. More voids and a disorganised flake-like topography were observed in specimens stored at 4 °C in comparison with those stored at 25 and 40 °C. Phase analysis evaluated by X-ray diffraction revealed differences in the material stored at low temperatures [48] with a reduction in peak intensity at 29.3° 2θ using a copper tube. The reduction in intensity was caused by a decreased amount of calcium silicate hydrate since the hydration process slows down at lower temperatures. Since calcium silicate hydrate is amorphous, a reduction in peak intensity at 29.3° 2θ would imply hydration of the tricalcium silicate to calcium silicate hydrate rather than the opposite. A reduction in temperature would in fact slow down the hydration process [15]. The slowing down of hydration was evident from the absence of the portlandite peak at 18° 2θ which was not reported by the authors [48]. The low temperatures also reduced the production of calcium hydroxide.

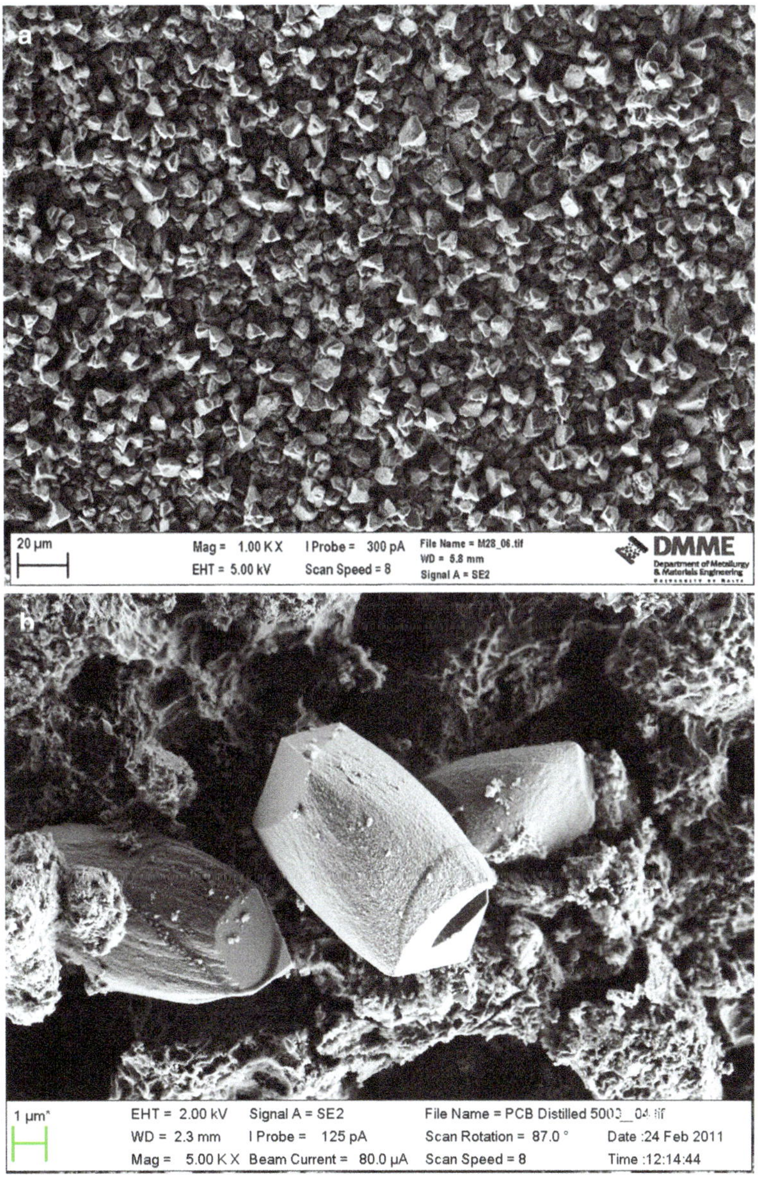

Fig. 5.9 Scanning electron micrographs showing carbonation of MTA surface. The calcium carbonate deposited on the material surface may take various distinctive shapes (**a**–**f**)

Fig. 5.9 (continued)

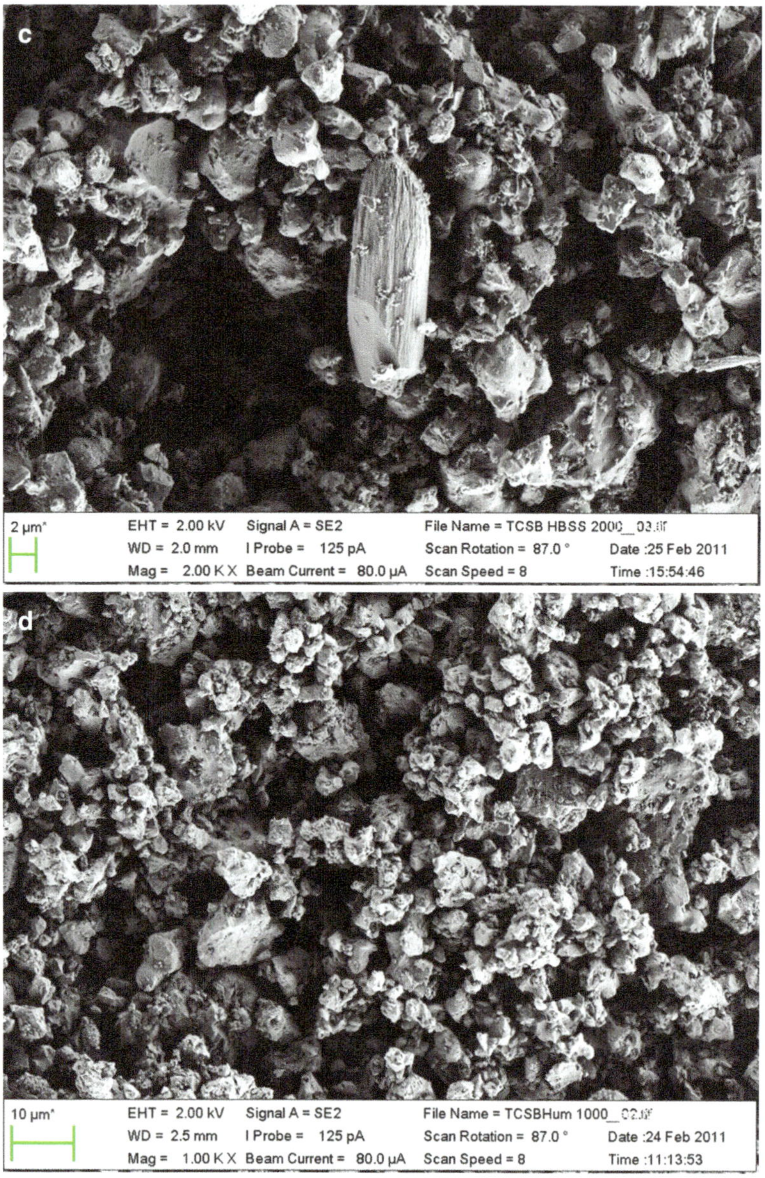

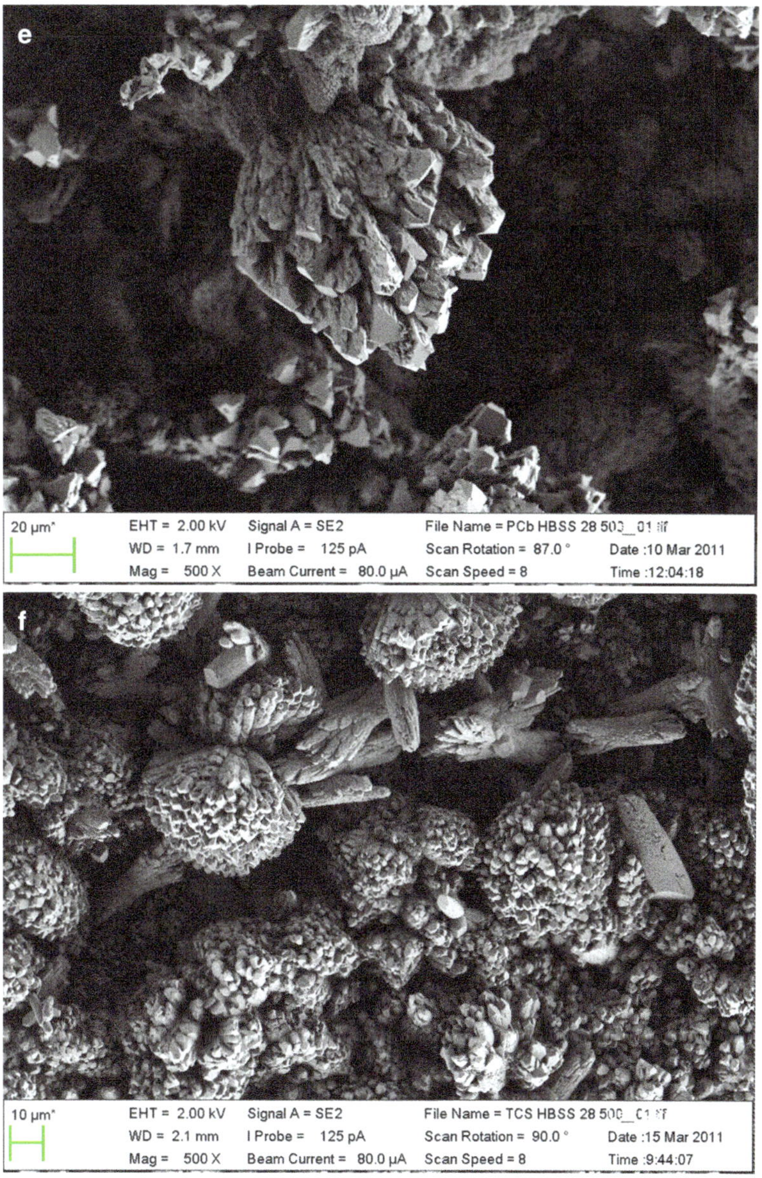

Fig. 5.9 (continued)

Conclusions

Set mineral trioxide aggregate is composed primarily of calcium silicate hydrate, calcium hydroxide and bismuth oxide with some minor inclusions of ettringite and monosulphate phases. Both the presence of calcium hydroxide and bismuth oxide present in the set material affect the reactivity of MTA. The multifaceted clinical use of MTA brings the material in contact with other materials used in both Restorative Dentistry and Endodontics together with the different environment it is placed in during use, namely, blood and tissue fluid when used as a root-end filling material and the temperature and pH of the environment. MTA is adversely affected mostly by the different environmental factors and contact with dental materials exhibiting reduced or incomplete hydration, increased porosity, retardation of setting, reduced strength and micro-hardness and reduced sealing ability. In turn, MTA reduces dentine toughness as it affects the integrity of the dentine collagen matrix. The bismuth oxide causes both material and tooth discolouration. MTA is also adversely affected by materials used in in vitro testing demonstrating retardation in setting and surface carbonation.

References

1. Aggarwal V, Jain A, Kabi D. In vitro evaluation of effect of various endodontic solutions on selected physical properties of white mineral trioxide aggregate. Aust Endod J. 2011;37(2):61–4.
2. Aggarwal V, Singla M, Miglani S, Kohli S. Comparative evaluation of push-out bond strength of ProRoot MTA, Biodentine, and MTA Plus in furcation perforation repair. J Conserv Dent. 2013;16(5):462–5.
3. Al-Hezaimi K, Naghshbandi J, Oglesby S, Simon JH, Rotstein IJ. Human saliva penetration of root canals obturated with two types of mineral trioxide aggregate cements. J Endod. 2005;31(6):453–6.
4. Asgary S, Eghbal MJ, Parirokh M, Ghoddusi J. Effect of two storage solutions on surface topography of two root-end fillings. Aust Endod J. 2009;35(3):147–52.
5. Ballal S, Venkateshbabu N, Nandini S, Kandaswamy D. An in vitro study to assess the setting and surface crazing of conventional glass ionomer cement when layered over partially set mineral trioxide aggregate. J Endod. 2008;34:478–80.
6. Bayrak S, Tunç ES, Saroğlu I, Eğilmez T. Shear bond strengths of different adhesive systems to white mineral trioxide aggregate. Dent Mater J. 2009;28(1):62–7.
7. Camilleri J. Characterization of hydration products of mineral trioxide aggregate. Int Endod J. 2008;41: 408–17.
8. Camilleri J. Evaluation of the effect of intrinsic material properties and ambient conditions on the dimensional stability of white mineral trioxide aggregate and Portland cement. J Endod. 2011;37:239–45.
9. Camilleri J. Scanning electron microscopic evaluation of the material interface of adjacent layers of dental materials. Dent Mater. 2011;27:870–8.
10. Camilleri J. The color stability of white mineral trioxide aggregate in contact with sodium hypochlorite solution. J Endod. 2014;40(3):436–40.
11. Camilleri J, Formosa L, Damidot D. The setting characteristics of MTA Plus in different environmental conditions. Int Endod J. 2013;46(9):831–40.
12. Camilleri J, Montesin FE, Brady K, Sweeney R, Curtis RV, Pitt Ford TR. The constitution of mineral trioxide aggregate. Dent Mater. 2005;21:297–303.
13. Camilleri J, Montesin FE, Papaioannou S, McDonald F, Pitt Ford TR. Biocompatibility of two commercial forms of mineral trioxide aggregate. Int Endod J. 2004;37:699–704.
14. Camilleri J, Pitt Ford TR. Evaluation of the effect of tracer pH on the sealing ability of glass ionomer cement and mineral trioxide aggregate. J Mater Sci Mater Med. 2008;19:2941–8.
15. Taylor HFW. Chapter 11: Admixtures and special uses of cements. In: Cement chemistry. 2nd ed. London: Thomas Telford Publishing; 1997. p. 341.
16. Formosa LM, Damidot D, Camilleri J. Mercury intrusion porosimetry and assessment of cement-dentin interface of anti-washout type mineral trioxide aggregate. J Endod. 2014. doi:10.1016/j.joen.2013.11.015.
17. Formosa LM, Mallia B, Bull T, Camilleri J. The microstructure and surface morphology of radiopaque tricalcium silicate cement exposed to different curing conditions. Dent Mater. 2012;28(5):584–95.
18. Formosa LM, Mallia B, Camilleri J. The effect of curing conditions on the physical properties of tricalcium silicate cement for use as a dental biomaterial. Int Endod J. 2012;45:326–36.
19. Gancedo-Caravia L, Garcia-Barbero E. Influence of humidity and setting time on the push-out strength of mineral trioxide aggregate obturations. J Endod. 2006;32(9):894–6.
20. Hachmeister DR, Schindler WG, Walker 3rd WA, Thomas DD. The sealing ability and retention characteristics of mineral trioxide aggregate in a model of apexification. J Endod. 2002;28:386–90.
21. Han L, Okiji T. Uptake of calcium and silicon released from calcium silicate-based endodontic materials into root canal dentine. Int Endod J. 2011;44(12):1081–7.
22. Han L, Okiji T, Okawa S. Morphological and chemical analysis of different precipitates on mineral trioxide aggregate immersed in different fluids. Dent Mater J. 2010;29(5):512–7.
23. Hashem AA, Wanees Amin SA. The effect of acidity on dislodgment resistance of mineral trioxide aggregate and bioaggregate in furcation perforations: an in vitro comparative study. J Endod. 2012;38(2):245–9.
24. Hasheminia M, Loriaei Nejad S, Asgary S. Sealing ability of MTA and CEM cement as root-end fillings of human teeth in dry, saliva or blood-contaminated conditions. Iran Endod J. 2010;5(4):151–6.
25. Hasheminia SM, Nejad SL, Dianat O, Modaresi J, Mahjour F. Comparing the sealing properties of mineral trioxide aggregate and an experimental ceramic based root end filling material in different environments. Indian J Dent Res. 2013;24(4):474–7.
26. Hong ST, Bae KS, Baek SH, Kum KY, Shon WJ, Lee W. Effects of root canal irrigants on the push-out strength and hydration behavior of accelerated mineral trioxide aggregate in its early setting phase. J Endod. 2010;36(12):1995–9.
27. Kang JS, Rhim EM, Huh SY, Ahn SJ, Kim DS, Kim SY, Park SH. The effects of humidity and serum on the surface microhardness and morphology of five retrograde filling materials. Scanning. 2012;34(4):207–14.
28. Kayahan MB, Nekoofar MH, Kazandağ M, Canpolat C, Malkondu O, Kaptan F, Dummer PM. Effect of acid-etching procedure on selected physical properties of mineral trioxide aggregate. Int Endod J. 2009; 42(11):1004–14.

29. Kayahan MB, Nekoofar MH, McCann A, Sunay H, Kaptan RF, Meraji N, Dummer PM. Effect of acid etching procedures on the compressive strength of 4 calcium silicate-based endodontic cements. J Endod. 2013;39(12):1646–8.
30. Kim Y, Kim S, Shin YS, Jung IY, Lee SJ. Failure of setting of mineral trioxide aggregate in the presence of fetal bovine serum and its prevention. J Endod. 2012;38(4):536–40.
31. Lee YL, Lin FH, Wang WH, Ritchie HH, Lan WH, Lin CP. Effects of EDTA on the hydration mechanism of mineral trioxide aggregate. J Dent Res. 2007;86: 534–8.
32. Leiendecker AP, Qi YP, Sawyer AN, Niu LN, Agee KA, Loushine RJ, Weller RN, Pashley DH, Tay FR. Effects of calcium silicate-based materials on collagen matrix integrity of mineralized dentin. J Endod. 2012;38(6):829–33.
33. Lenherr P, Allgayer N, Weiger R, Filippi A, Attin T, Krastl G. Tooth discoloration induced by endodontic materials: a laboratory study. Int Endod J. 2012;45(10): 942–9.
34. Loxley EC, Liewehr FR, Buxton TB, McPherson 3rd JC. The effect of various intracanal oxidizing agents on the push-out strength of various perforation repair materials. Oral Surg Oral Med Oral Pathol Oral Radiol Endod. 2003;95(4):490–4.
35. Marciano MA, Camilleri J, Hungaro Duarte MA. Assessment of color stability of white MTA Angelus and bismuth oxide in contact with tooth structure. J Endod. 2014. doi:10.1016/j.joen.2014.01.044.
36. Montellano AM, Schwartz SA, Beeson TJ. Contamination of tooth-colored mineral trioxide aggregate used as a root-end filling material: a bacterial leakage study. J Endod. 2006;32(5):452–5.
37. Namazikhah MS, Nekoofar MH, Sheykhrezae MS, Salariyeh S, Hayes SJ, Bryant ST, Mohammadi MM, Dummer PM. The effect of pH on surface hardness and microstructure of mineral trioxide aggregate. Int Endod J. 2008;41:108–16.
38. Nandini S, Ballal S, Kandaswamy D. Influence of glass-ionomer cement on the interface and setting reaction of mineral trioxide aggregate when used as a furcal repair material using laser Raman spectroscopic analysis. J Endod. 2007;33:167–72.
39. Nekoofar MH, Davies TE, Stone D, Basturk FB, Dummer PM. Microstructure and chemical analysis of blood-contaminated mineral trioxide aggregate. Int Endod J. 2011;44(11):1011–8.
40. Nekoofar MH, Namazikhah MS, Sheykhrezae MS, Mohammadi MM, Kazemi A, Aseeley Z, Dummer PM. pH of pus collected from periapical abscesses. Int Endod J. 2009;42:534–8.
41. Nekoofar MH, Oloomi K, Sheykhrezae MS, Tabor R, Stone DF, Dummer PM. An evaluation of the effect of blood and human serum on the surface microhardness and surface microstructure of mineral trioxide aggregate. Int Endod J. 2010;43(10):849–58.
42. Nekoofar MH, Stone DF, Dummer PM. The effect of blood contamination on the compressive strength and surface microstructure of mineral trioxide aggregate. Int Endod J. 2010;43(9):782–91.
43. Oloomi K, Saberi E, Mokhtari H, Mokhtari Zonouzi HR, Nosrat A, Nekoofar MH, Dummer PM. Evaluation of the effect of blood contamination on the compressive strength of MTA modified with hydration accelerators. Restor Dent Endod. 2013;38:128–33.
44. Oskoee SS, Kimyai S, Bahari M, Motahari P, Eghbal MJ, Asgary S. Comparison of shear bond strength of calcium-enriched mixture cement and mineral trioxide aggregate to composite resin. J Contemp Dent Pract. 2011;12(6):457–62.
45. Rahimi S, Ghasemi N, Shahi S, Lotfi M, Froughreyhani M, Milani AS, Bahari M. Effect of blood contamination on the retention characteristics of two endodontic biomaterials in simulated furcation perforations. J Endod. 2013;39(5):697–700.
46. Ramachandran VS. Chapter 1: Interaction of admixtures in the cement-water system. In: Paillere AME, Spon FN, editors. Application of admixtures in concrete. 1st ed. Rilem report no. 10. London: CRC Press; 1992.
47. Ramachandran VS. Interaction of chemical admixtures in the cement – water system by research on the manufacture and use of cements. In: Proceedings of the Engineering Foundation Conference. Henniker, July 28–Aug 2, 1985. p. 121–31.
48. Saghiri MA, Lotfi M, Joupari MD, Aeinehchi M, Saghiri AM. Effects of storage temperature on surface hardness, microstructure, and phase formation of white mineral trioxide aggregate. J Endod. 2010;36(8): 1414–8.
49. Saghiri MA, Lotfi M, Saghiri AM, Vosoughhosseini S, Aeinehchi M, Ranjkesh B. Scanning electron micrograph and surface hardness of mineral trioxide aggregate in the presence of alkaline pH. J Endod. 2009;35(5):706–10.
50. Saghiri MA, Lotfi M, Saghiri AM, Vosoughhosseini S, Fatemi A, Shiezadeh V, Ranjkesh B. Effect of pH on sealing ability of white mineral trioxide aggregate as a root-end filling material. J Endod. 2008;34(10):1226–9.
51. Saghiri MA, Shokouhinejad N, Lotfi M, Aminsobhani M, Saghiri AM. Push-out bond strength of mineral trioxide aggregate in the presence of alkaline pH. J Endod. 2010;36(11):1856–9.
52. Salem Milani A, Rahimi S, Froughreyhani M, Vahid Pakdel M. Effect of blood contamination on marginal adaptation and surface microstructure of mineral trioxide aggregate: a SEM study. J Dent Res Dent Clin Dent Prospects. 2013;7(3):157–63.
53. Sato EY, Svec T, Whitten B, Sedgley CM. Effects of bone graft materials on the microhardness of mineral trioxide aggregate. J Endod. 2012;38(5):700–3.
54. Sawyer AN, Nikonov SY, Pancio AK, Niu LN, Agee KA, Loushine RJ, Weller RN, Pashley DH, Tay FR. Effects of calcium silicate-based materials on the flexural properties of dentin. J Endod. 2012;38(5):680–3.
55. Shemesh H, Souza EM, Wu MK, Wesselink PR. Glucose reactivity with filling materials as a limitation for using the glucose leakage model. Int Endod J. 2008;41(10):869–72.

56. Shokouhinejad N, Nekoofar MH, Iravani A, Kharrazifard MJ, Dummer PM. Effect of acidic environment on the push-out bond strength of mineral trioxide aggregate. J Endod. 2010;36(5):871–4.
57. Smith JB, Loushine RJ, Weller RN, Rueggeberg FA, Whitford GM, Pashley DH, Tay FR. Metrologic evaluation of the surface of white MTA after the use of two endodontic irrigants. J Endod. 2007;33:463–7.
58. Stefopoulos S, Tsatsas DV, Kerezoudis NP, Eliades G. Comparative in vitro study of the sealing efficiency of white vs grey ProRoot mineral trioxide aggregate formulas as apical barriers. Dent Traumatol. 2008;24: 207–13.
59. Storm B, Eichmiller FC, Tordik PA, Goodell GG. Setting expansion of gray and white mineral trioxide aggregate and Portland cement. J Endod. 2008;34(1): 80–2.
60. Tingey MC, Bush P, Levine MS. Analysis of mineral trioxide aggregate surface when set in the presence of fetal bovine serum. J Endod. 2008;34:45–9.
61. Tomson PL, Grover LM, Lumley PJ, Sloan AJ, Smith AJ, Cooper PR. Dissolution of bio-active dentine matrix components by mineral trioxide aggregate. J Dent. 2007;35(8):636–42.
62. Torabinejad M, Chivian N. Clinical applications of mineral trioxide aggregate. J Endod. 1999;25(3): 197–205.
63. Torabinejad M, Higa RK, McKendry DJ, Pitt Ford TR. Dye leakage of four root end filling materials: effects of blood contamination. J Endod. 1994;20(4):159–63.
64. Tsujimoto M, Ookubo A, Wada Y, Matsunaga T, Tsujimoto Y, Hayashi Y. Surface changes of mineral trioxide aggregate after the application of bleaching agents: electron microscopy and an energy-dispersive X-ray microanalysis. J Endod. 2011;37(2):231–4.
65. Tsujimoto M, Tsujimoto Y, Ookubo A, Shiraishi T, Watanabe I, Yamada S, Hayashi Y. Timing for composite resin placement on mineral trioxide aggregate. J Endod. 2013;39(9):1167–70.
66. Uyanik MO, Nagas E, Sahin C, Dagli F, Cehreli ZC. Effects of different irrigation regimens on the sealing properties of repaired furcal perforations. Oral Surg Oral Med Oral Pathol Oral Radiol Endod. 2009; 107(3):e91–5.
67. Vallés M, Mercadé M, Duran-Sindreu F, Bourdelande JL, Roig M. Influence of light and oxygen on the color stability of five calcium silicate-based materials. J Endod. 2013;39(4):525–8.
68. Vallés M, Mercadé M, Duran-Sindreu F, Bourdelande JL, Roig M. Color stability of white mineral trioxide aggregate. Clin Oral Investig. 2013;17(4):1155–9.
69. Vanderweele RA, Schwartz SA, Beeson TJ. Effect of blood contamination on retention characteristics of MTA when mixed with different liquids. J Endod. 2006;32(5):421–4.
70. Watts JD, Holt DM, Beeson TJ, Kirkpatrick TC, Rutledge RE. Effects of pH and mixing agents on the temporal setting of tooth-colored and gray mineral trioxide aggregate. J Endod. 2007;33(8):970–3.
71. Zakizadeh P, Marshall SJ, Hoover CI, Peters OA, Noblett WC, Gansky SA, Goodis HE. A novel approach in assessment of coronal leakage of intraorifice barriers: a saliva leakage and micro-computed tomographic evaluation. J Endod. 2008;34(7):871–5.

Clinical Applications

6

Marco Antonio Hungaro Duarte,
Clóvis Monteiro Bramante,
and Gustavo De Deus

6.1 Introduction

Following the introduction of MTA in 1993, its use has broadened considerably and is nowadays used in several clinical situations in which calcium hydroxide was employed. Initially, MTA was employed in cases of root perforations and as a retrograde filling material [82]; eventually, other indications for the use of the material evolved, and it is being used in cases of direct or indirect pulp capping, pulpotomy, root perforation, repair internal and external root resorptions, endodontic treatment, incomplete root formation, apical plug, deciduous teeth, dens invaginatus, and revascularization. For its effective use, it is important to know the mechanism of action and the correct way of employing the material.

M.A. Hungaro Duarte, PhD (✉)
Department of Dentistry, Endodontics and Dental Materials, Bauru Dental School, University of Sao Paulo, Al Octavio Pinheiro Brisola 9-75, Bauru, SP 17012-901, Brazil
e-mail: mhungaro@fob.usp.br

C. Monteiro Bramante, PhD
Department of Dentistry, Endodontics and Dental materials, Bauru Dental School, University of Sao Paulo, Al Octavio Pinheiro Brisola 9-75, Orlando Cardoso 1-40 Apto 22, Bauru, SP 17016-260, Brazil
e-mail: bramante@fob.usp.br, clobra@uol.com.br

G. De Deus, DDS, MSc, PhD
Department of Endodontics, Grande Rio University (UNIGRANRIO), Av. Henrique Dodsworth 85 apto 808 Lagoa, Rio de Janeiro RJ 22061-030, Brazil
e-mail: endogus@gmail.com

The mechanism of action of MTA is similar to that of calcium hydroxide. The calcium hydroxide produced as a by-product of hydration of MTA is leached out in solution and dissociates into Ca^{++} and OH^- ions. The Ca^{++} ions, when in contact with the connective tissue, form an area of necrosis, forming carbon dioxide which in turn together with the calcium hydroxide forms calcite crystals (calcium carbonate), which serve as the core of calcification. The alkalinity of the medium stimulates the tissue to secrete a glycoprotein named fibronectin, which together with the calcite crystals stimulate the formation of collagen type I, which together with the calcium, induces mineralization [43].

6.2 Mode of Use

6.2.1 Manipulation

MTA is mixed with distilled water in a 3:1 ratio. The ratio can be changed according to the area where the material will be utilized [32]. In the pulp chamber, MTA may be mixed to a stiffer mix, while in the root canal, where access is difficult, and it can also be more fluid (Fig. 6.1).

6.2.2 Insertion

The MTA should be inserted in place immediately after handling, avoiding its dehydration.

J. Camilleri (ed.), *Mineral Trioxide Aggregate in Dentistry*,
DOI 10.1007/978-3-642-55157-4_6, © Springer-Verlag Berlin Heidelberg 2014

A Lentulo spiral can be used for its insertion or alternatively a micro amalgam carrier, gutta-percha plugger, Map system, Dovgan applicator, or ultrasound (Fig. 6.2).

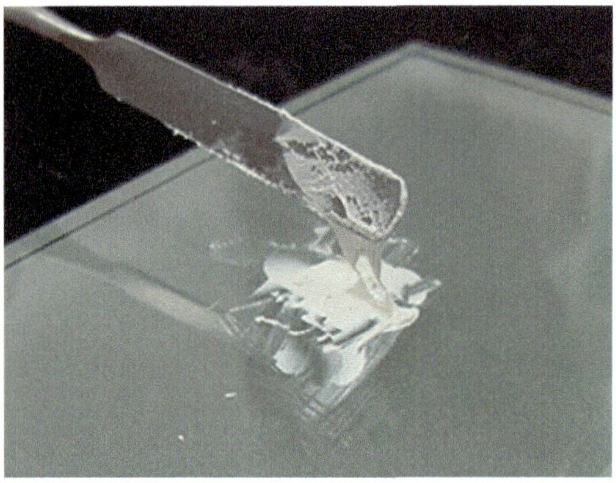

Fig. 6.1 The MTA mix. Note the consistency of the paste

6.3 Clinical Applications of MTA

The variety of MTA uses include:

(a) Direct or indirect pulp capping
(b) Pulpotomy
(c) Incomplete root formation
(d) Perforation
(e) Canal obturation
(f) Endodontic surgery
(g) Internal or external tooth resorption
(h) Root fracture
(i) Revascularization

6.3.1 Direct Pulp Capping

Direct pulp capping is performed when there is accidental exposure of the pulp, with the goal of maintaining pulp vitality and facilitating the formation of mineralized tissue, thus sealing the exposure.

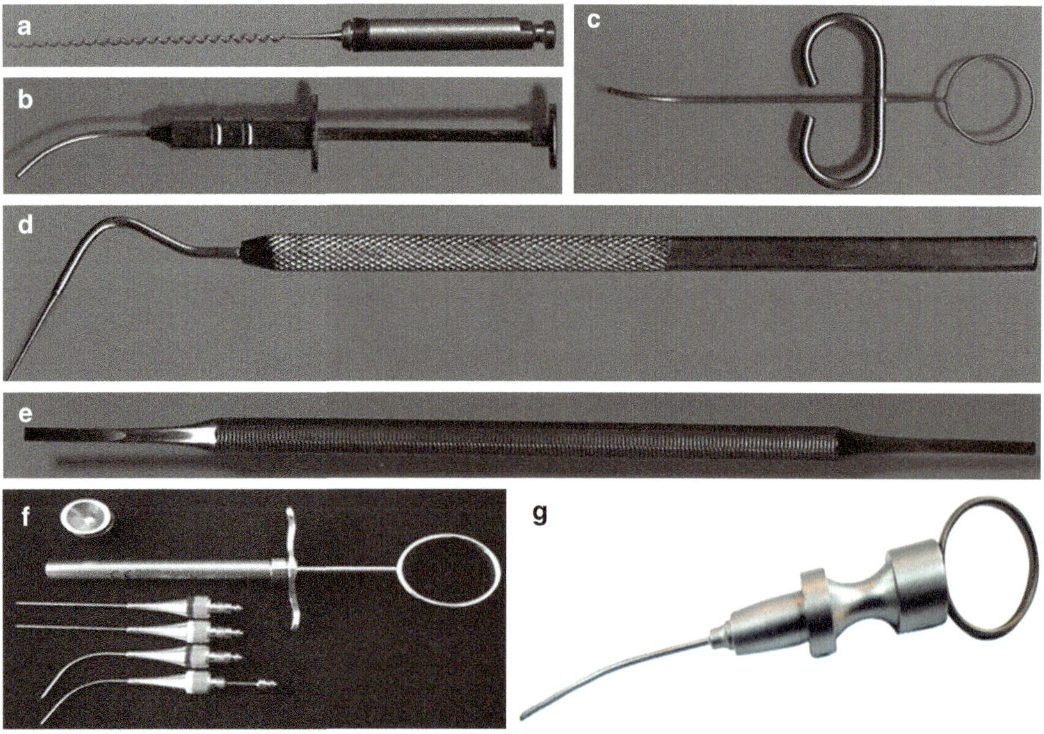

Fig. 6.2 Insertion devices for MTA: (**a**) Lentulo spiral, (**b**) amalgam micro-carrier, (**c**) MTA carrier, (**d**) gutta-percha plugger, (**e**) chisel, (**f**) Map system, and (**g**) Dovgan applicator

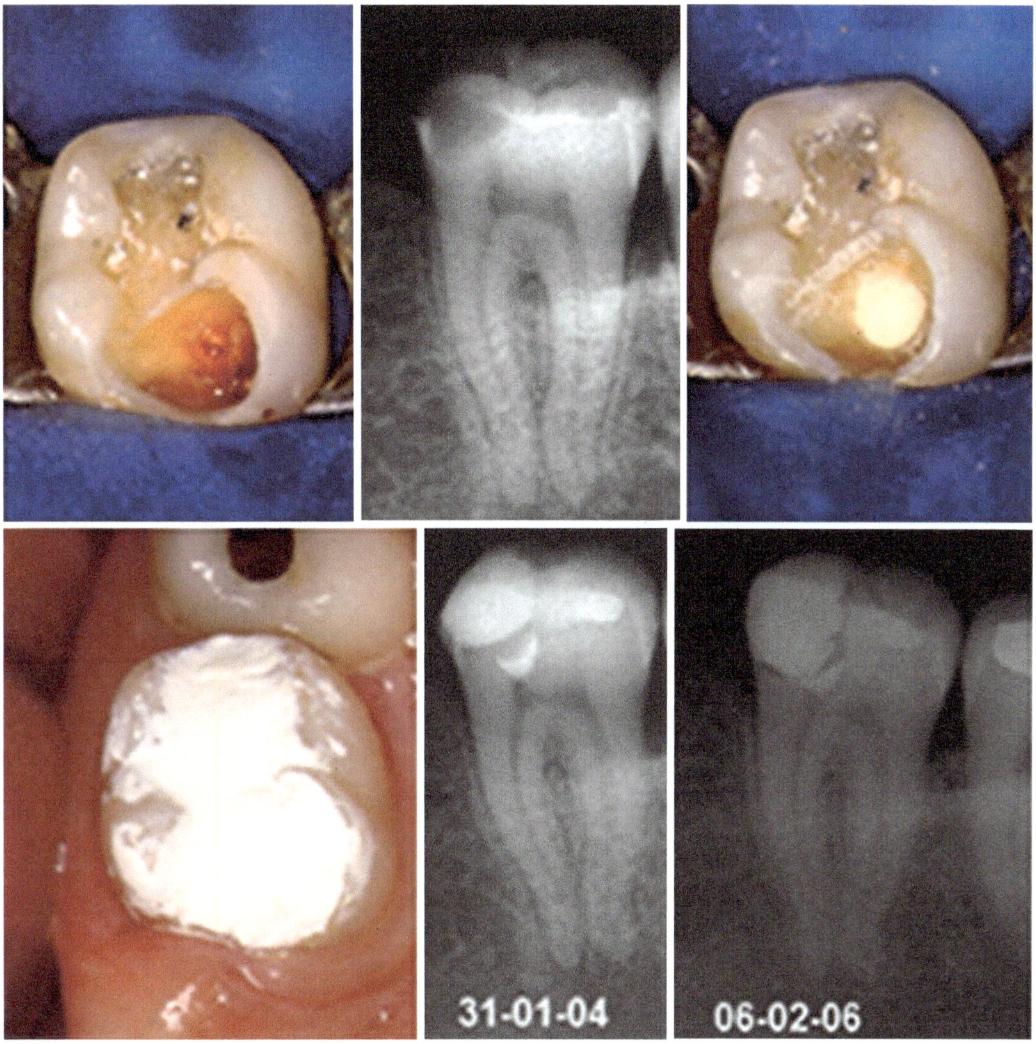

Fig. 6.3 Direct pulp capping with MTA

MTA used for direct pulp capping has exhibited a similar or superior response to calcium hydroxide, leading to formation of a mineralized barrier, in addition to its sealing ability [1, 2, 21, 28, 41, 43, 48, 58, 71, 75, 83]. In one study [58], 69 direct pulp protections performed with MTA and 53 with calcium hydroxide were assessed, and a higher success rate was demonstrated with MTA.

After confirmation of the exposure of the pulp tissue and the conditions thereof, the cavity is irrigated with saline solution to remove dentinal pulp waste and achieve pulp hemostasis. The MTA should be applied with care so as to not compress the material into the pulp cavity. All material that is on the surrounding walls should be removed with a curette and the cavity sealed with a restorative material (Fig. 6.3).

6.3.2 Pulpotomy

Pulpotomy involves the removal of the coronal pulp, maintaining the radicular, and is indicated when there is irreversible inflammation of the coronal pulp, and particularly indicated in the teeth with incomplete root formation.

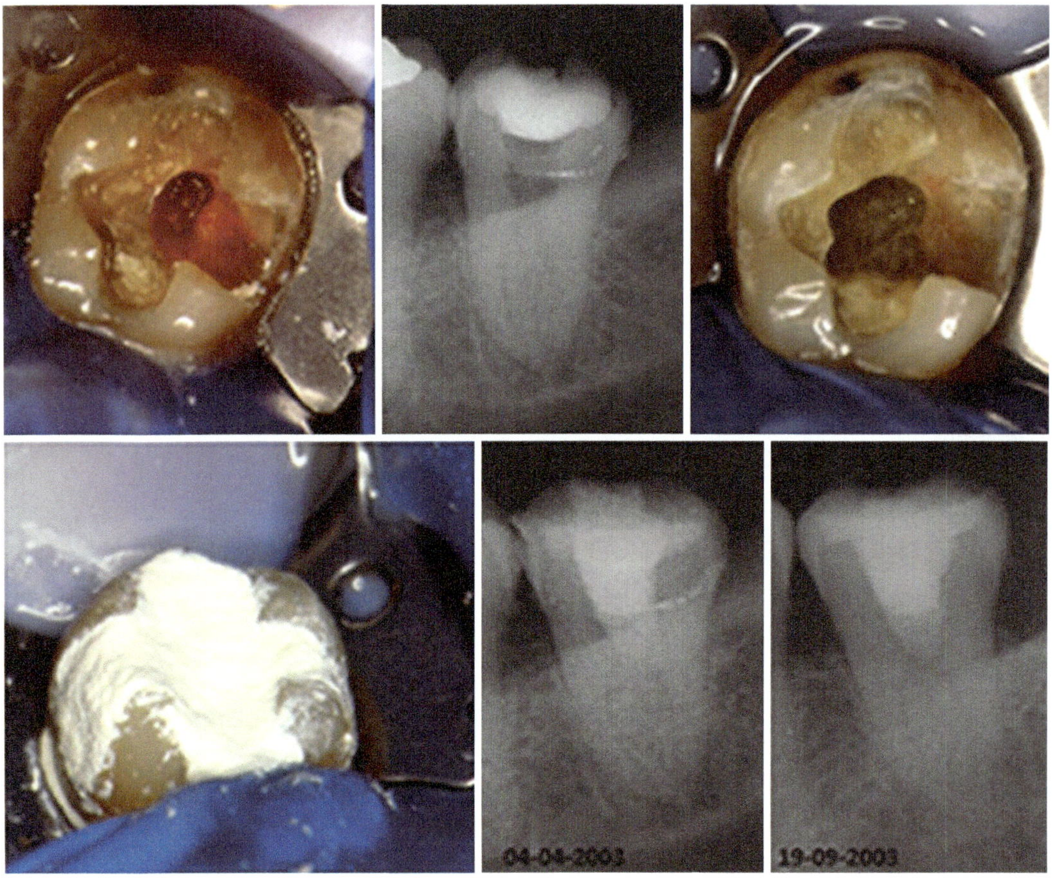

Fig. 6.4 Pulpotomy with MTA

In a histological study [41] where pulpotomy procedures were performed on dog teeth, a better dentine bridge formation occurred with cases treated with MTA than in those where calcium hydroxide was employed. Other authors also confirmed the efficiency of the MTA in the pulpotomy procedure [11, 15, 41, 56, 74].

After the coronal opening, the coronal pulp is removed with a curette, followed by irrigation with saline solution. The MTA is placed over the pulp tissue without pressure, at a thickness of approximately 3 mm. Calcium hydroxide paste can be placed over it, consistently well, and the cavity closed with a restorative material (Fig. 6.4). The calcium hydroxide paste is placed over the MTA in order to avoid direct contact of the sealant with the MTA, especially when the restoration is performed in the same session.

The repair occurs by the formation of a mineralized tissue on the remaining radicular pulp (Fig. 6.5).

6.3.3 Incomplete Root Formation

The tooth with incomplete root formation constitutes a problem for endodontic treatment. Because the apex is not completely formed, there is difficulty in instrumentation and obturation of the canal, and there is a great risk of extrusion of material from the apical region. Apexification is defined as a method to induce formation of the mineralized barrier on the open root apex or the continued apex development of the tooth. Calcium hydroxide has been the material of choice for this procedure with periodic changes

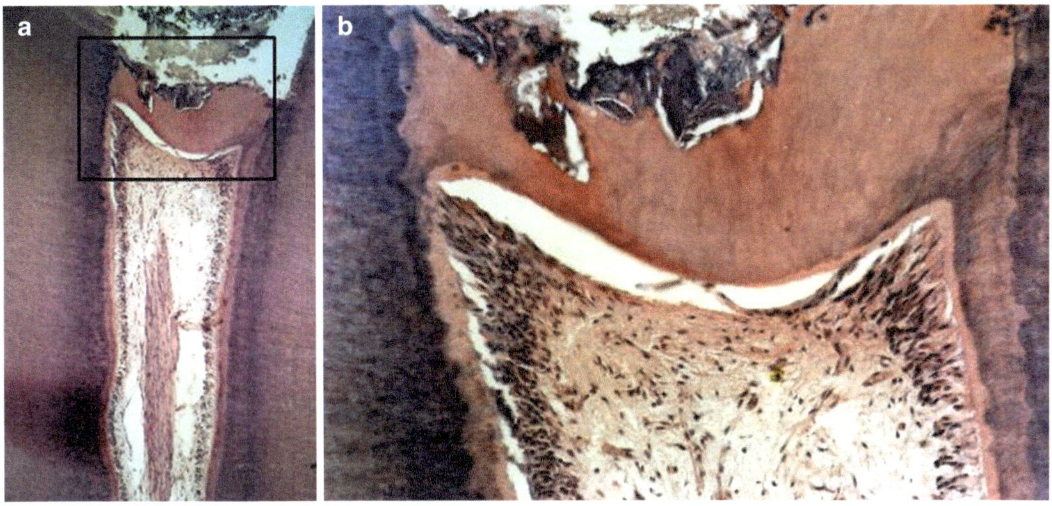

Fig. 6.5 (**a**) Mineralized tissue formed after pulpotomy with MTA; (**b**) largest increase in the marked area

lasting from 5 to 20 months in order to induce the formation of the mineralized barrier. The process is slow with vulnerability to the temporary sealing, with a possible occurrence of recontamination, tooth fracture, and an unpredictable outcome [5, 6, 69]. For these reasons, apexification in one or two sessions using MTA has been proposed [61, 62], with the goal of a more rapid completion of the case.

After instrumentation of the canal, the MTA is placed in small portions in the apical region with the aid of a Lentulo spiral. The Map system or Dovgan applicator is used to obtain the apical plug which must be 3–5 mm (ideally 5 mm). With a K file or Hedstrom file wrapped in cotton compatible with the canal size, the vertical compaction of the MTA is performed. Alternatively, the compaction can be performed with a gutta-percha plugger. The radiograph is taken to confirm the presence of the apical plug, and if it is not satisfactory, the MTA is removed by irrigation with saline solution and the procedure is repeated. The canal obturation follows with gutta-percha and sealer. If the obturation is not performed in the same session, the canal can be filled with a slurry of calcium hydroxide dressing which remains as a temporary dressing for a maximum of 30 days (Fig. 6.6).

A success rate of 90 % was observed when the MTA apical plug was placed via the canal [59, 61]. Other studies have also observed a complete root formation in the teeth with open apices treated with MTA [4, 24, 25, 27, 30, 35, 38, 44, 49, 55, 61, 63, 77, 78].

The apical plug can also be placed by completely filling the canal with MTA to then immediately removing it to the desired length with a K file, leaving only the part corresponding to the apical plug. Next, with a K file wrapped in cotton, the MTA is compacted (Fig. 6.7). All the material that is on the walls of the canal should be removed in the same session that the MTA is inserted in the canal as after it sets MTA is difficult and sometimes impossible to remove. The apical plug should ideally be 5 mm [84] and may be greater depending on the foramen opening of the root.

If the apical plug provides adequate resistance, the obturation of the canal could be done in the same session; otherwise the remainder of the canal should be filled with calcium hydroxide paste, leaving the obturation to be completed in successive treatment session when the MTA setting is complete (Figs. 6.8 and 6.9).

If the foraminal opening is too wide, extrusion of the MTA from the periapical region can occur,

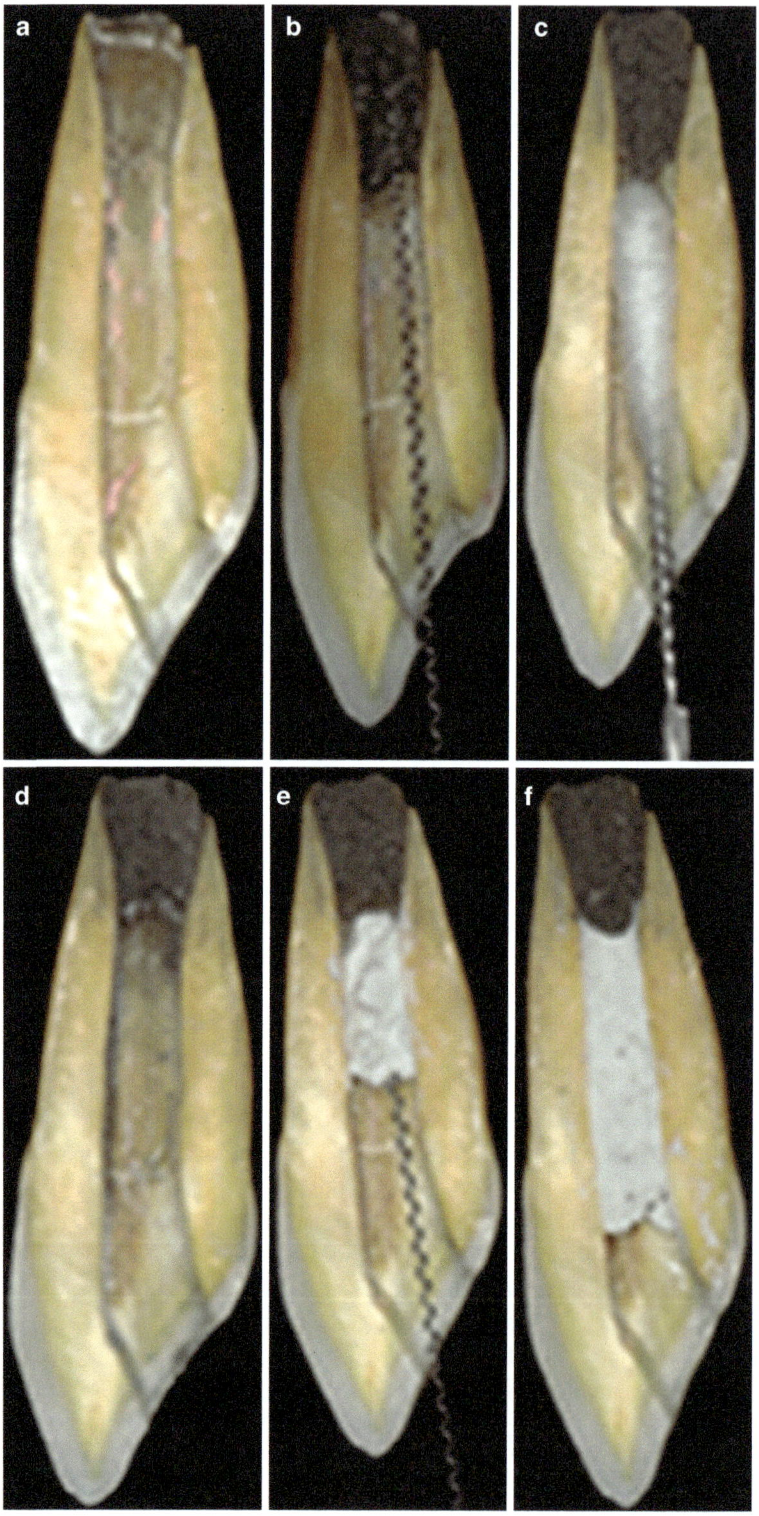

Fig. 6.6 Fabricating the apical plug with the aid of a Lentulo spiral and endodontic file. (**a**) Tooth with incomplete apices; (**b**) Insertion of MTA; (**c**) Compactation of MTA; (**d**) Tooth with MTA in the apical portion; (**e**) Filling the other canal portions with callcium hydroxide; (**f**) Tooth with the canal filled with MTA and calcium hydroxide paste

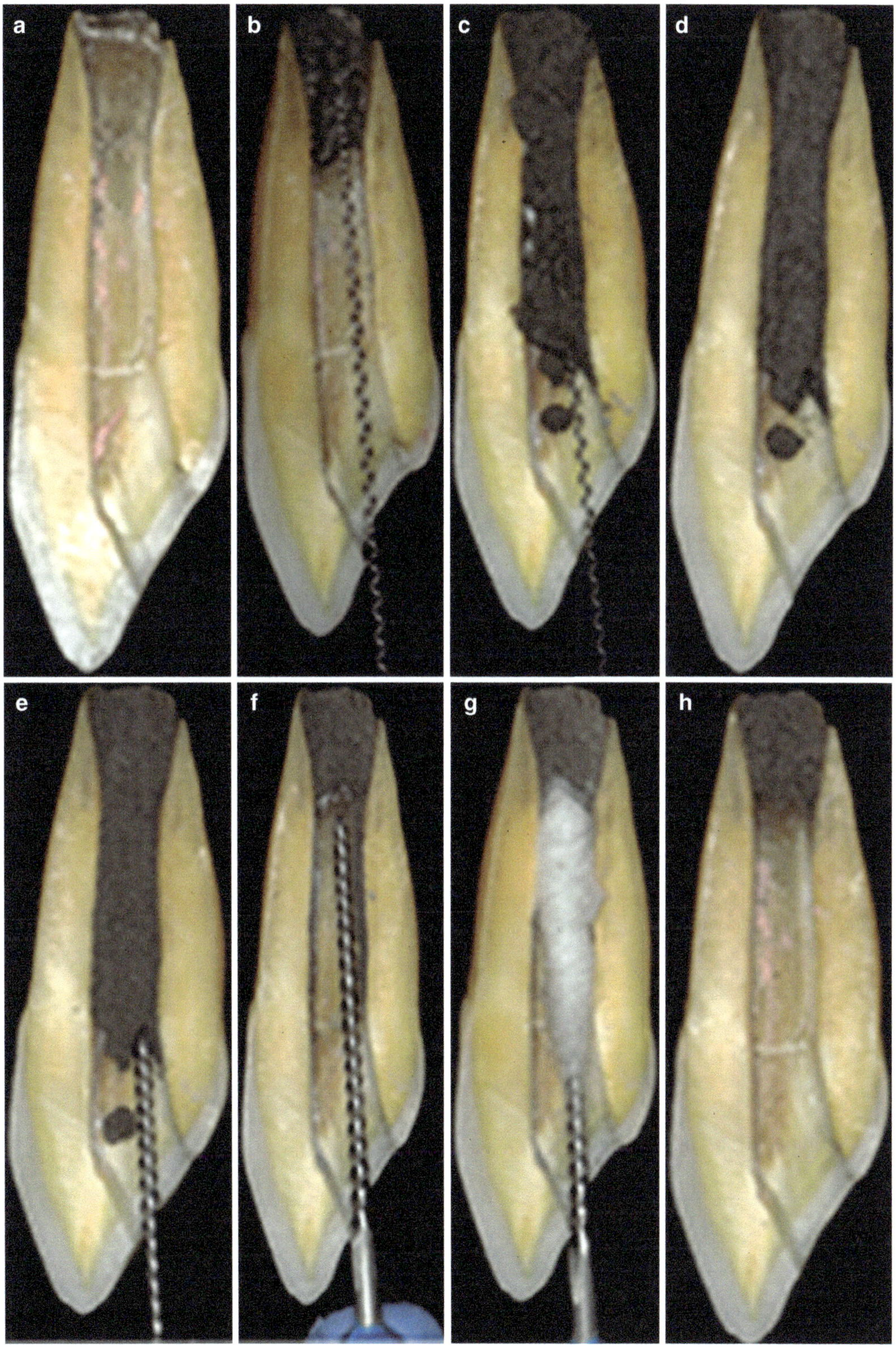

Fig. 6.7 Fabricating the apical "plug" by filling the entire canal with MTA and then adjusting the desired length with a file. (**a**–**d**) Sequence of entire root canal filled with MTA; (**e**–**g**) remotion of the MTA in the cervical and medium portion of the canal; (**h**) Tooth with the apical portion filled with MTA

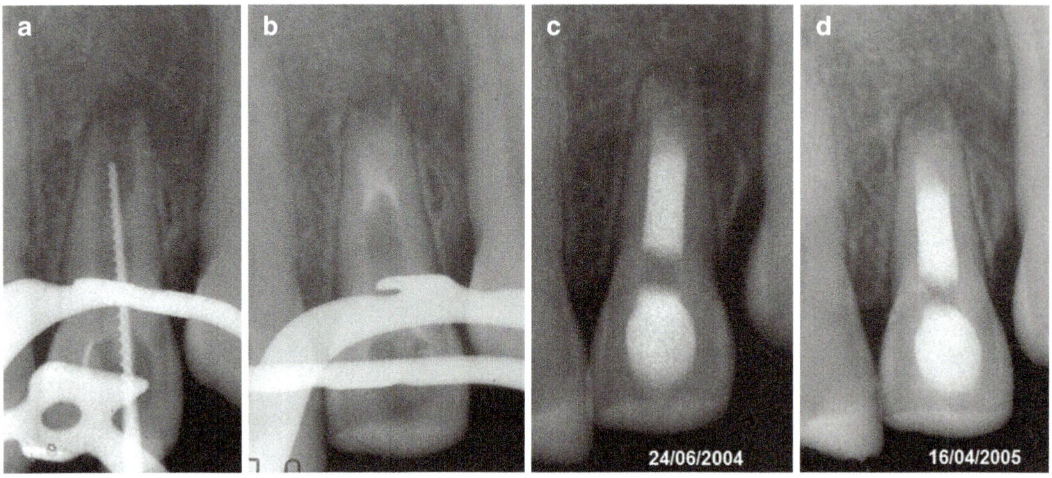

Fig. 6.8 The MTA apical plug in the treatment of the teeth with incomplete root formation

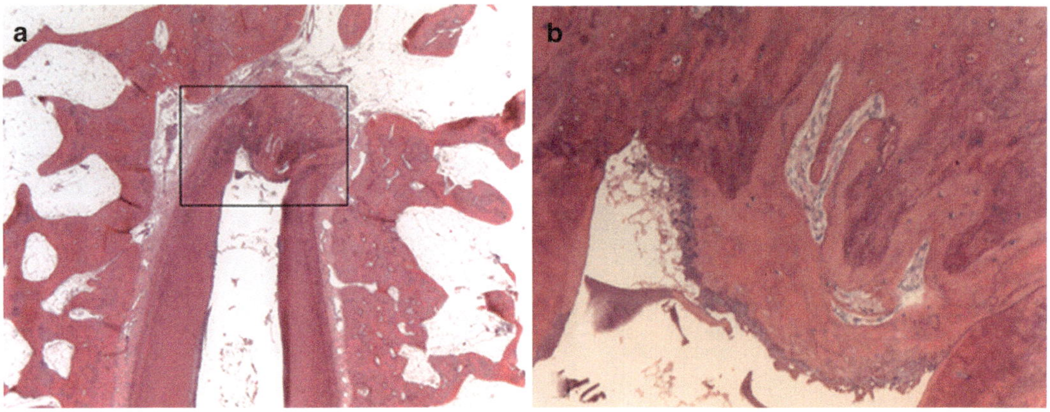

Fig. 6.9 (**a**) Mineralized tissue formed at the apex of a tooth with incomplete root formation, treated with MTA; (**b**) largest increase in the marked area

which is not recommended [19, 34, 39, 59, 65]. Placement of a matrix (barrier) of calcium hydroxide, calcium sulfate, or collagen to minimize the extrusion of material into the periapical tissues has been recommended [19, 34]. The extra root matrix (barrier), aside from preventing extrusion of the MTA, prevents contact with tissue fluids or blood during its insertion (Fig. 6.10). These materials are easy to use, are well tolerated by the periodontal tissues, provide a dry field against which the MTA will condensate, and are reabsorbed in a few days, without interfering with the repair process in the region.

After instrumentation of the canal, the matrix material is brought to the apical region via the canal using a gutta-percha plugger compatible with the diameter of the canal. After the insertion of the apical matrix, the MTA is introduced in the canal with the aid of a Lentulo spiral, Map system, or Dovgan applicator obtaining the apical plug. A root canal filling composed of gutta-percha and sealer completes the final obturation (Figs. 6.11 and 6.12).

6.3.4 Root Perforation

Root perforation is a common accident occurring during endodontic treatment, resulting in a communication between the pulp cavity and the

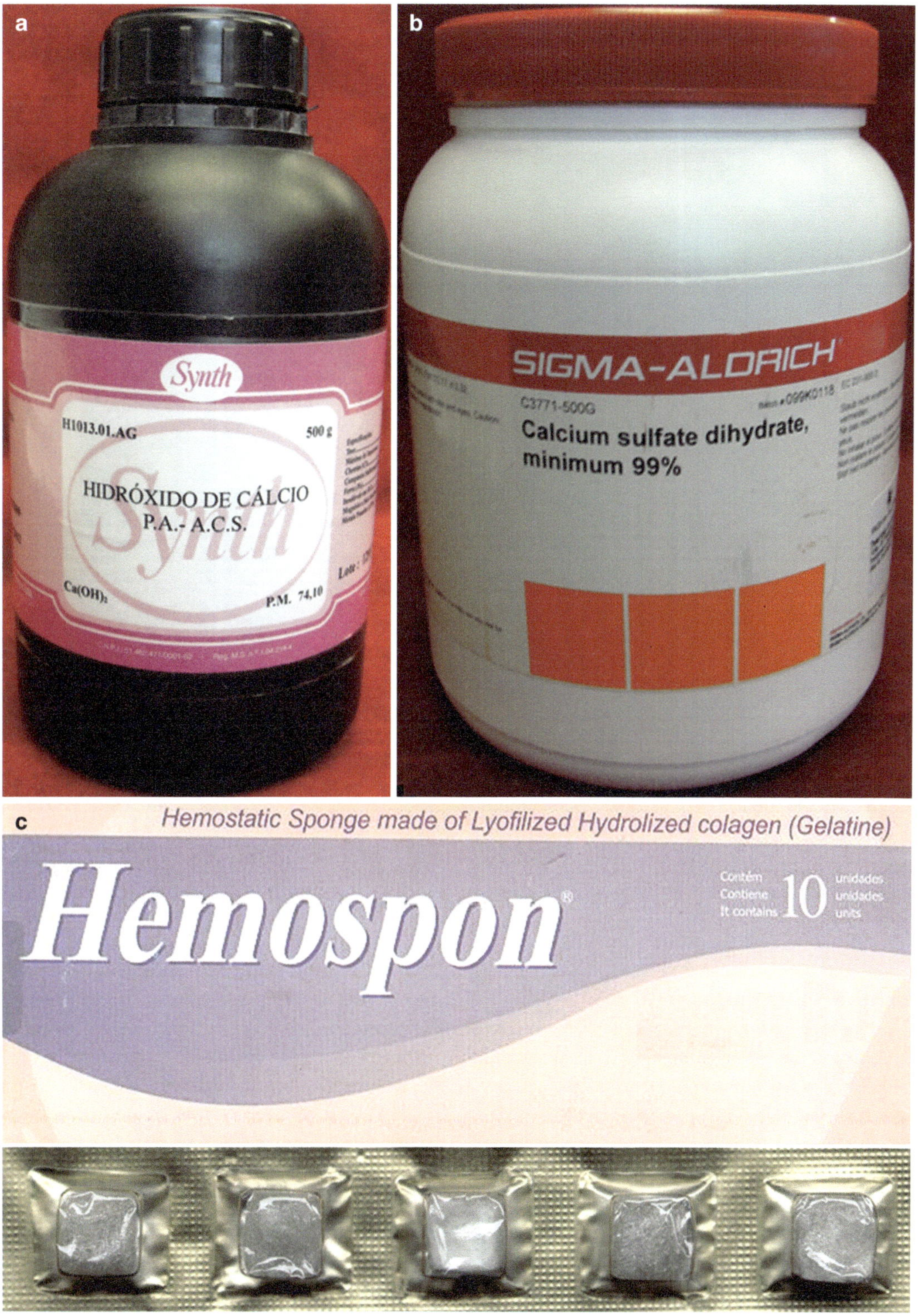

Fig. 6.10 Materials used for extra root matrix (barrier): (**a**) calcium hydroxide, (**b**) calcium sulfate, and (**c**) hemostatic collagen

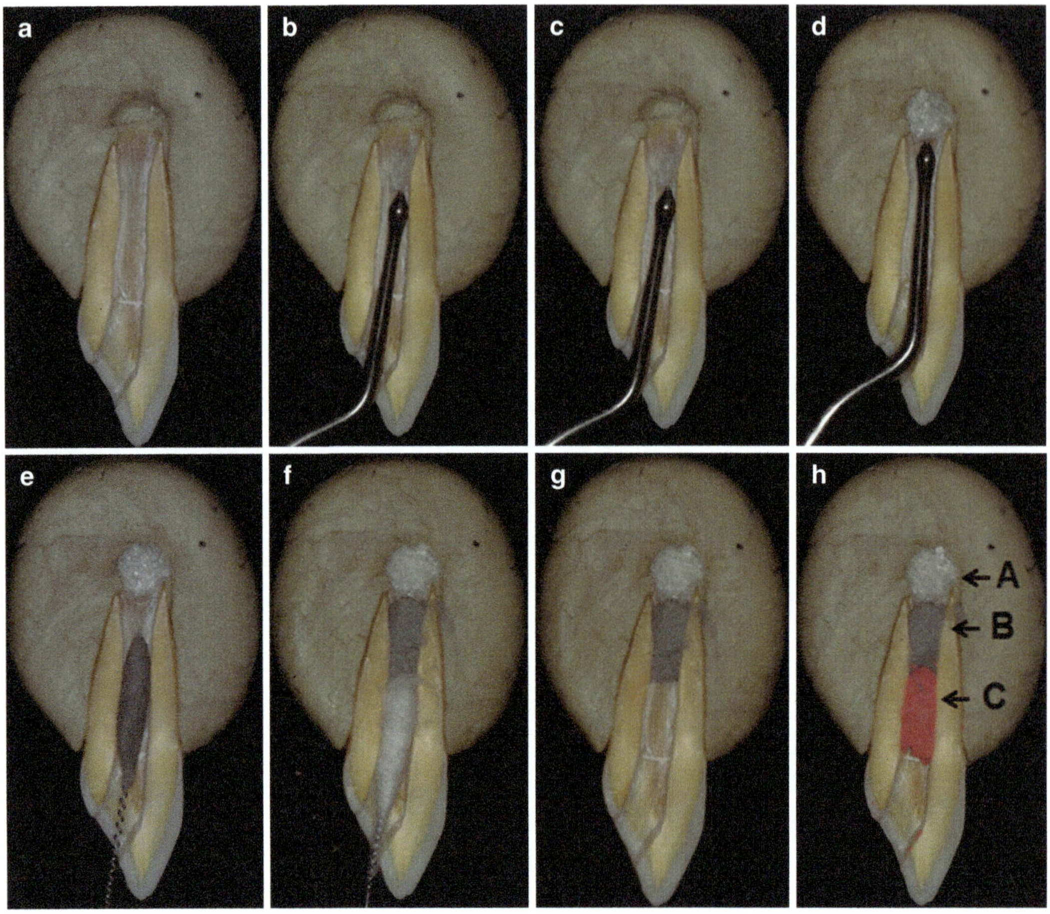

Fig. 6.11 Fabrication of the extra root apical matrix (barrier) with collagen: (**A**) matrix, (**B**) MTA, and (**C**) canal obturation. (**a**–**d**) Insertion of the collagen matrix in the periapical tissue; (**e**–**h**) Insertion of the MTA in the apical portion and obturation of the remaining portion of the canal

periodontium and can occur at any stage of treatment and can be located at the level of the pulp chamber and root canal.

The repair of the root perforation occurs with the formation of a mineralized tissue sealing itself, the neoformation of bone tissue, and periodontal ligament reinsertion (Fig. 6.13)

Root perforations have classically been treated using calcium hydroxide, but the large perforations did not respond well to this treatment. With the introduction of MTA, this treatment has become easier and faster, and with predictable results even in large perforations [3, 8, 10, 20, 31, 36–38, 40, 47, 52, 54, 57, 60, 76, 87].

The successful treatment of a root perforation depends on factors such as level, location, size, and presence or absence of contamination. The root perforation treatment with MTA or with calcium hydroxide is indicated in the intra-osseous perforations.

When the root perforation occurs, the sooner the treatment is carried out, the greater is the likelihood of success. The root perforation at the level of the pulp chamber is irrigated with saline solution to clean and control bleeding in order to apply the MTA. A sufficient amount of material is required to seal the root perforation with the gutta-percha plugger. If the tooth is exposed and the root perforation is contaminated, it is important to insert an antiseptic medication before sealing the tooth; in the second session, the medication is removed, and the chamber is irrigated by inserting

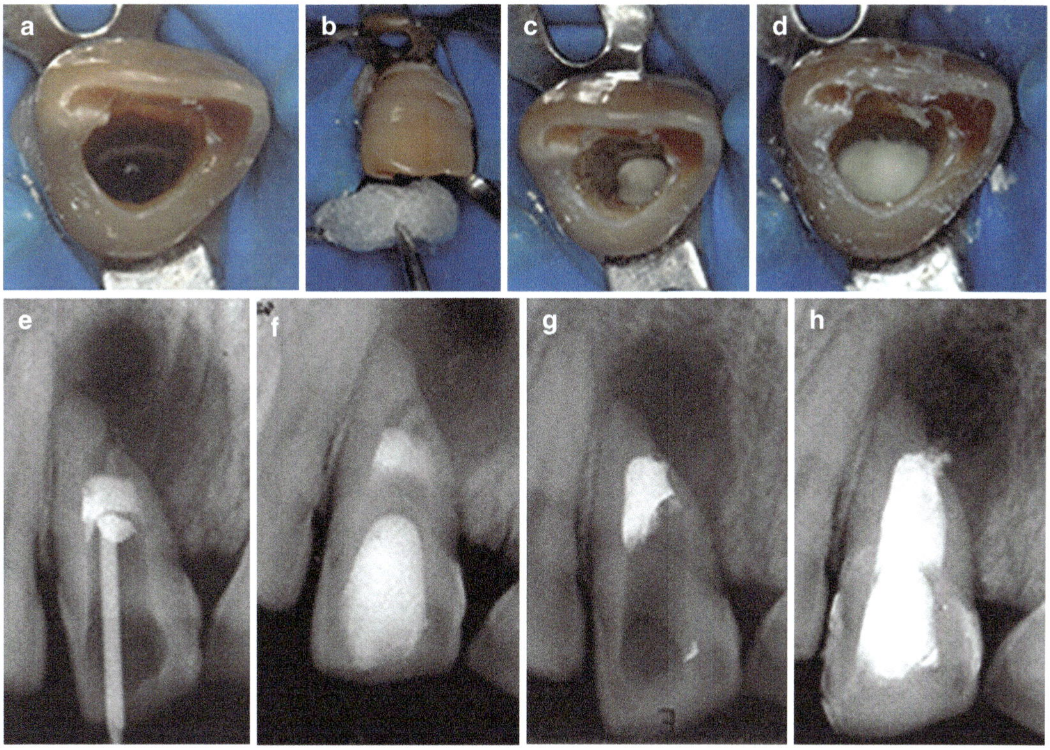

Fig. 6.12 Fabrication of the apical collagen matrix for placement of MTA in the teeth with incomplete root formation

a calcium hydroxide paste in the root perforation, followed by inserting MTA in the third session.

If the root perforation is intra-canal, after instrumentation, it is filled with calcium hydroxide paste. In the second session, the calcium hydroxide is removed from the canal, hence proceeding with obturation. The obturation is immediately cut to expose the root perforation, proceeding with the sealing with MTA (Fig. 6.14).

Extrusion of the MTA may occur if the root perforation is too large, hindering its resorption and repair area. In this case, it is convenient to make use of the extra root barrier with calcium hydroxide, calcium sulfate, and collagen, which must be placed, via the root perforation in the bone cavity ahead of the MTA. The excess barrier material is removed from the path of the root perforation with a K file, compatible with the diameter of the root perforation, followed by insertion of MTA (Figs. 6.15 and 6.16). The importance of the use of the matrix was highlighted by some authors [3, 10, 20, 39, 47, 76].

6.3.5 Canal Obturation

During the root canal preparation, over-instrumentation can occur which may favor the occurrence of over-obturation. In this situation, MTA can be used as an apical plug, with a similar way to the method described for the tooth with incomplete root formation. The larger the size of the instrument past the apex, the greater should be the thickness of the apical plug [23].

After the canal preparation, the apical plug is fabricated with the MTA, inserting it only in the apical region or alternatively completely filling the root canal with the MTA, to then remove part of it, leaving only the portion corresponding to the apical plug (Fig. 6.17), which must be at least 3 mm thick [4, 23, 51, 69].

The root canal filling can be done in the same session or on a consecutive visit, depending on the consistency and strength of the apical plug. During the obturation, the cone should be well adjusted to the canal, so as not to exert strong

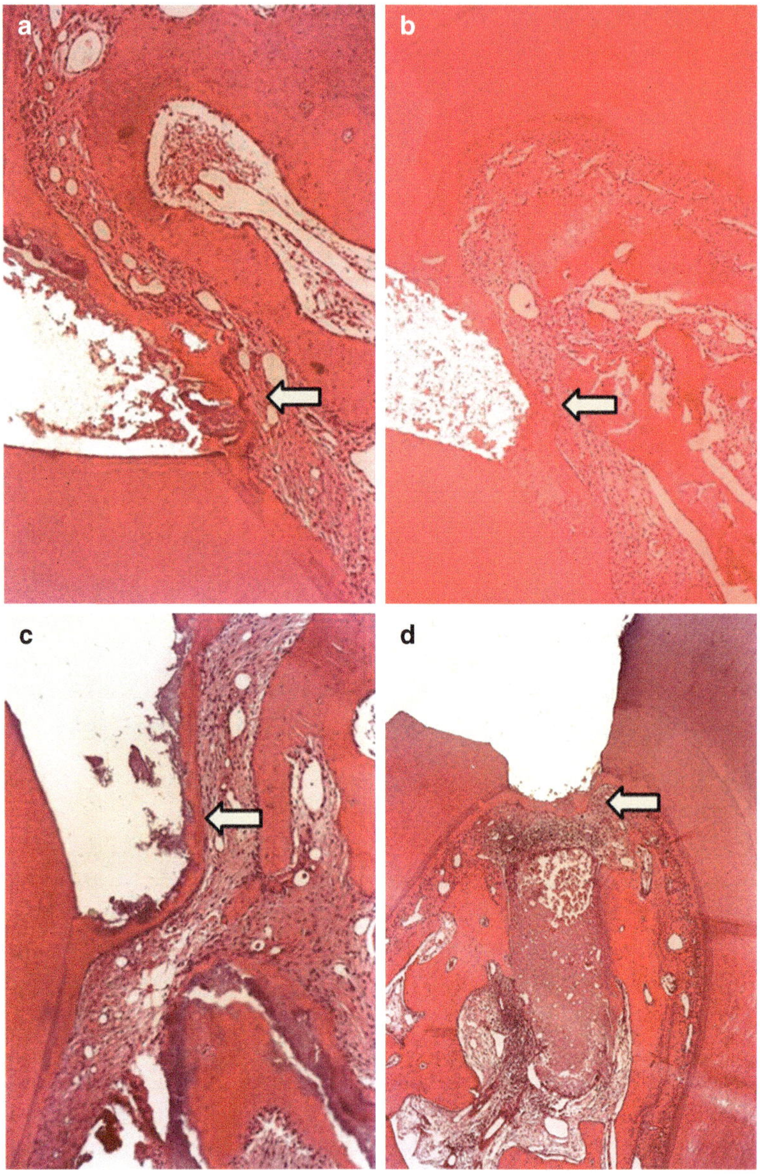

Fig. 6.13 Microscopic aspects of the repair of root perforations treated with MTA (*white arrow*)

pressure on the apical plug during the obturation, leading to leakage of the material (Fig. 6.18).

The canal can also be obturated with gutta-percha and cement-based MTA, such as MTA Fillapex. MTA has been shown to be effective in the physical and biological point of views when used in the obturation of the root canal with or without gutta-percha [42, 86].

6.3.6 Endodontic Surgery

When endodontic treatment fails or retreatment is not possible, endodontic surgery is indicated. Among the different types of surgery is the retrograde filling, which consists of the preparation of an apical cavity and its filling with retro-obturation material. The MTA is highly indicated

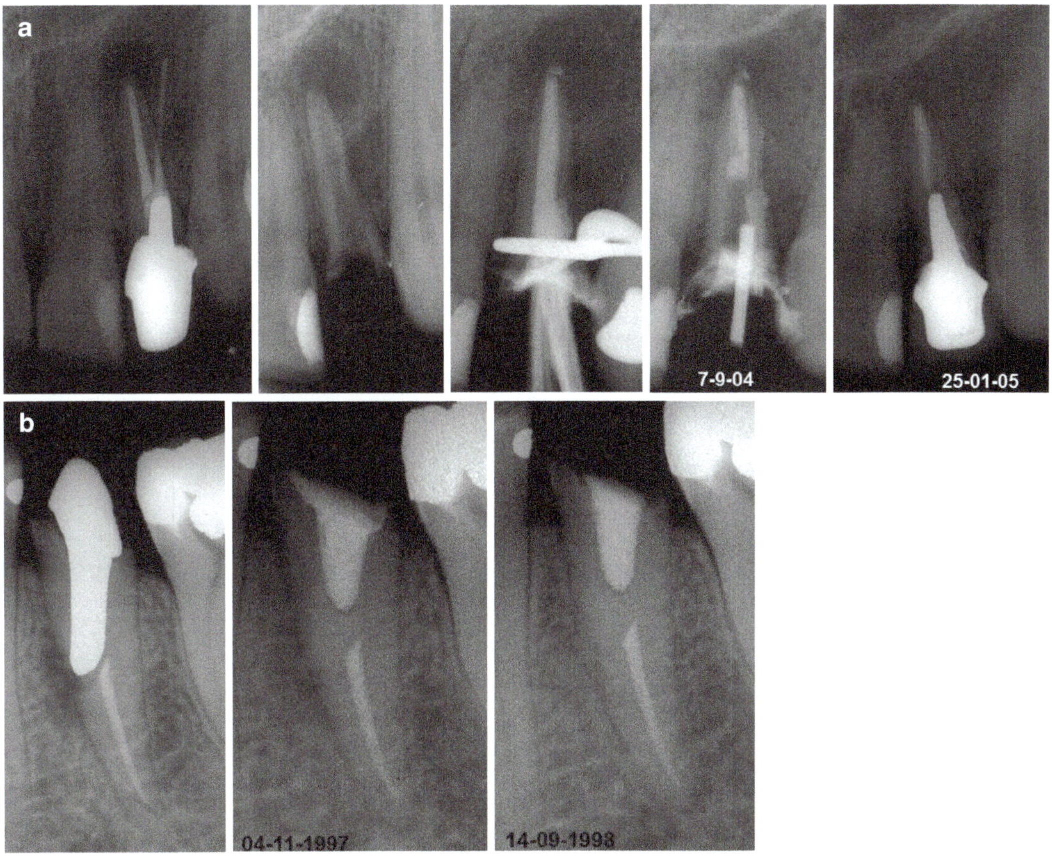

Fig. 6.14 Root perforations sealed with MTA: (**a**) upper lateral incisor; (**b**) lower premolar. Observe the repaired area

for retrograde filling [7, 9, 13, 16, 22, 26, 51, 72, 79–82].

The retro apical cavity is prepared with ultrasound, trying to follow the direction of the canal, with a depth of 3–5 mm, maintaining retention and regularity. The MTA should have a consistency that facilitates its insertion into the cavity by means of a Lucas curette, Map system, or Dovgan applicator.

After placement of the MTA, the surgical wound should not be irrigated, since this can result in dislodgement of the material from the retro-cavity. Excess material should be removed with Gracey or Lucas curettes or gauze moistened with saline solution (Fig. 6.19).

6.3.7 Tooth Resorption

External or internal tooth resorption is a multifactorial pathology and may be caused by pulp necrosis, dental trauma, orthodontic tooth movement, tooth whitening, and more. The internal and external resorption can cause communication of the canal with the periodontium, and in this case, the treatment is more difficult with a doubtful prognosis.

The resorption has classically been treated with calcium hydroxide, and more recently with MTA [45, 68]. If the internal resorption is perforated and there is invaginated tissue, it is removed with a K file with its tip bent, followed by irrigation

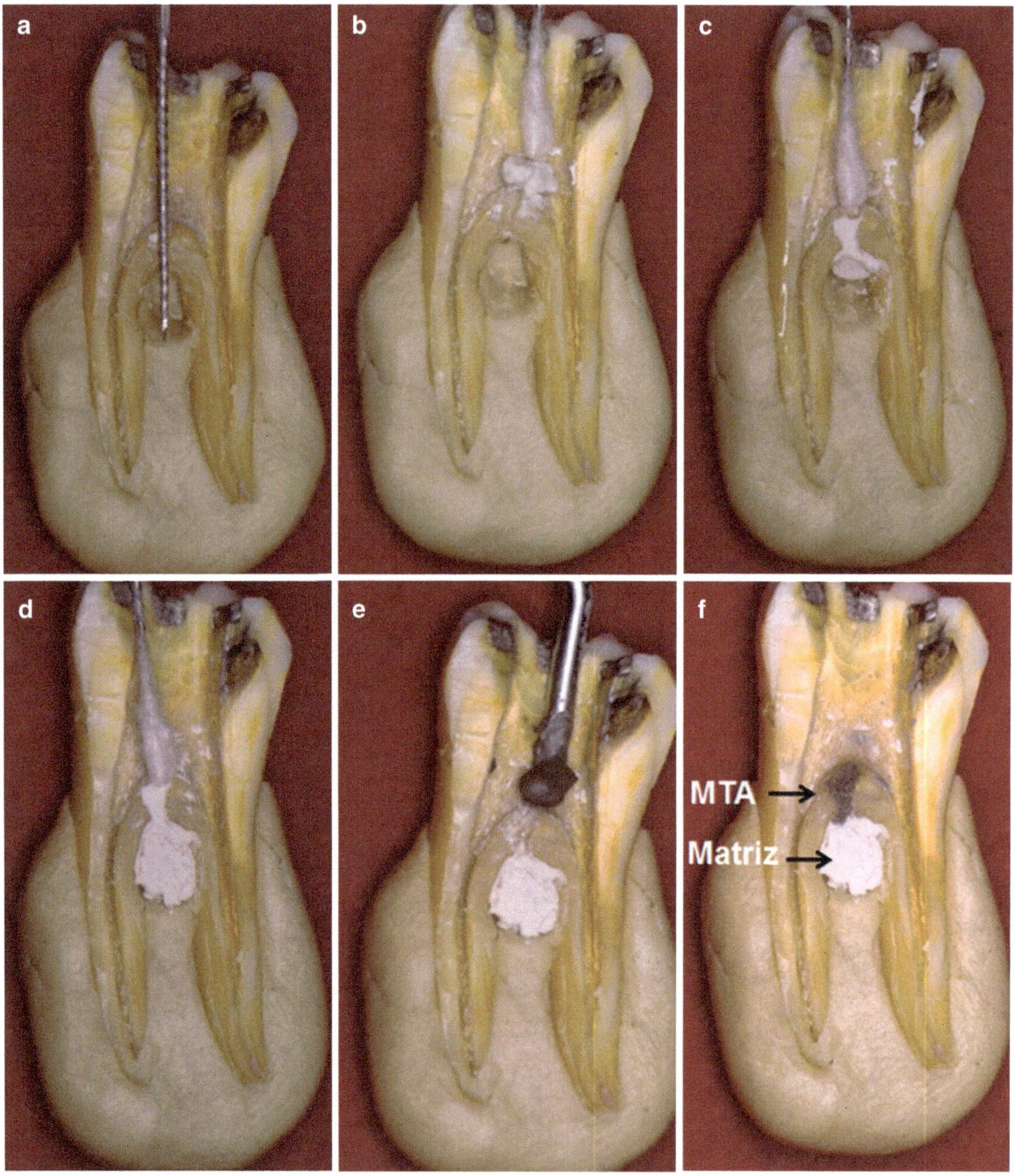

Fig. 6.15 Fabrication of the calcium sulfate matrix and MTA in the root perforation. (**a–c**) Confection of the matrix with calcium sulphate in the furcal region; (**d–f**) Insertion of MTA in the furcal perforation

with sodium hypochlorite solution. It is important to use a dressing with calcium hydroxide, until all the invaginated tissue is totally eliminated. The MTA is delivered to the canal with a Lentulo spiral, Map system, or Dovgan applicator, filling the entire area of resorption (Fig. 6.20).

6.3.8 Root Fractures

Dental fractures with a traumatic etiology can occur in the crown, root, or crown/root. When in the root, it can be vertical or transversal, and the vertical fracture presents a very poor prognosis.

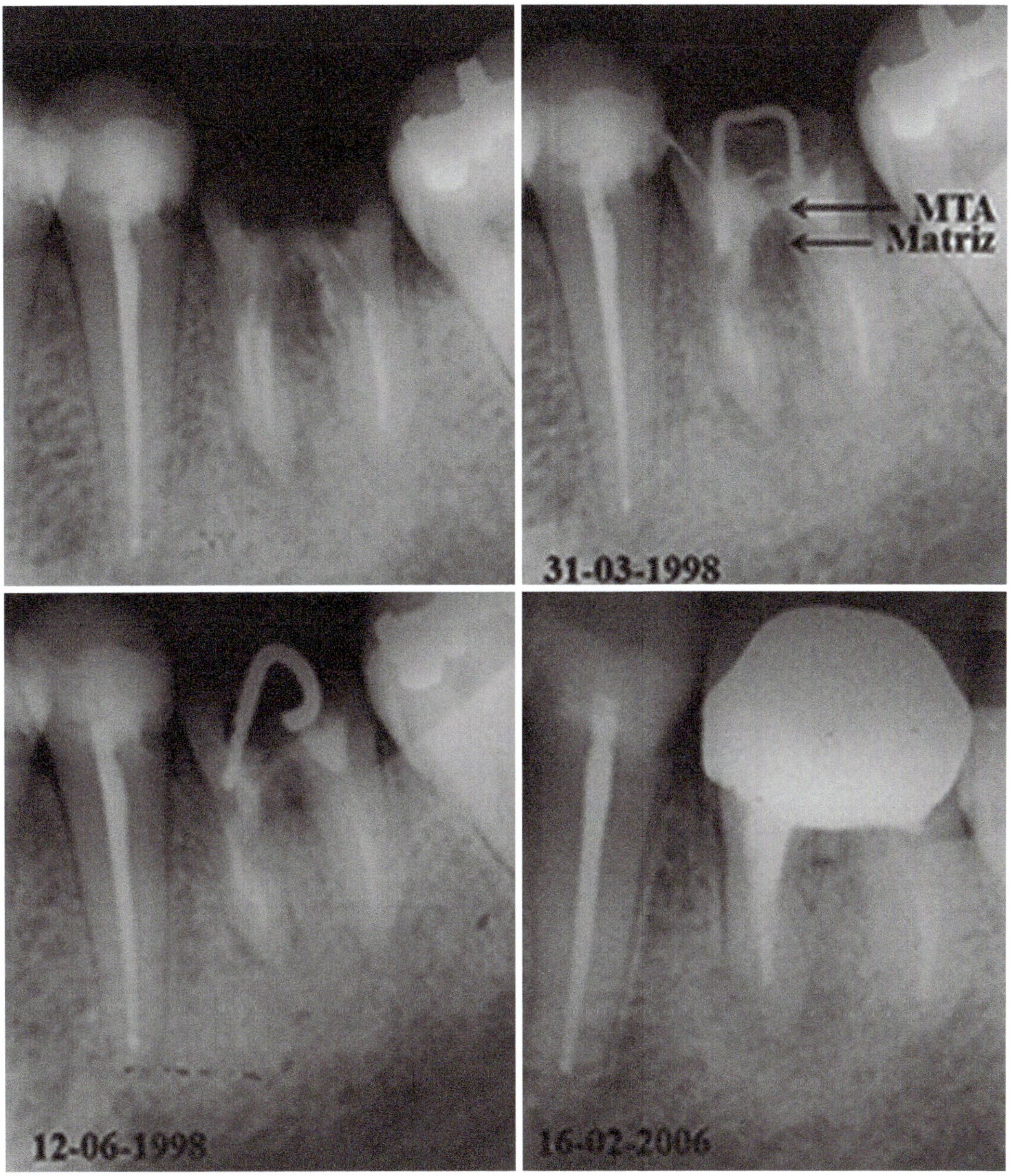

Fig. 6.16 Root perforation treatment with the calcium sulfate matrix and MTA

The transversal, depending on their location (cervical, middle, and apical), can have a success outcome in the treatment. The root fracture located in the cervical and middle thirds causes difficulty for treatment because it is difficult for dental immobilization, leading to injury or even preventing the consolidation of the fragments. For these cases, it is possible to strengthen the tooth with an intra-canal pin cemented with MTA [18].

The canal is instrumented, and then an apical plug with MTA is performed. A metal pin is selected in order to remain adjusted in the canal, which is filled with MTA, seating the pin inside.

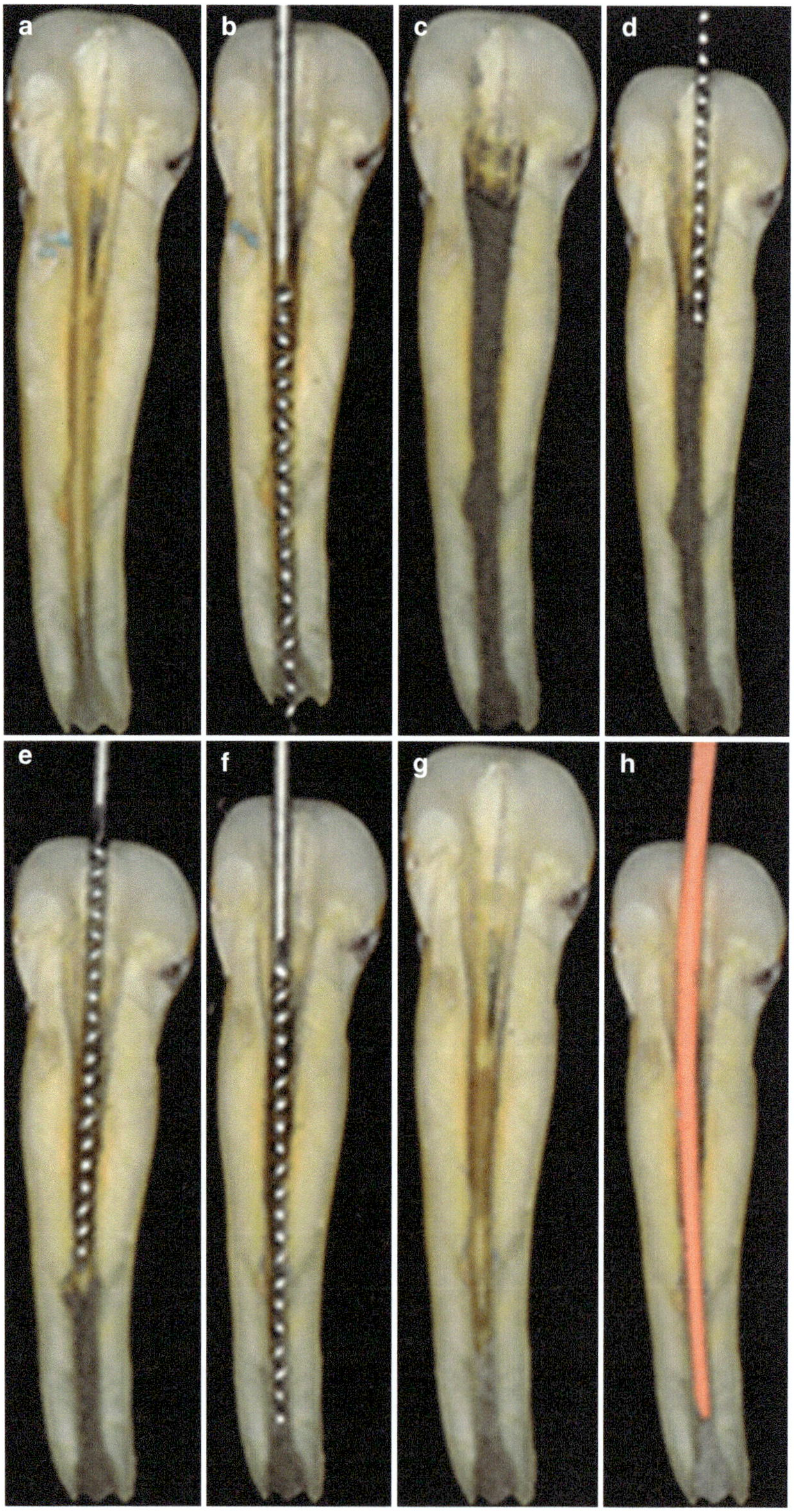

Fig. 6.17 Fabrication of the apical plug with MTA in an over-instrumented canal. (**a**–**d**) Root canal preparation and obturation wth MTA; (**e**–**h**) Remotion of MTA in the cervical and medium portions of the root canal and insertion of a gutta-percha cone

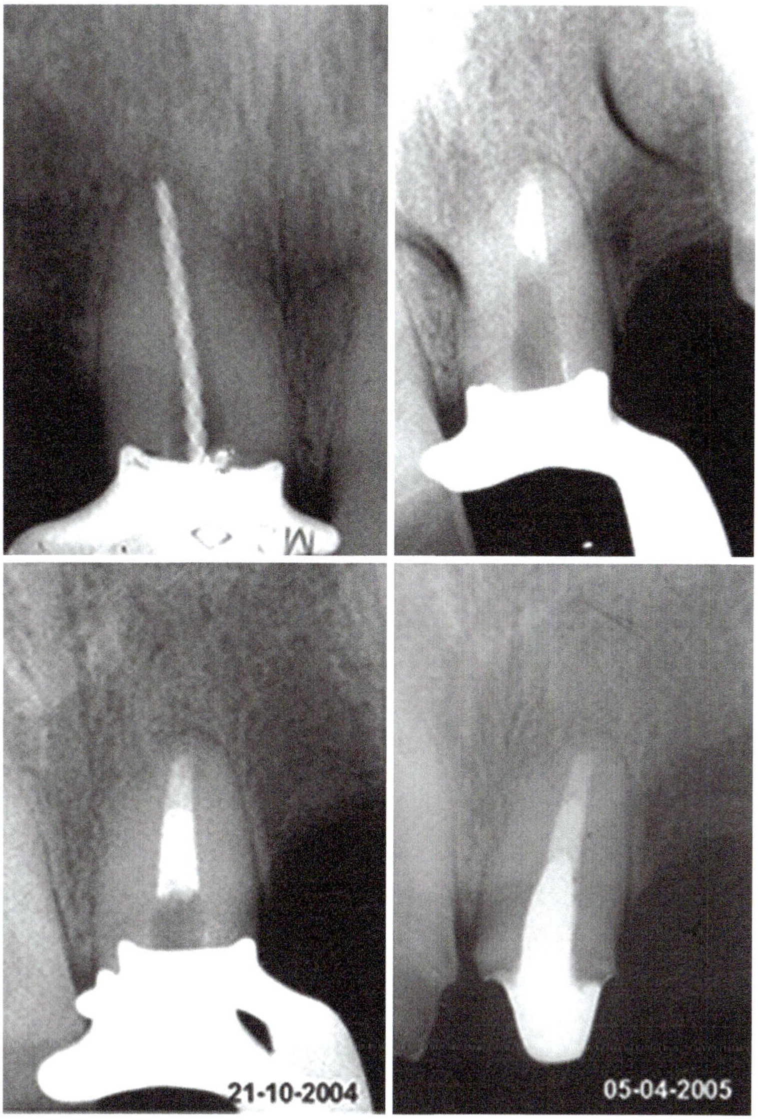

Fig. 6.18 Apical plug with MTA and obturation of the canal with gutta-percha and sealer

Thus, there is reinforcement for the root, preventing mobility of the coronary segment (Fig. 6.21).

6.3.8.1 Other Applications

In addition to the applications mentioned above, MTA can also be used in other clinical situations, such as dens invaginatus, maintenance of the primary teeth, reimplantation, and more recently revascularization.

The dens invaginatus is a developmental anomaly of the tooth, modifying both the crown and the tooth root, complicating endodontic treatment [46, 66]. It is more frequent in the maxillary lateral incisor, and can also be found in other teeth. The invagination caused by dens invaginatus may reach different root thirds, having been classified by Oehler [66] as type I, cervical third; II, middle third; and III, apical third. This invagination can communicate with the pulp cavity, compromising the pulp and leading to the periapical lesion. Treatment of dens invaginatus may be prophylactic, conventional endodontic treatment, endodontic surgery, or an association of the latter. Management of dens invaginatus

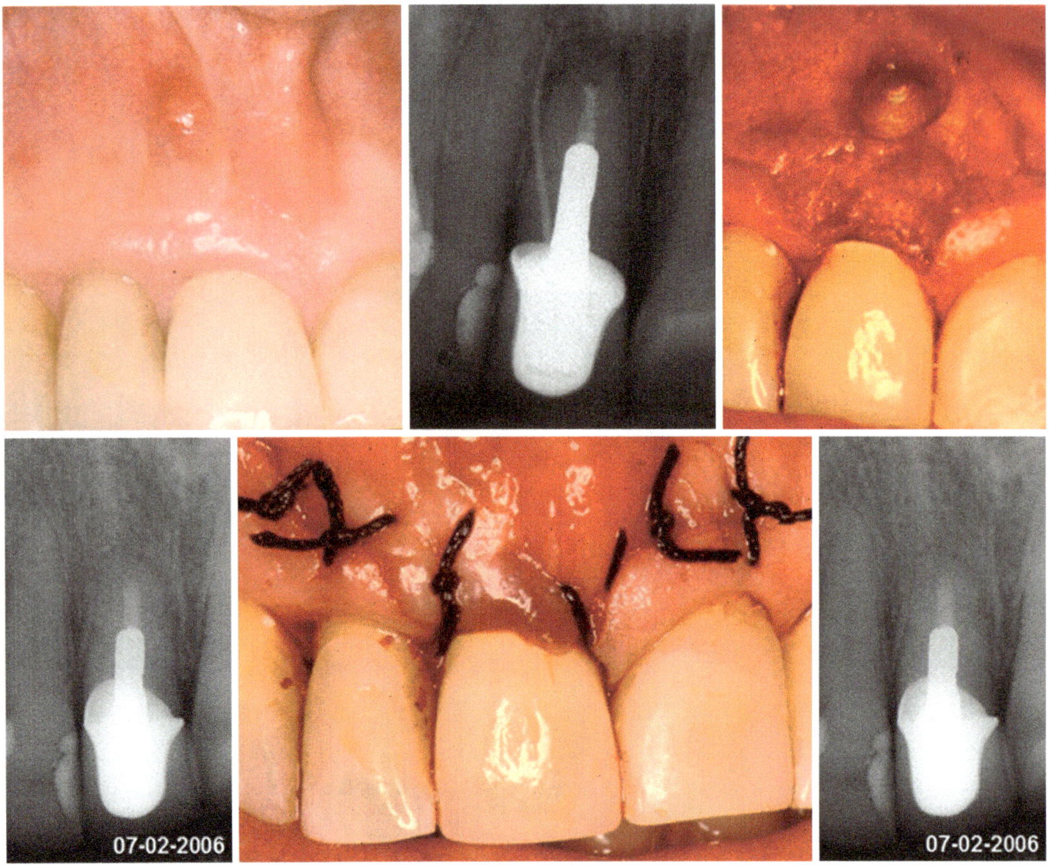

Fig. 6.19 Retrograde filling in the maxillary central incisor with the use of MTA

types I and II, when the apex is still open, can be performed with an apical plug with MTA and the root canal filling with gutta-percha and sealer (Fig. 6.22) or, in a more complex situation, filling the whole canal with MTA [34, 50, 53].

MTA can also be used when the primary tooth does not have its permanent successor and needs to be kept in the mouth to maintain the patient's occlusal harmony. After instrumentation, irrigation, and medication of the canal, it is completely filled with MTA avoiding the extrusion of material to the periapical region (Fig. 6.23). MTA has been used in the maintenance of the primary teeth [67].

Dental trauma may also result in tooth avulsion, which often leads to resorption and tooth loss. An alternative treatment is the filling of the entire canal with MTA [70], with the goal of continuing root formation and maintenance of the tooth (Fig. 6.24).

In 1971, Nygaard-Ostby [64] proposed a procedure for the teeth with necrotic pulps which consisted in promoting the filling of the canal with blood, inducing clot formation and a new pulp tissue. The advantage of this procedure was to promote a root complement and the deposition of mineralized tissue on the walls of the canals, making the teeth more resistant.

For many years, this treatment was forgotten and recently returned to be utilized, especially in the teeth with incomplete root formation and pulp necrosis, being named

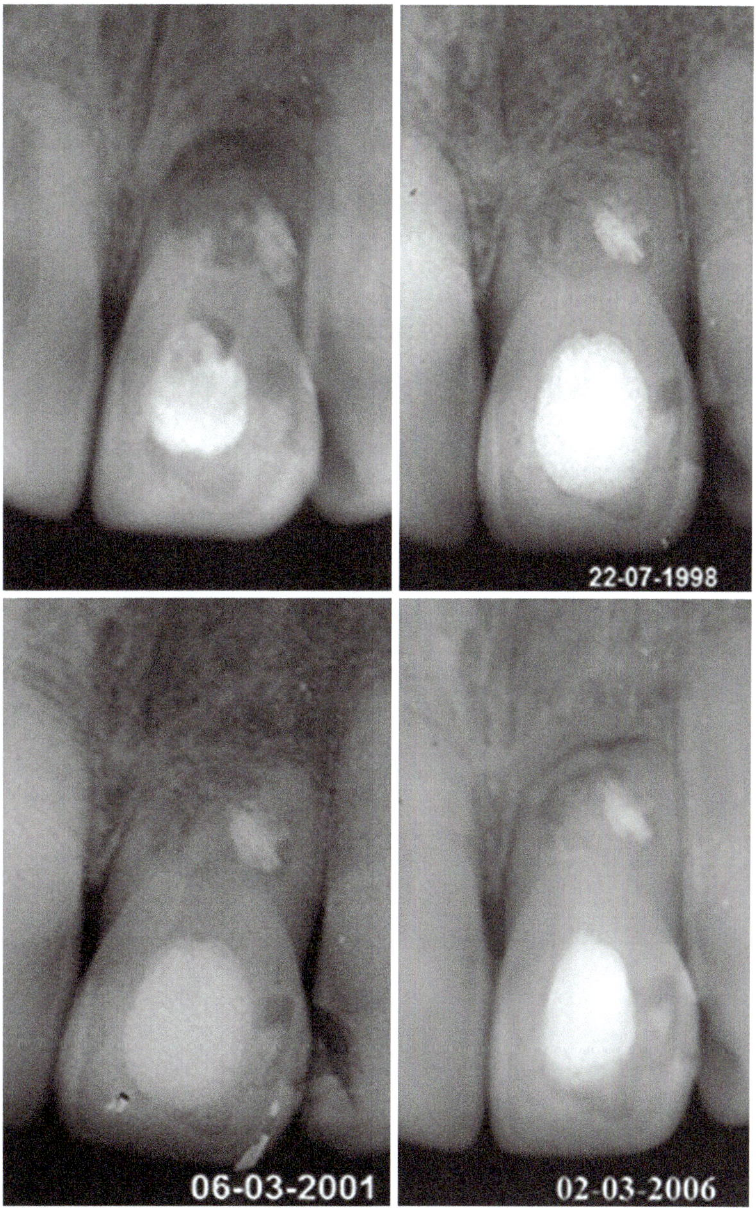

Fig. 6.20 Apical resorption treated with MTA

revascularization or regenerative endodontic procedure [17, 33, 73].

After the instrumentation and medication of the canal (tri-antibiotic or calcium hydroxide pastes), the foramen is exceeded in order to obtain the bleeding to fill the canal. With a cotton ball, the blood is compressed, typically in the cervical level, until the clot is obtained. The MTA plug is fabricated on top of this, sealing the tooth with a glass ionomer (Fig. 6.25). Clinical controls and radiographs demonstrate the completed root formation as well as the mineralized tissue formed by decreasing the diameter of the canal.

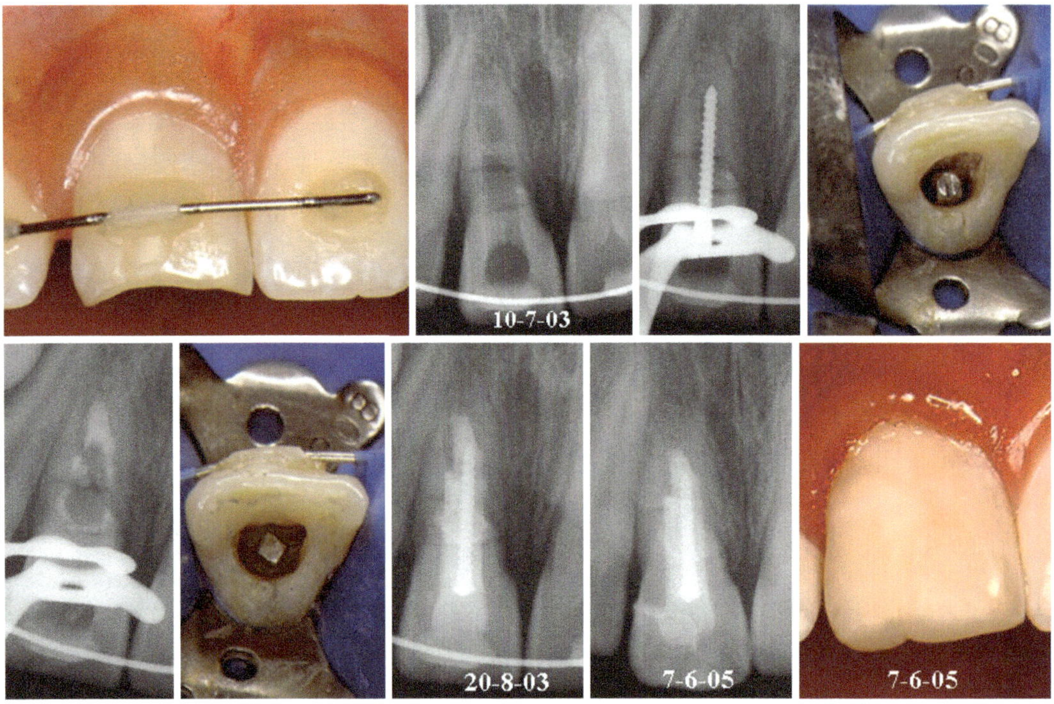

Fig. 6.21 Treatment of root fracture with MTA, reinforced with an intra-canal pin

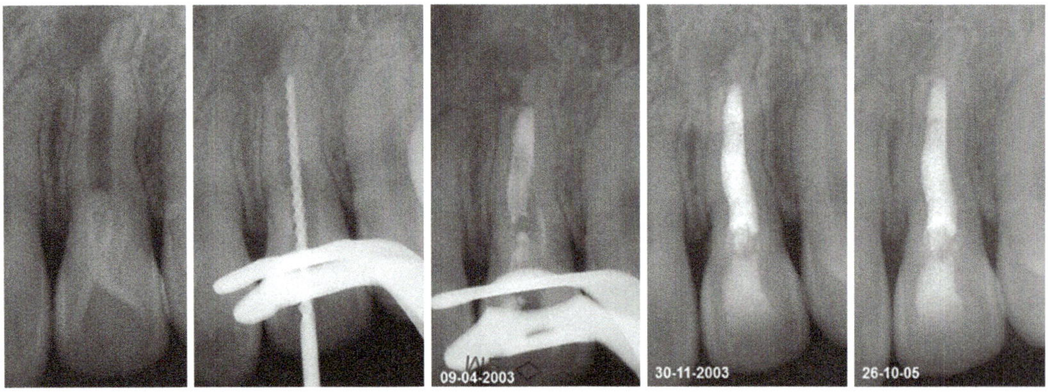

Fig. 6.22 Dens invaginatus treated with an MTA apical "plug" and canal obturation with gutta-percha and sealer

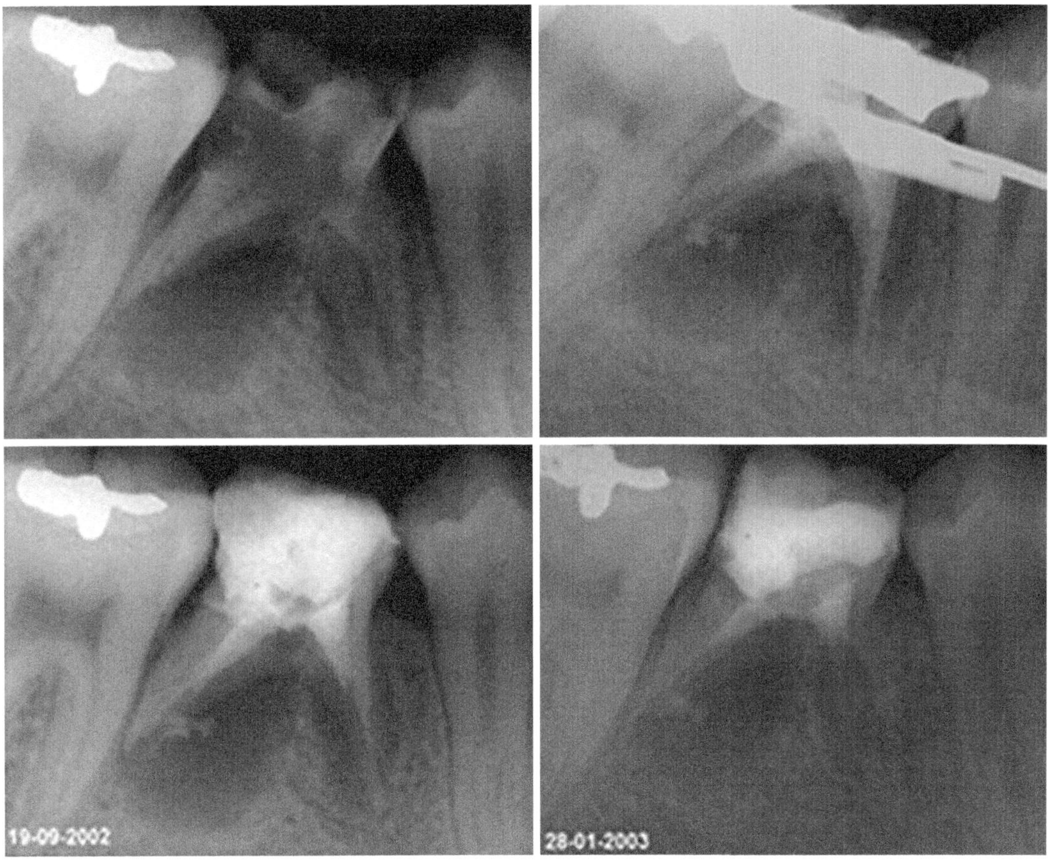

Fig. 6.23 Maintenance of the primary tooth with the canal filled with MTA

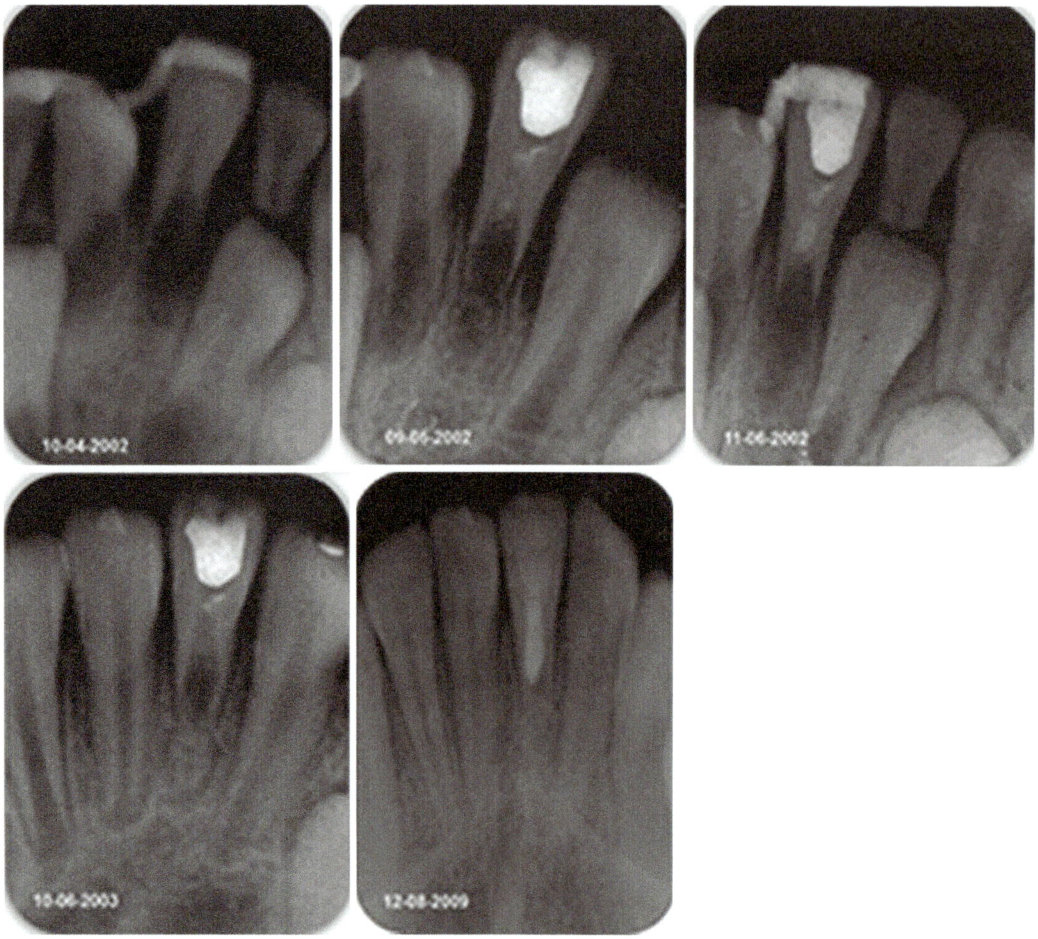

Fig. 6.24 Avulsed and reimplanted incisor and the canal filled with MTA (Images courtesy of Luiz Gonzales Navarro)

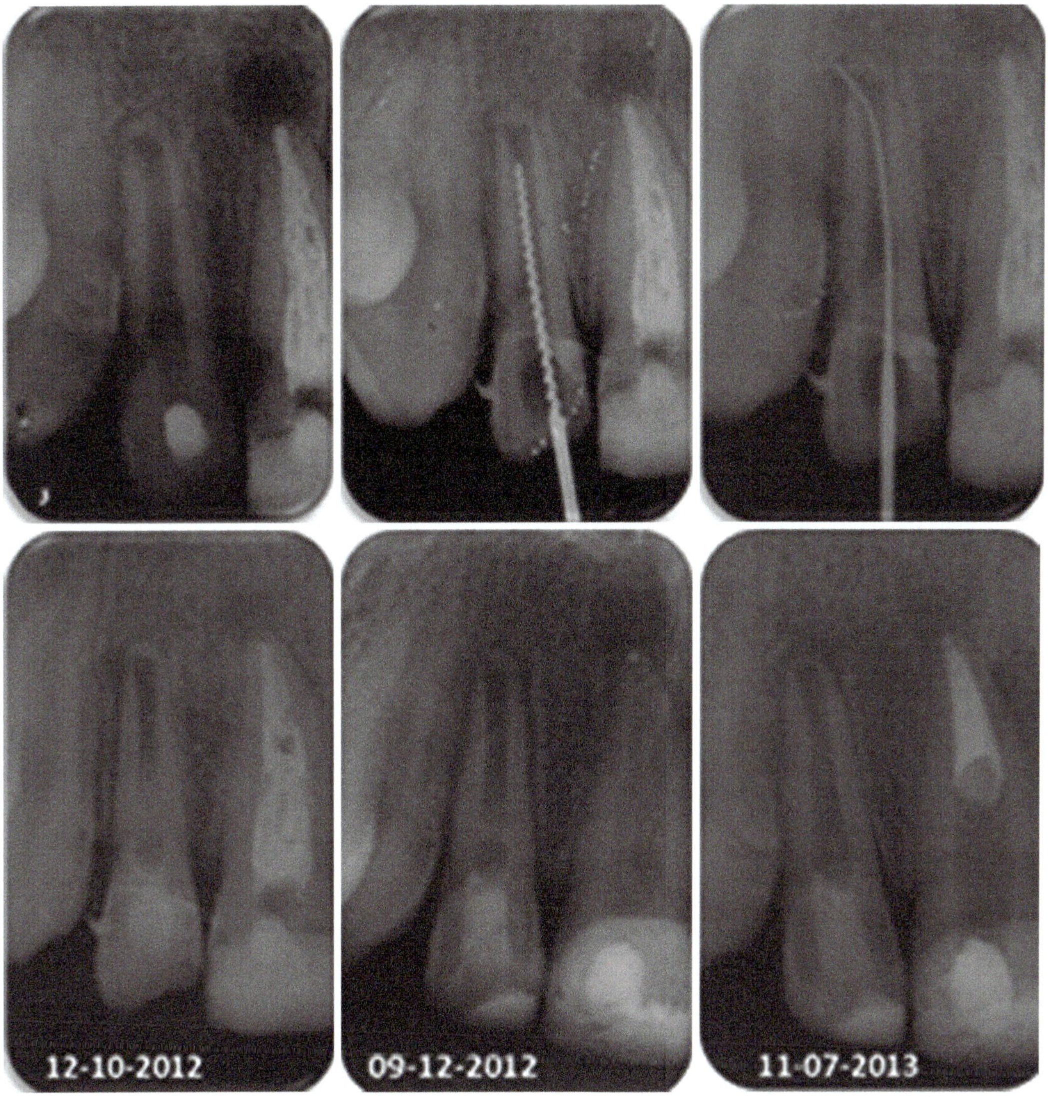

Fig. 6.25 Revascularization with the use of MTA

Conclusions

MTA was introduced in dentistry, initially for the treatment of perforations and dental and endodontic surgery due to its physicochemical and biological properties. It came to be used for the same indications where calcium hydroxide was once used, but with greater advantages. To be performed successfully, the correct diagnosis is important for these treatment modalities, thereby instituting the planning and appropriate treatment for each clinical situation.

When using MTA, it is important to note the following requirements:

(a) Following the powder-liquid ratio recommended by the manufacturer, it can be changed slightly to achieve the proper consistency depending on where the material will be used in the pulp chamber, the canal, or endodontic surgery. A too thick or too fluid consistency makes the material difficult to work with.

(b) Small leakage of the material for the periodontium is reabsorbed, but large amounts should be avoided because the material can harden, hindering its resorption by interfering in the repair process.

(c) When there is a risk of extravasation (drilling on instrumentation, incomplete apex, apical resorption, dens invaginatus), it is advisable to use the extra root matrix with calcium hydroxide, calcium sulfate, or collagen before the use of MTA.

(d) MTA can discolor the tooth by the function of the cement components, the contamination by blood or contact with photoactivated resin. Leaving the MTA in the pulp chamber should be avoided, mainly in the anterior teeth, and placement of a restorative material on the MTA is recommended.

(e) MTA can harden if it remains in the canal in an unwanted area, making it difficult or even impossible to remove, so any waste material must be removed immediately.

(f) In the retrograde filling, the excess MTA must be removed by means of a curette or gauze moistened with saline solution. The use of irrigation is not recommended because it washes out all the material, including that present in the retrograde cavity.

(g) The use of the microscope facilitates the visualization of the correct placement of the MTA and the surgical procedures.

(h) MTA can be inserted at the desired location through the amalgam micro-carrier or instruments developed for this purpose (Map system, Dovgan, Messinger, MTA-Angelus applicator) greatly facilitating its placement.

(i) Ultrasound provides a better adaptation for the MTA plug.

References

1. Accorinte MLR, Holland R, Reis A, Bortoluzzi M, Murata SS, Dezan Jr E, Souza V, Alessandro LD. Evaluation of mineral trióxide aggregate and calcium hydroxide cement as pulp-capping agents in human teeth. J Endod. 2008;34:1–6.
2. Aeinehchi M, Eslami B, Ghanbariha M, Saffar AS. Mineral trioxide aggregate (MTA) and calcium hydroxide as pulp-capping agents in human teeth: a preliminary report. Int Endod J. 2003;36:225–31.
3. Al-Daafas A, Al Nazhan S. Histological evaluation of contaminated furcal perforation in dog's teeth repaired with MTA with or without internal matrix. Oral Surg Oral Med Oral Pathol Oral Radiol Endod. 2007;103: 92–9.
4. Al-Kahtani A, Shostad S, Schifferle R, Bhambhani S. *In vitro* evaluation of microleakage of an orthograde apical plug of mineral trioxide aggregate in permanent with simulated immature apices. J Endod. 2005;31:117–9.
5. Andreasen JO, Munksgaard EC, Bakland LK. Comparison of fracture resistance in root canals of immature sheep teeth after filling with calcium hydroxide or MTA. Dent Traumatol. 2006;22:154–6.
6. Andreasen JO, Farik B, Munksgaard EC. Long-term calcium hydroxide as a root canal dressing may increase risk of root fracture. Dent Traumatol. 2002;18:134–7.
7. Aqrabawi J. Sealing ability of amalgam, super EBA cement, and MTA when used as retrograde filling materials. Br Dent J. 2000;188:266–8.
8. Arens DE, Torabinejad M. Repair of furcal perforations with mineral trioxide aggregate-two case reports. Oral Surg Oral Med Oral Pathol Oral Radiol Endod. 1996;82:84–8.
9. Baek SH, Plenk H, Kiom S. Periapical tissue responses and cement regeneration with amalgam, super EBA and MTA as root-end filling materials. J Endod. 2005;31:444–9.
10. Bargholz C. Perforation repair with mineral trioxide aggregate a modified matrix concept. Int Endod J. 2005;38:59–69.
11. Barrieshi-Nusair KM, Qudeimat MA. A prospective clinical study of mineral trioxide aggregate for partial pulpotomy in cariously exposed permanent teeth. J Endod. 2006;32:731–5.
12. Belobrov I, Parashos P. Treatment of tooth discoloration after the use of white mineral trioxide aggregate. J Endod. 2011;37:1017–20.
13. Bernabé PFE, Gomes-Filho JE, Rocha WC, Nery MJ, Otoboni Filho JA, Dezan Junior E. Histological evaluation of MTA as a root-end filling material. Int Endod J. 2007;40:758–65.
14. Bortoluzzi EA, Araújo GS, Tanomaru JMG, Tanomaru Filho M. Marginal gingiva discoloration by gray MTA: a case report. J Endod. 2007;33:325–7.
15. Bortoluzzi EA, Broon NJ, Bramante CM, Consolaro A, Garcia RB, Moraes IG, Bernardineli N. Mineral Trioxide Aggregate with or without calcium chloride in pulpotomy. J Endod. 2008;34(2):172–5.
16. Bortoluzzi EA, Broon NJ, Bramante CM, Garcia RB, Moraes IG, Bernardineli N. Sealing ability of MTA and radiopaque Portland cement with or without calcium chloride for root-end filling. J Endod. 2006; 32:897–900.
17. Bose R, Nummikoski P, Hargreaves K. A retrospective evaluation of radiographic outcome in immature teeth with necrotic root canal systems treated with

regenerative endodontic procedures. J Endod. 2009; 35:1343–9.

18. Bramante CM, Menezes RS, Moraes IG, Bernardineli N, Garcia RB, Letra A. Use of MTA and intracanal post reinforcement in a horizontally fractured tooth: a case report. Dent Traumatol. 2006;22:275–8.
19. Bramante CM, Moraes IG, Bernardineli N, Garcia RB, Broon N, Bramante AS. Is a matrix required for treatment of root perforation with MTA? ENDO Endod Pract Today. 2007;1:295–300.
20. Broon NJ, Bramante CM, Assis GF, Bortoluzzi EA, Bernardineli N, Moraes IG, Garcia RB. Healing of root perforations treated with mineral trioxide aggregate (MTA) and Portland cement. J Appl Oral Sci. 2006;14:305–11.
21. Cho SY, Seo DG, Lee SJ, Lee J, Lee SJ, Jung IJ. Prognostic factors for clinical outcomes according to time after direct pulp capping. J Endod. 2013;39: 327–31.
22. Chong BS, Pitt Ford TR, Hudson MB. A prospective clinical study of Mineral Trioxide Aggregate and IRM when used as root-end filling materials in endodontic surgery. Int Endod J. 2003;36:520–6.
23. Coneglian PZA, Orosco FA, Bramante CM, Moraes IG, Garcia RB, Bernardineli N. In vitro sealing ability or white and gray mineral trioxide aggregate (MTA) and white Portland cement used as apical plug. J Appl Oral Sci. 2007;15:181–5.
24. D'Arcângelo C, D'Amario M. Use of MTA for orthograde obturation of nonvital teeth with open apices: report of two cases. Oral Surg Oral Med Oral Pathol Oral Radiol Endod. 2007;104:e98–e101.
25. DeDeus G, Coutinho Filho T. The use of white Portland cement as an apical plug in the tooth with a necrotic pulp and wide-open apex: a case report. Int Endod J. 2007;40:653–60.
26. Economides N, Pantelidou O, Kokkas A, Tziafas D. Short-term periradicular tissue response to mineral trioxide aggregate (MTA) as root-end filling material. Int Endod J. 2003;36:44–8.
27. El Meligy OAS, Avery DR. Comparison of apexification with mineral trioxide aggregate and calcium hydroxide. Pediatr Dent. 2006;28(3):248–53.
28. Faraco Júnior IM, Holland R. Response of the pulp of dogs to capping with mineral trioxide aggregate or a calcium hydroxide cement. Dent Traumatol. 2001;17: 163–6.
29. Felman D, Parashos P. Coronal tooth discoloration and white mineral trioxide aggregate. J Endod. 2013;39:484–7.
30. Felippe WT, Felippe MCS, Rocha MJC. The effect of mineral trioxide aggregate on the apexification and periapical healing of teeth with incomplete root formation. Int Endod J. 2006;39:2–9.
31. Ferris DM, Baumgartner JC. Perforation repair comparing two types of mineral trioxide aggregate. J Endod. 2004;30:422–4.
32. Fridland M, Rosado R. Mineral trioxide aggregate (MTA) solubility and porosity with different water-to-powder ratios. J Endod. 2003;29:814–7.
33. Geisler TM. Clinical considerations for regenerative endodontic procedures. Dent Clin North Am. 2012;56: 603–26.
34. Gharechahi M, Ghoddusi J. A nonsurgical endodontic treatment in open apex and immature teeth affected by dens invaginatus using a collagen membrane as an apical barrier. J Am Dent Assoc. 2012;143:144–8.
35. Ham KA, Witherspoon DE, Gutmann JL, Ravindranath S, Gait TC, Opperman LA. Preliminary evaluation of BMP-2 expression and histological characteristics during apexification with calcium hydroxide and mineral trioxide aggregate. J Endod. 2005;31:275–9.
36. Hamad HA, Tordik PA, Mcclanahan SB. Furcation perforation repair comparing gray and white MTA: a dye extraction study. J Endod. 2006;32:337–40.
37. Hashem AAR, Hassanien EE. ProRoot MTA, MTA-Angelus and IRM used to repair large furcation perforations: sealability study. J Endod. 2008;34:59–61.
38. Hayashi M, Shimizu A, Ebisu S. MTA for obturation of mandibular central incisors with open apices: case report. J Endod. 2004;30(2):120–2.
39. Holland R, Mazuqueli L, Souza V, Murata SS, Dezan Junior E. Influence of the type of vehicle and limit of obturation on apical and periapical tissue response in dogs teeth after root filling with mineral trioxide aggregate. J Endod. 2007;33:693–7.
40. Holland R, Otoboni Filho JA, Souza V, Nery MJ, Bernabé PFE, Dezan Junior E. Mineral trioxide aggregate repair of lateral root perforations. J Endod. 2001;27:281–4.
41. Holland R, Souza V, Murata SS, Nery MJ, Bernabé PFE, Otoboni Filho JA. Healing process of dog dental pulp after pulpotomy and pulp covering with mineral trioxide aggregate or Portland cement. Braz Dent J. 2001;12:109–13.
42. Holland R, Souza V, Nery MJ, Otoboni Filho JA, Bernabé PFE, Dezan Junior E. Reaction of dog's teeth to root canal filling with mineral trioxide aggregate or a glass ionomer sealer. J Endod. 1999;25:728–30.
43. Holland R. Histochemical response of the pulp of dogs to capping with mineral trioxide aggregate or a calcium hydroxide cement. Dent Traumatol. 2001;17: 163–6.
44. Hong ST, Bae KS, Baek SH, Kum KY, Lee WC. Microleakage of accelerated mineral trioxide aggregate and Portland cement an *in vitro* apexification model. J Endod. 2008;34:56–8.
45. Hsien H, Cheng YA, Lee YL, Lan NH, Lin CP. Repair of perforating internal resorption with mineral trioxide aggregate: a case report. J Endod. 2003;29:538–9.
46. Hulsmann M. Dens invaginatus: etiology, classification, prevalence, diagnosis and treatment considerations. Int Endod J. 1997;30:79–90.
47. Jantarat J, Daspher SJ, Messer HH. Effect of matrix placement on furcation perforation repair. J Endod. 1999;25:192–5.
48. Karabucak B, Li L, Lim J, Iqbal M. Vital pulp therapy with mineral trioxide aggregate. Dent Traumatol. 2005;21:240–3.

49. Karp J, Bryk J, Menke E, McTigue D. The complete endodontic obturation of an immature permanent incisor with mineral trioxide aggregate: a case report. Pediatr Dent. 2006;28:273–8.
50. Koh ET, Pitt Ford TR, Kariyawasam SP, Chen NN, Torabinejad M. Prophylactic treatment of dens evaginatus using mineral trioxide aggregate. J Endod. 2001;27:540–2.
51. Lamb EL, Loushine RJ, Weller RN, Kimbrough WF, Pashley DH. Effect of resection on the apical sealing ability of mineral trioxide aggregate. Oral Surg Oral Med Oral Pathol Oral Radiol Endod. 2003;95:732–5.
52. Lee SJ, Monsef M, Torabinejad M. Sealing ability of a mineral trioxide aggregate for repair of lateral root perforations. J Endod. 1993;19:541–4.
53. Lima MV, Bramante CM, Garcia RB, Moraes IG, Bernardineli N. Endodontic treatment of dens in dente associated with a chronic periapical lesion using an apical plug of mineral trioxide aggregate. Quintessence Int. 2007;38:41–5.
54. Main C, Mirzayan N, Shabahang S, Torabinejad M. Repair of root perforations using mineral trioxide aggregate: a long-term study. J Endod. 2004;30: 80–3.
55. Martin RL, Monticelli F, Brackett WW, Loushine RJ, Rockman RA, Ferrari M, Pashley DH, Tay FR. Sealing properties of mineral trioxide aggregate orthograde apical plugs and root filling an *in vitro* apexification model. J Endod. 2007;33:272–5.
56. Menezes RS, Bramante CM, Letra A, Carvalho VGG, Garcia RB. Histologic evaluation of pulpotomies in dog using two types of mineral trioxide aggregate and regular and white Portland cement as wound dressings. Oral Surg Oral Med Oral Pathol Oral Radiol Endod. 2004;98:376–9.
57. Menezes RS, Silva Neto UX, Carneiro E, Letra A, Bramante CM, Bernardineli N. MTA repair of a subcrestal perforation: a case report. J Endod. 2005;31: 212–4.
58. Mente J, Geletneky B, Ohle M, Koch MJ, Ding PGF, Wolf D, Dreyhaupt J, Martin N, Staehle HJ, Pfefferle T. Mineral trioxide aggregate or calcium hydroxide direct pulp capping: an analysis of clinical treatment outcome. J Endod. 2010;36:806–13.
59. Mente J, Hage N, Pfefferle T, Koch MJ, Dreyhaupt J, Staehle HJ, Friedman S. Mineral trioxide aggregate apical plugs in teeth with open apical foramina: a retrospective analysis of treatment outcome. J Endod. 2009;35:1354–8.
60. Mente J, Hage N, Pfefferle T, Koch MJ, Geletneky B, Dreyhaupt J, Martin N, Staehle HJ. Treatment outcome of mineral trioxide aggregate: repair of root perforations. J Endod. 2010;36:208–13.
61. Mente J, Leo M, Panagidis D, Ohle M, Schneider S, Bermejo JL, Pfefferle T. Treatment outcome of mineral trioxide aggregate in open apex teeth. J Endod. 2013;39:20–6.
62. Mooney GC, North S. The current opinions and use of MTA for apical barrier formation of non-vital immature permanent incisors by consultants in pediatric dentistry in the UK. Dent Traumatol. 2008;24:65–9.
63. Moroto M, Barberia E, Planells P, Vera V. Treatment of a non-vital immature incisor with mineral trioxide aggregate (MTA). Dent Traumatol. 2003;19: 165–9.
64. Nygaard-Ostby B, Hjortdal O. Tissue formation in the root canal following pulp removal. Scand J Dent Res. 1971;79:333–43.
65. Nosrat A, Nekoofar MH, Bolhari B, Dummer PMH. Unintentional extrusion of mineral trioxide aggregate: a report of three cases. Int Endod J. 2012;45: 1165–76.
66. Oehler FAC. Dens invaginatus (dilated composite odontome) I-variations of the invagination process and associated anterior crows form. Oral Surg Oral Med Oral Pathol. 1957;10:1204–18.
67. O'Sullivan SM, Hartwell GR. Obturation of retained primary mandibular second molar using mineral trioxide aggregate: a case report. J Endod. 2001;27: 703–5.
68. Ozdemir HO, Ozçelik B, Karabucak B, Cehreli ZC. Calcium ion diffusion from mineral trioxide aggregate through simulated root resorption defects. Dent Traumatol. 2008;24:70–3.
69. Pace R, Giuliani V, Pini Prato L, Baccetti T, Pagavino G. Apical plug technique using mineral trioxide aggregate; results from a case series. Int Endod J. 2007; 40:478–84.
70. Panzarini SR, Holland R, Souza V, Poi WR, Sonoda CK, Pedrini D. Mineral trioxide aggregate as a root canal filling material in reimplanted teeth. Microscopic analysis in monkeys. Dent Traumatol. 2007;23: 265–72.
71. Pariroki M, Asgary S, Eghbal MJ, Stowe S, Eslami B, Eskandarizade A, Shabahang S. A comparative study of white and grey mineral trioxide aggregate as pulp capping agents in dog's teeth. Dent Traumatatol. 2005;21:150–4.
72. Pelliccioni GA, Vellani CP, Gatto MRA, Gandolfi MG, Marchetti C, Prati C. Proroot mineral trioxide aggregate cement used as retrograde filling without addition of water: an *in vitro* evaluation of its microleakage. J Endod. 2007;33:1082–5.
73. Petrins JA, Boda KK, Shambarger S, Bowles WR, Mc Clanahan SB. Challenges in regenerative endodontics: a case series. J Endod. 2010;36:536–41.
74. Pitt Ford TR, Torabinejad M, Abedi HR, Bakland LK, Kariyawasam SP. Using mineral trioxide aggregate as a pulp-capping material. J Am Dent Assoc. 1996;127: 1491–4.
75. Queiroz AM, Assed S, Leonardo MR, Nelson Filho P, Silva LAB. MTA and calcium hydroxide for pulp capping. J Appl Oral Sci. 2005;13:126–30.
76. Rafter M, Baker M, Alves M, Daniel J, Remeikis N. Evaluation of healing with use of an internal matrix to repair furcation perforations. Int Endod J. 2002;36: 775–83.
77. Sarris S, Tahmassebi JF, Duggal MS, Croos IA. A clinical evaluation of mineral trioxide aggregate for root-end closure of non-vital immature permanent incisors in children-a pilot study. Dent Traumatol. 2008;24:79–85.

78. Simon S, Rilliard F, Berdal A, Machtou P. The use of mineral trioxide aggregate in one-visit apexification treatment: a prospective study. Int Endod J. 2007;40: 186–97.
79. Torabinejad M, Hong CU, Lee SJ, Monsef M, Pitt Ford TR. Investigation of mineral trioxide aggregate for root-end filling in dogs. J Endod. 1995;21: 603–8.
80. Torabinejad M, Lee SJ, Hong UC. Apical marginal adaptation of orthograde and retrograde root-end fillings: a dye leakage and scanning electron microscopic study. J Endod. 1994;20:402–7.
81. Torabinejad M, Pitt Ford TR, McKendry DJ, Abedi HR, Miller DA, Kariyawasam SP. Histologic assessment of mineral trioxide aggregate as a root end filling in monkeys. J Endod. 1997;23:225–8.
82. Torabinejad M, Watson TF, Pitt Ford TR. Sealing ability of a mineral trioxide aggregate when used as a root-end filling material. J Endod. 1993;19: 591–5.
83. Tziafas D, Pantelidou O, Alvanou A, Belibasakis G, Papadimitriou S. The dentinogenic effect of mineral trioxide aggregate (MTA) in short-term capping experiments. Int Endod J. 2002;35:245–54.
84. Valois CRA, Costa ED. Influence of the thickness of mineral trioxide aggregate on sealing ability of root-end fillings *in vitro*. Oral Surg Oral Med Oral Pathol Oral Radiol Endod. 2004;97:108–11.
85. Vivan RR, Ordinola-Zapata R, Zeferino MA, Bramante CM, Bernardineli N, Garcia RB, Duarte MA, Tanomaru-Filho M, Moraes IG. Evaluation of the physical and chemical properties of two commercial and three experimental root-end filling materials. Oral Surg Oral Med Oral Pathol Oral Radiol Endod. 2010;110:250–6.
86. Vizgirda PJ, Liewehr FR, Patton WR, McPherson JC, Buxton TB. Comparison of laterally condensed gutta-percha, thermoplasticized gutta-percha and mineral trioxide aggregate as root canal filling materials. J Endod. 2004;30:103–6.
87. Yildrim T, Gençoglu N, Firat I, Guzel O. Histologic study of furcation perforation treated with MTA or Super EBA in dog teeth. Oral Surg Oral Med Oral Pathol Oral Radiol Endod. 2005;100:120–4.

7 Material Modifications and Related Materials

Jamileh Ghoddusi

7.1 Introduction

During the past decades, the introduction of biocompatible sealing materials has facilitated performing an effective and efficient endodontic procedure. Although this revolutionary phase has not necessarily made endodontic treatment easy, better materials and improved technology have enabled the clinician to provide a better treatment in a wide range of complicated cases.

Since 1993, the basic principles of endodontic therapy have been strictly followed, and introduction of *mineral trioxide aggregate* (MTA) [110] maximizes the predictability of optimal treatment outcomes in compromised cases such as sealing the open apex or perforated area, retrograde filling, and also covering the vital pulp tissue during the endodontic procedure [72].

However, it should be noted that MTA has some drawbacks that have made it difficult to use in some cases. A questionnaire-based study [64] on postgraduate students in operative dentistry in the UK revealed that factors preventing the use of MTA in permanent and primary dentition are related to the material cost and the lack of evidence, respectively.

Another survey conducted in Turkey among the senior members of the endodontic departments of fourteen dental schools revealed that they used MTA in their clinical practice, apexification, perforations, retrograde fillings, and root resorption as the most common treatment procedure. Financial limitation was the main reason for negative responses, followed by other factors such as the difficult handling properties and low radiopacity of the material [158].

MTA has been used for several applications such as root perforation repair, root-end filling, and vital pulp therapy and as an apical plug; therefore, its essential properties for each treatment are expected to be different. For example, serving as a suitable retrograde filling material, apical plug, and perforation repair materials requires intimate sealing capacity, insolubility, biocompatibility, and promotion of tissue regeneration without provoking inflammation and mechanical strength; the latter however will not be an important factor for capping materials in vital pulp therapies.

To improve the undesirable properties of MTA (i.e., setting time, handling, antibacterial effect, discoloration), researchers have attempted to add some materials to its formulation. As some of the essential properties of MTA have been negatively changed, it is important to note that for gaining a suitable modification, all essential properties of the new material should be taken into consideration.

J. Ghoddusi, DDS, MSc
Department of Endodontics, Dental Research Center, School of Dentistry, Mashhad University of Medical Sciences, 984, Vakilabad Blvd, Mashhad 91735, Iran
e-mail: ghoddusij@mums.ac.ir

J. Camilleri (ed.), *Mineral Trioxide Aggregate in Dentistry*,
DOI 10.1007/978-3-642-55157-4_7, © Springer-Verlag Berlin Heidelberg 2014

7.2 Modifications

7.2.1 Improving the Setting Time

The materials used in oral cavity should ideally have a rather short setting time to avoid being washed away by saliva and to reduce the possibility of the unset materials present in the mouth which may cause oral tissue irritation [2]. Being very grainy and having a poor consistency make it difficult to use MTA in some of the clinical applications. Unfortunately, MTA is assumed as a difficult material to handle because of its granular consistency [106], slow setting time [44], and low compressive strength [67, 106] compared to other materials and being loose early after mixing [162]. To improve its application in endodontics, the development of a new formulation(s) of MTA is necessary to optimize both the strength and the setting time without compromising its other advantages [31].

Kao et al. [100] used reagent grade SiO_2, CaO, and Al_2O_3 powders as matrix materials and MgO, ZnO, and Fe_2O_3 powders as additives to produce an MTA-like cement. These cements exhibited a significantly faster setting time (14 min) than MTA when mixed with water, although there was a significant decrease in diametric tensile strength, ranging from 0.9 to 3.1 MPa in comparison with MTA (4.4 MPa). The addition of ZnO, MgO, and Fe_2O_3 to the MTA-like cement led to significantly higher strength compared to the original MTA. The pH values of the MTA-like cements were changed from 11 to 13, similar to the results obtained with MTA.

7.2.1.1 Excluding the Gypsum

In industry, the setting time of the *Portland cement* is modified at the end stage of the manufacturing process by grinding the cement with calcium sulfate (gypsum). All dental materials using Portland cement as the main cementitious phase will thus include some gypsum in the formulation. This inadvertently retards the material set. Removal of the gypsum results in a flash set, which may be controlled by the application of a superplasticizing admixture to increase the effectiveness of the material.

A novel cement *Proto A* was produced by inter-grinding the cement clinker without gypsum and mixing it with water and superplasticizer. It has been shown that both Proto A and MTA were made from similar constituent elements and phases, namely, tricalcium and dicalcium silicate. The setting time of a Portland cement may be reduced by excluding the gypsum during the final stage of the manufacturing process without affecting its other properties. The new prototype cement has improved workability and a reduced setting time. This could reduce a chairside time and the number of visits [32]. A new technique for biocompatibility evaluation was employed for testing of these new prototypes [44]. The biocompatibility of the test materials was assessed by a direct test method using Alamar Blue dye, which quantitatively evaluated the cell viability. Indirect test method was also used for evaluation of cells grown on material elution. The results showed the presence of no toxic leachable substances from the experimental materials. Cell growth was poor when seeded in direct contact with cements. Both cements were shown to have similar biocompatibility.

7.2.1.2 Addition of Calcium Aluminate

Mixtures of calcium aluminate cement and Portland cement result in a fast setting material with an associated reduction in compressive strength of the resultant material [43]. The compressive strength and setting time can be improved by adding calcium sulfate in the anhydrous form to the mixture of Portland cement and calcium aluminate cement thus creating a calcium sulfoaluminate. The physical properties and handling properties can be improved further by a reduction in the water to cement ratio. This is achieved through an application of the superplasticizing admixture. The physical and mechanical properties of two experimental types of Portland cement (calcium sulfoaluminate and calcium flouro-aluminate cement) when mixed with the superplasticizer were compared [31]. They showed satisfactory setting times and compressive strength values in comparison with glass ionomer cement.

7.2.1.3 Hydration Accelerators

Many studies have been conducted on $CaCl_2$ as a hydration accelerator mixed with MTA. A dental Portland cement accelerated with calcium chloride was initially introduced by Aquilina in 1999 at Guy's Hospital, London. This was followed by an investigation to evaluate the biocompatibility of the accelerated Portland cement [2]. An addition of 10 or 15 % $CaCl_2$ to the Portland cement as an accelerant has no adverse effect on the biocompatibility of MTA mixture. This study indicated that acceleration of Portland cement by adding the $CaCl_2$ stimulates the proliferation of SaOS-2 cells in vitro and actively supports a biological response in these cells through the production of cytokines like IL-1β, IL-6, IL-18, and osteocalcin. Many researchers have shown that modified ProRoot MTA has lower setting time [6, 18, 109, 173] and better handling, but lower compressive strength [106, 109] in comparison with unmodified MTA. Improvement in the sealing ability of the MTA and Portland cement mixed with calcium chloride has also been demonstrated [25, 90].

Some researchers used calcium nitrate and calcium formate as an accelerator mixed with the MTA and gained similar findings [173]. One of the most important criteria for using materials in contact with human tissues is biocompatibility. The biocompatibility of the MTA mixed with calcium chloride, calcium nitrate, or calcium formate was assessed, and these accelerators may be a biocompatible alternative when a rapid set is indicated [118]. The addition of calcium chloride to the MTA did not change the biological properties in the formation of mineralized barrier after pulpotomy [24]. Conversely, other researchers demonstrated that the addition of $CaCl_2$ to MTA as a pulp capping biomaterial has a deteriorating effect on calcific bridge formation, inflammation, and necrosis in dogs' teeth [134].

The early application of the endodontic irrigants may weaken the bond strength in the interface between accelerated MTA and dentin [91]. Therefore, after using MTA mixed with $CaCl_2$ for perforation repair, its exposure to the NaOCl irrigation during early setting phase caused an improvement in the push-out strength of the accelerated MTA and an increase in formation of calcium hydroxide crystals on the surface of accelerated MTA.

Calcium lactate gluconate (CLG) has also been mixed with MTA in order to improve the setting time and handling properties. A reduced setting time, inferior compressive strength, and lower pH in MTA mixed with CLG [109] were reported, although its sealing ability was improved [92] and adequate biocompatibility [98] was observed. The biocompatibility of MTA mixed with different hydration accelerators such as calcium chloride, calcium lactate gluconate, and citric acid was assessed [99]. The most favorable biocompatibility was observed in 0.1 wt% citric acid group. In addition, 10 wt% $CaCl_2$ showed poor cell viability and indicated less cell attachment in SEM evaluation.

In other studies, disodium hydrogen orthophosphate (Na_2HPO_4) was used instead of water to be mixed with MTA [56, 93]. A significant reduction in the setting time (26 min) was shown when 15 % Na_2HPO_4 was added to the MTA without adverse effects on the diametric tensile strength. Ding et al. [56] observed biocompatibility of Na_2HPO_4 solution mixed MTA on L929 cells.

For increasing the working time of MTA, some researchers added an alternative delivery vehicle, KY Jelly (Johnson and Johnson, New Brunswick, NJ) [106]. Its cellular toxicity appears to be acceptable [102]; however, the most important issue that needs to be ruled out is whether this composition offers suitable biological activity for routine clinical use. To date, no documents have supported other important properties of this material.

7.2.1.4 Finer Particle Size Modification

A novel mineral trioxide aggregate (MTA Plus; Avalon Biomed Inc., Bradenton, FL, USA) has been introduced which has a similar composition to MTA but is ground finer; thus, the material has a higher specific surface area [39]. MTA Plus is provided with either a hydrosoluble gel or water ampoules for mixing. When used with anti-washout gel, its washout was reduced [65]. The high specific surface area increases the rate of reaction but does not necessarily reduce the setting time. The high rate of reaction was demonstrated by an increased release of calcium hydroxide in solution [39].

A new version of MTA has been patented in the USA and claimed to set faster with acceptable resistance to acidic environmental conditions by adding a small amount of strontium and reducing the particle size (US Patent application No. 13/211.880). Based on previous investigations [145–147], the nano-modification of the MTA with nanoparticles of strontium has resulted in reduction in the setting time and the surface porosity and increase in acid resistance, microhardness, and compressive strength.

7.2.2 Handling Improvement

The hardened MTA mixture is influenced by several factors: quantity of water during mixing, the procedure for mixing, pressure used for compaction, environment humidity, and temperature [162]. Many clinicians subjectively have reported that the handling properties of MTA are not ideal thus creating an apical plug, or perforation repair and obturation of the tooth in a single visit were not possible [5].

MTA is difficult to manipulate due to its dry consistency [30]. To improve this consistency, propylene glycol has been proposed and added to MTA Angelus [57]. The mixture of MTA with the ratio of 80 % distilled water and 20 % propylene glycol is favorable, but increasing the PG proportion interfered with setting time. The effect(s) of using the volume of 100 % on setting time has yet to be observed.

7.2.3 Enhancement of the Antibacterial Properties

The antibacterial and antifungal properties of the MTA have been extensively evaluated and conflicting results have been reported [62, 89, 121, 155, 163, 176, 180]. Several investigations reported that MTA has limited antimicrobial effect against some microorganisms [62, 121, 176]. MTA has an antibacterial effect on some facultative bacteria and no effect on any species of strict anaerobes [163]. To enhance the antimicrobial properties of MTA, some investigators replaced distilled water with some antimicrobial reagents such as chlorhexidine [86, 89, 106, 120, 152, 155, 156, 174], iodoform [52, 144], sodium hypochlorite [97, 106, 174], and silver zeolite [129].

Although many studies showed that substituting 0.12 % chlorhexidine gluconate with water enhanced the antimicrobial properties of MTA [120, 155], it should be noted that this mixture may cause cell apoptosis [86] and a decrease in the compressive strength of MTA [89]. Conversely, the implantation of a mixture of MTA and chlorhexidine subcutaneously resulted in no adverse effect on the tissue response [156]. In addition, MTA mixed with chlorhexidine leads to antibacterial effects against *E. faecalis* for at least 48 h [120].

The use of 3 % NaOCl gel mixed MTA resulted in freshly mixed MTA having a lower cell viability than the set one [97]. Iodoform in combination with MTA has been used for enhancing the antibacterial effect and showed no improvement in antimicrobial properties of MTA [144]. No significant difference in inflammatory tissue responses between MTA and Portland cement when mixed with iodoform was observed [52].

According to the results of the aforementioned investigations, it seems that improving selective properties of MTA such as setting time and antibacterial properties, by adding some liquids, may adversely affect other advantages of the material. New compositions of MTA should be evaluated comprehensively before their recommendation for clinical application.

7.2.4 Reducing the Discoloration

Although white MTA was developed to solve the problem of tooth discoloration produced by gray MTA, several studies have reported tooth discoloration after using both kinds of MTA [27, 96, 101, 135, 166]. This effect limits the application of MTA in aesthetically sensitive areas for treatment of perforations, pulp capping, and pulpotomy and as an apical barrier recommended to seal the dentinal tubules by dentin bonding agents before using both types of MTA is recommended to prevent further tooth discoloration [4]. Removing the discolored dentin and internal bleaching has also been recommended to improve the aesthetic following the use of MTAs [17].

7.2.5 Elimination of the Heavy Metals

A major concern regarding the use of cements like MTA which are made from naturally occurring minerals is the amount of leachable arsenic and lead present in material components. According to the ISO 9917, the leachable lead and arsenic must be less than 100 and 2 ppm, respectively [140]. Many researchers [54, 58, 117] reported that MTA and Portland cement displayed very low amount of arsenic release; hence, no contraindication was demonstrated for its use in clinical practice regarding the presence of this chemical element. It has been recommended to use in a very small amount, e.g., less than 1 g, in clinical endodontic procedure [123]. Thus, the recorded amount of 34.27 mg arsenic per kilogram of material for gray Portland cement leads to 34.27 μg of arsenic per gram of MTA cement which is less than the toxic dose (140–210 mg for an individual weighing 70 kg).

A water-based cement labeled as MTA Bio (Angelus, Londrina, PR, Brazil) has been marketed with the aim of avoiding the presence of arsenic and lead. MTA Bio have been claimed to be fully synthesized in a laboratory under controlled, clean, and segregated conditions to ensure that the final product is free of contamination. According to the manufacturer, as a consequence of high-quality control of the cement production, the final cement is free of undesirable contaminant substances, in particular, arsenic. Compared to the original MTA, its similar sealing ability [55], shorter setting time [169], and low cytotoxic effects [113] on cultures of odontoblast-like cells have been demonstrated.

Novel formulations of root-end filling materials are based mostly on tricalcium silicate. Tricalcium silicate cement exhibited a similar microstructure and hydration characteristics to Portland cement [36]. Tricalcium silicate cement and materials based on this latter cement, namely, Biodentine and Bioaggregate, exhibited a low-level release of acid-extractable trace elements [42]. Thus, tricalcium silicate can be a suitable substitution to the Portland component in MTA.

7.2.6 Light-Curable MTA-Like Materials

The use of a number of resin systems has been reported with the main ones being light-curing systems Bis-GMA and a biocompatible resin [73, 74]; 2-hydroxyethyl methacrylate (HEMA), tetraethylene glycol dimethacrylate (TEGDMA), camphorquinone, and ethyl-4-(dimethylamino) benzoate (EDMAB) and with and without polyacrylic co-maleic acid [69, 70]; Bis-GMA and TEGDMA [66]; and Bis-GMA, pyromellitic acid diethylmethacrylate (PMDM), and HEMA [141]. The light-curing systems proposed so far have exhibited alkalinizing pH, calcium ion release, formation of apatite [66, 69], and functional groups able to chelate calcium ions [69]. Furthermore, therapeutic remineralization of dentin was observed [69, 70, 141, 150]. The light-cure MTA was well accepted by the alveolar tissue of rats, with the formation of mineralized tissue close to the materials [74]. It presented a moderate chronic inflammatory response at 30 days that decreased at 60 days but was more intense than with MTA Angelus and without dystrophic calcifications. It was possible to conclude that light-cure MTA was similar to MTA at 60 days, but it did not stimulate mineralization [73]. Regardless the calcium-releasing ability and the bioactivity, little or no hydration was exhibited by resin-modified MTA. Reaction rims around the cement particles were absent, and the formation and leaching of calcium hydroxide was shown to be negligible [66].

7.2.7 Replacement the Radiopacifiers

Bismuth oxide was added in 1:4 proportions as radiopacifier to the MTA so the material could easily be distinguished from the surrounding anatomical structures on a radiograph. Bismuth oxide in MTA does not act as inert material. The bismuth replaces the silicon in the calcium silicate structure [33]. Furthermore, only 8 % of bismuth in the oxide form was present in the set material, while the un-hydrated MTA presented 21.6 % bismuth oxide. Leaching in increasing amounts was also shown for bismuth in ProRoot MTA [33]. Studies reported that the cytotoxicity of Portland cement containing bismuth oxide (BPC) was higher than that of PC after a short-term culture period of 1 day, whereas this cytotoxic effect was recovered during the long-term culturing [119]. Bismuth oxide induces cell death [45]. On the contrary, other researchers showed that BPC exhibited greater radiopacity and similar biocompatibility to PC in human periodontal ligament cells [105]. Bismuth oxide is used in a number of dental materials particularly root canal sealers. It has always been associated with tooth discoloration. Reports of discoloration of MTA with resultant tooth discoloration are found in the literature. The discoloration of MTA has been associated with a lack of oxygen in the root canal [166, 167] and also as a result of reaction with sodium hypochlorite used for root canal irrigation [38].

The bismuth oxide in MTA can be replaced by other radiopacifying materials. Ideally, an alternative radiopacifier should only impart the necessary radiopacity to the cement and should be inert, free from any contaminants, colorless, and nontoxic and be added in minimal amounts. Addition of gold powder, silver/tin alloy [40], barium sulfate [26, 40, 95], iodoform [26], zirconium oxide [26, 49], zinc oxide [40, 95], lead oxide, bismuth subnitrate, bismuth carbonate, and calcium tungstate [95] results in a radiopacity value of more than 3 mm of the aluminum scale. The gold powder was completely inert and was not leached out in solution [35]. The main disadvantages with using gold to replace the bismuth oxide in MTA include the cost of the gold and also the resultant color of the cement imparted by the gold. A filler loading of 30 % zirconium oxide to Portland cement mixed at a water to cement proportion of 0.3 resulted in a material with comparable properties to mineral trioxide aggregate. Addition of zirconium oxide powder as radiopacifying material did not seem to affect the compressive strength of the resultant material [49].

7.3 Related Materials

Root-end filling material is placed in contact with the periradicular tissue and thus requires biocompatibility as its main property. Therefore, an ideal root-end filling material should be nontoxic, noncarcinogenic, biocompatible with the host tissue, dimensionally stable, insoluble in tissue fluids, antibacterial, radiopaque, easy to manipulate, have adequate working time with fast setting time, and adhere to the tooth structure.

Some examples of the endodontic materials are gutta-percha, zinc oxide eugenol-based cements, composite resin, glass ionomer cements, gold foil, polycarboxylate cements, polyvinyl cements, and amalgam. Unfortunately, most of them have shown different levels of weakness in biocompatibility, leakage, solubility, handling properties, moisture incompatibility, and cost.

Although nowadays MTA has been thoroughly examined and revealed promising results, the ideal root-end filling material has yet to be found. New materials have claimed to have all the advantages of MTA without any of its drawbacks. More evidence is required to support these materials as an improved MTA or as its new alternatives. In this section, new products with new formulation, with similar application to MTA, are discussed (summarized in Table 7.1). According to the findings from Owadally and Pitt Ford's investigation [132], newly formulated products should be evaluated to determine whether they have compatible properties even when the majority of its constituents are similar to those of MTA.

7.3.1 Tricalcium Silicate-Based Endodontic Repair Cements

7.3.1.1 Bioaggregate

Bioaggregate (Innovative BioCeramic, Vancouver, Canada) is a relatively new product containing calcium silicate hydrate, calcium hydroxide,

Table 7.1 Characteristics of some related materials

Base materials	Derivatives	Composition	Properties
Tricalcium silicate-based endodontic materials	Bioaggregate	Calcium silicate hydrate + calcium hydroxide + hydroxyapatite + tantalum oxide + amorphous silicon oxide	Nontoxic [53, 175, 177, 182], nontoxic [104], antibacterial effect [180], sealing ability [59, 108], fracture resistant [164]
	EndoSequence root repair material	Calcium silicate + monobasic calcium phosphate + zirconium oxide + tantatum oxide + filler agent	Bioactive [5, 88, 115, 153], not bioactive [122], sealing ability [127], not sealing ability [87], antibacterial [114]
	Biodentine	Tricalcium silicate + calcium carbonate + zirconium oxide + calcium chloride	Remineralization induction [81], odontoblast differentiation [107], adverse effect on the dentin toughness [111, 151], not sealing ability [37], low porosity [41]
	Calcium-enriched mixture (CEM)	Calcium hydroxide + calcium oxide + calcium phosphate + calcium sulfate + calcium silicate + calcium carbonate	Hydroxyapatite formation [13], sealing ability [11, 84, 103], antimicrobial [14, 83], acceptable cytotoxicity [15, 125], suitable biocompatibility [1, 136], induce hard tissue formation [142], suitable for vital pulp therapy [8–10, 12, 63, 116, 128, 157]
	Generex A	Calcium silicate + unique gels + hydroxyapatite	Suitable compressive strength, washout resistant and setting time [139]
	Capasio	Calcium aluminosilicate + dental glass + bismuth oxide	Adequate physical and chemical properties [139], promote apatite deposition [138], osteoblast growth and nodule formation [171]
	Theracal	CaO + calcium silicate particles + strontium glass + fumed silica + barium sulfate + barium zirconate + resin containing Bis-GMA and PEGDMA	Calcium ion release and hydroxyapatite formation [68], decreasing cell metabolism [85]
Endodontic cements not based on tricalcium silicate	Calcium aluminate cement	Calcium aluminate + calcium dialuminate	Rapid setting, good flow, improved handling properties, high mechanical strength, reduced porosity [131]
	EndoBinder	Calcium aluminate based	Adequate physical and chemical properties [130], biocompatible [3, 48]
	Castor oil	Polymer derived from the castor oil plant (triglyceride of ricinoleic acid)	Antibacterial [165], biocompatible [22, 112], acceptable cytotoxicity and genotoxicity [28, 29], sealing ability [51]
	Ceramicrete D	Phosphosilicate ceramic + hydroxyapatite + cerium oxide + deionized water	Sealing ability [108], clinical handling and washout resistant [139]

hydroxyapatite, tantalum oxide, and amorphous silicon oxide, which is intended to be used for perforation repair and as a retrograde filling material. In a study using X-ray diffraction analysis [137], the absence of aluminum-based compounds was demonstrated. Furthermore, tantalum oxide has been included as a radiopacifier. The hydrated material released less calcium in solution than Biodentine [79]. In vitro studies [53, 175, 177, 182] revealed that Bioaggregate is nontoxic to human fibroblasts and osteoblasts. In addition, it may induce fibroblast differentiation and expression of the mineralization-association gene in osteoblasts.

On evaluation of the systemic toxic effect of MTA and Bioaggregate on the kidney and liver, some adverse effects on liver and kidney cells in rats were demonstrated. The effect of MTA was significantly more severe than the Bioaggregate [104]. Evaluation of an antibacterial activity of this cement against *E. faecalis* revealed comparable results with MTA which was even enhanced after addition of the dentin powder [180]. Its sealing ability has been assessed by dye [59] and glucose [108] leakage, and results indicated similar ability to MTA as a root-end filling material. In one study [164], fracture resistance of immature teeth filled with Bioaggregate was higher than MTA, suggesting this cement can be used in immature teeth, as a root canal filling material.

7.3.1.2 EndoSequence Root Repair Material

Recently, a new root repair material has been introduced to the market: *EndoSequence Root Repair Material* (ERRM; Brasseler, Savannah, GA). According to the manufacturer, it is composed of calcium silicate, monobasic calcium phosphate, zirconium oxide, tantatum oxide, and filler agents and is available as paste in preloaded syringes and also in a moldable putty form. The preloaded syringe also has intracanal tips that can be bent to facilitate its placement in clinical situations. According to the manufacturer instruction, it has a working time of 30 min and a setting reaction initiated by moisture with a final set achieved approximately 4 h thereafter.

Although in one study, elutes of ERRM significantly reduced the bioactivity and alkaline phosphatase activity of human osteoblast-like cells [122], the results of other studies conducted on its bioactivity revealed that it may have cell viability similar to MTA in both set and fresh conditions [5, 88, 115, 153]. Sealing ability of this novel material was compared with MTA, and the results showed no significant difference in bacterial leakage between either of them [127]. In contrast, by using a bacterial leakage model [87], it was concluded that samples in ERRM group leaked significantly more than those in MTA group.

Antibacterial activity of ERRM was compared with MTA, and results demonstrated similar antimicrobial properties during their setting reaction against ten clinical strains of *E. faecalis* [114]. In an in vitro study [82], simulated root resorption defects were prepared, and after filling the root canal with either ERRM or MTA, the pH at the root surface of the teeth was measured. In the ERRM group, pH values declined during the first 24 h, and its 1-week evaluation was comparable with MTA during the 1st and 2nd weeks [82].

7.3.1.3 Biodentine

Biodentine is manufactured by Septodont (Septodont, Saint-Maur-Fosses Codex, France) and is composed of tricalcium silicate, calcium carbonate, and zirconium oxide as the radiopacifier, while its liquid form contains calcium chloride as the setting accelerator and water-reducing agent. This composition has been verified in a recent publication [46]. The calcium chloride accelerates the setting time of Biodentine, while the other additives enhance the physical properties [80]. According to the manufacturer, Biodentine is produced using a novel technological platform called Active Biosilicate Technology, which guarantees the purity of the material. An investigation of the presence of leachable arsenic, lead, and chromium from Biodentine exhibited the low levels of toxic heavy elements in this material [42]. The fine particle size [46] accompanied by the presence of calcium carbonate which enhances the material hydration results in the release of calcium hydroxide in solution [79]. A study demonstrated the formation of a silicate- and calcium-rich layer in dentin in contact with Biodentine and MTA. Silicon is known to enhance the rate of new bone growth and also induce remineralization of demineralized dentin when released from bioactive materials [81].

When Biodentine is applied directly onto the pulp, it induces an early odontoblast differentiation and the initiation of mineralization, probably due to a modulation of TGF-β1 secretion from the dental pulp cell [107]. Prolonged contact of mineralized dentin with calcium silicate-based materials, such as Biodentine, has an adverse effect on the dentin toughness and integrity of the dentin collagen matrix; therefore, caution is recommended when these materials are applied to the thin dentinal walls [111, 151].

When Biodentine was used as a dentin replacement material in the sandwich technique overlaying with composite, significant leakage occurred at the dentin-material interface [37]. Drying of Biodentine results in cracking and micro-leakage. Biodentine exhibits very low porosity when compared to MTA Bioaggregate and intermediate restorative material (IRM) (Dentsply Caulk, Milford, Delaware) [41].

7.3.1.4 Calcium-Enriched Mixture

Asgary et al. [16] introduced a new endodontic cement in 2008 to combine the superior biocompatibility of MTA with appropriate setting time (less than 1 h), handling characteristics, chemical properties, and reasonable price. This newly formulated biomaterial, named *calcium-enriched mixture* (CEM) cement (BioniqueDent, Tehran, Iran), was made using different calcium compounds; the patent is granted from US Patent and Trademark Office (USPTO) (endodontic filling material; USA, 7,942,961, 2011 May 17).

The manufacturer claimed that the mixed paste of CEM is not sticky; it does not tend to adhere to the applicator and can be easily condensed by the operator. In addition, some calcium compounds in CEM such as calcium sulfate and calcium silicate may cause a slight expansion of the material through continuous hydration after initial setting of the material and further crystalline maturation.

The results of recent investigations revealed that CEM comprises water-soluble calcium and phosphate ions and forms hydroxyapatite after setting [13]. Its sealing ability as a root-end filling material has been also evaluated and comparable results with MTA have been shown [11, 84, 103]. In presence of saliva contaminations, CEM showed superior sealing ability compared to MTA [84].

Antimicrobial properties of CEM against gram-negative, gram-positive, and cocci/bacilli bacteria were compared with MTA and calcium hydroxide (CH) using *agar diffusion test*. Results showed comparable antibacterial effects with CH and significantly better results than MTA [14, 83]. In addition, recent studies in cell culture revealed its cytotoxicity to be within acceptable range [15, 125], suitable biocompatibility [1, 136], and ability to induce hard tissue formation [142]. The results of in vivo studies on dogs showed that as pulp capping materials, MTA and CEM showed similar favorable biological outcomes, and both better than CH especially in terms of inducing the formation of the dentinal bridge [12, 157]. In several clinical trials in primary and permanent teeth [8–10, 63, 116, 128], CEM was used as a vital pulp therapy agent, and results indicated that the performance of new biomaterials may trend toward more biological treatments.

7.3.1.5 Generex A

Generex A (Dentsply Tulsa Dental Specialties, Tulsa, OK) is a calcium silicate-based material with similarities to ProRoot MTA. However, Generex A is mixed with unique gels instead of water and, together with a powder consistency, results in improved material handling and shorter setting time. Generex A powders contain hydroxyapatite to nucleate the production of hydroxyapatite in vivo which might be responsible for acceleration of osteoblastic activity in rats [170]. In addition, in an in vitro study, its compressive strength, washout resistance, and setting time were found to be better than MTA [139].

7.3.1.6 Capasio

Capasio (Primus Consulting, Bradenton, FL) is the new calcium aluminosilicate-based material which has been introduced in an effort to improve the weaknesses of previous materials. It is composed primarily of bismuth oxide, dental glass, and calcium aluminosilicate with a water-based gel. Upon the final setting (e.g., 9 min), this material is slightly more acidic (pH = 10.9) than WMTA (pH = 11.6). Moreover, it has demonstrated similar or improved physical characteristics such as setting time, radiopacity, compressive strength, pH, and washout resistance [139].

When used as a root-end filling material, Capasio is more likely to penetrate dentinal tubules, and similar to MTA, it promotes apatite deposition when exposed to synthetic tissue fluid [138]. In a comparative study, Capasio has not been shown to support the primary osteoblast growth and facilitate nodule formation in comparison with MTA and Generex A [21]. Recently,

Capasio powder has been refined and renamed as *Quick-Set* (Primus Consulting), and the cationic surfactant was removed from the liquid gel component, which was proposed to interfere with cell cytocompatibility. In a study, Quick-Set demonstrated similar cytotoxicity profile to MTA [171].

7.3.1.7 TheraCal

TheraCal (Bisco Inc., Schaumburg, IL, USA) is a new light-cured resin-modified paste containing CaO, calcium silicate particles (type III Portland cement), strontium glass, fumed silica, barium sulfate, barium zirconate, and resin containing Bis-GMA and poly(ethylene glycol) dimethacrylate (PEGDMA) (International Patent A61K33/42), which has been introduced as a pulp capping material. It has the ability to release calcium ions and create an environmental pH close to physiological pH after 7 days. The latter characteristic favors the formation of apatite and induces the differentiation of new odontoblasts, thus resulting in the formation of new dentin. Its ability to polymerize to a depth of 1.7 mm may eliminate the risk of untimely dissolution [68]. Although bioactive and calcium-releasing properties have been demonstrated for TheraCal, decreased cell metabolism when compared to the control has been demonstrated [85].

7.3.2 Endodontic Cements Not Based on Tricalcium Silicate

7.3.2.1 Calcium Aluminate Cement

A novel *calcium aluminate endodontic cement* was developed at the Federal University of São Carlos, Brazil, by Pandolfelli et al. [133] (Patent registration INPI 0704502–6). This cement aims to preserve the positive properties and clinical applications of MTA while increasing the possibility of extended applications without the disadvantages of the original material. The calcium aluminate cement is comprised of calcium aluminate ($CaO{\cdot}Al_2O_3$) and calcium dialuminate ($CaO.2Al_2O_3$) phases, which are responsible for the hydraulic setting process [138]. In one study, the chemical, physical, and mechanical properties of the cement were assessed, and results showed more rapid setting, better flow, improved handling properties, rather high mechanical strength, and reduced porosity with lower pore size compared to MTA Angelus [131]. On the other hand, on the surface of this cement in combination with accelerator, stoichiometric hydroxyapatite was detected after immersion in simulated body fluid solution [130].

7.3.2.2 EndoBinder

A new calcium aluminate-based endodontic cement (Patent Number PI0704502-6-2007) called EndoBinder (Binderware, São Carlos, SP, Brazil) has been developed, with the aim of preserving the properties and clinical applications of MTA without its negative characteristics. The cement is produced by the process of aluminum oxide and calcium carbonate calcination at temperatures between 1,315 and 1,425 °C. The formed calcium aluminate is cooled and then triturated until an adequate particle size is obtained. Free magnesium oxide and calcium oxide, which are responsible for the undesired expansion, and ferric oxide which leads to tooth darkening have been eliminated. This material has been shown to present adequate physical and chemical properties [130] and induce a higher rate of osteogenic cells differentiation compared to those exposed to MTA [48]. In addition, when tested on rat subcutaneous tissues, it proved to be biocompatible [3]. In a 1-year in vitro study, GMTA, WMTA, and EndoBinder with and without radiopacifying agent displayed color alteration after 360 days [71].

7.3.2.3 Castor Oil Cement

Recently, a material-based polymer derived from the *castor oil plant* (*Ricinus communis*) was introduced to endodontics, also known as *castor bean polyurethane cement* (COB, Poliliquil, Araraquara, SP, Brazil), is composed of 81–96 % triglyceride of ricinoleic acid, and is considered as a natural polyol containing three hydroxyl radicals.

This cement has been reported to have antibacterial activity against *E. coli* [165] and is progressively integrated into the alveolar bone in the wound-healing process [47]. Aiming at

Table 7.2 Properties of MTA-based sealers

Sealers	Composition	Biocompatibility	Antibacterial	Sealing ability	Calcium ion release
Endo-CPM-Sealer	MTA + calcium chloride + calcium carbonate	(+) [76, 77]	(+) [159] (−)[124]	(+)[50]	(+) [160]
iRoot SP Sealer	Calcium silicate based (unknown)	(+) [181]	(+) [179]	(+) [61, 178]	(+) [23]
MTA Fillapex	MTA + salicylate resin + natural resin + silica nanoparticles + bismuth oxide + dehydrated calcium sulfate	(+) [78, 149] (−) [20]	(+) [124]	(+) [75] (−) [154]	(+) [23]
MTA Obtura	White MTA + viscous fluid	N/Y/E[a]	N/Y/E[a]	(−) [168]	N/Y/E[a]
ProRoot Endo Sealer	Tricalcium silicate + dicalcium silicate + calcium sulfate + calcium aluminate + bismuth oxide	N/Y/E[a]	N/Y/E[a]	(+) [172]	N/Y/E[a]

[a]Not yet evaluated

evaluation of its cytotoxicity and genotoxicity, this material proved to be biocompatible when used in maxillary sinus floor augmentation [22] and is well osseo-integrated [112], without any negative influence on the cell survival [28, 29]. The sealing ability of this cement has been evaluated by the dye leakage method, and results have shown an efficient sealing ability [51].

7.3.2.4 Ceramicrete

Ceramicrete is a self-setting phosphate ceramic developed at the Argonne National Laboratory that sets in an ambient condition formed by acid-base reaction between an acid phosphate (KH_2PO_4) and a negligible soluble basic metal oxide (calcined MgO). More recently, a biocompatible, radiopaque Ceramicrete-based dental/bone material has been created by incorporating hydroxyapatite powder and cerium oxide radiopaque filler into the phosphosilicate ceramic. The Ceramicrete-based material has an initial setting time of 6 min and a final setting time of 12 min, it can also be rolled into a sausage-like formation for easier manipulation with dental instruments and sets under water with minimal washout [143]. A modified version of the material (Ceramicrete D) was introduced by mixing the powder with deionized water. The sealing ability of Ceramicrete D was reported to be favorable [161].

In another study by Leal et al. [108], two endodontic bioceramic repair cements (Bioaggregate and Ceramicrete D) displayed similar leakage results to white MTA when used as root-end fillings materials. Ceramicrete D had significantly lower glucose penetration. Physical and chemical analyses showed that the clinical handling and washout resistant of the Ceramicrete D were superior to those of MTA; however, it was weaker, less radiopaque, and initially more acidic than Generex A and Capasio [139].

7.3.3 MTA-Based Sealers

Despite favorable characteristics, MTA presented some physical properties that hinder its application for root canal filling. An appropriate material for using as a root canal filling should be biocompatible, induce mineralized tissue formation, has suitable flow rate and manipulation. Recently, in an effort to incorporate the desirable biological properties of MTA into an easy to manipulate and insert material, some manufacturers have added specific components to MTA-based cements. Materials resulting from this attempt are listed in Table 7.2.

7.3.3.1 Endo-CPM-Sealer

The *Endo-CPM-Sealer* (Egeo S.R.L., Buenos Aires, Argentina) was introduced in an attempt to combine the physicochemical properties of a root canal sealer with the biological properties of MTA. According to the manufacturer, CPM Sealer is composed of MTA, SiO_2, $CaCO_3$, Bi_2O_3, $BaSO_4$, propylene glycol alginate, propylene glycol, sodium citrate, and calcium chloride after mixing. Calcium carbonate, as a component that reduces the pH of the mixture, restricts the surface necrosis of cells in contact with the material and thus allows the action of the alkaline phosphatase and, consequently, the deposition of mineralized tissue [76]. Hydroxyl and calcium ions have also been shown to release from this cement similar to MTA, and therefore, they may act as an alternative root-end filling material [160]. Researchers demonstrated that Endo-CPM-Sealer has a good antimicrobial activity [159]. In addition, fibroblast cultures revealed that Endo-CPM-Sealer is not cytotoxic [77]. According to the manufacturer and study results [50], Endo-CPM-Sealer can be considered as an alternative sealing material in the treatment of root perforations. When used as an apical plug, the CPM and MTA had similar adaptation to the dentin walls.

7.3.3.2 iRoot SP Sealer

A new bioceramic-based sealer *iRoot SP* (Innovative Bioceramix, Vancouver, Canada) is described by the manufacturer as a convenient, premixed, ready-to-use, injectable, white hydraulic cement paste. This material uses the natural moisture of the dentinal tubules to initiate and complete its setting reaction. According to the manufacturer, iRoot SP is an aluminum-free, hydrophilic, calcium silicate-based material that requires the water to set and harden. In addition to its antibacterial activity and biocompatibility [179, 181], it showed good sealing ability [61, 178] and bonding to root canal dentin even under different degrees of dentin moisture [60, 126]. Intracanal placement of calcium hydroxide seems to improve the dislodgment resistance of the iRoot SP [7].

7.3.3.3 MTA Fillapex

MTA Fillapex (Angelus, Londrina PR, Brazil) is a new double paste MTA-based root canal sealer. Its composition after mixing is basically mineral trioxide aggregate, salicylate resin, natural resin, bismuth oxide, and dehydrated calcium sulfate. This material has excellent radiopacity, easy handling, and good working time. MTA Fillapex showed antibacterial activity against *E. faecalis* before setting [124]. According to the manufacturer, this is the only root canal sealer that promotes cementum regeneration. However, one study showed lower cell viability rates when compared with the control group [20]. On the contrary, other investigations on human osteoblast-like cells and rat tissues showed the sealer presents suitable bioactivity [78, 149]. In some studies, MTA Fillapex presented lower sealing ability than MTA [154] and lower push-out bond values to root dentin compared with other sealers [148].

7.3.3.4 MTA Obtura

MTA Obtura (Angelus, Solucoes Odontologicas, Londrina, PR, Brazil) is a mixture of white MTA with a proprietary viscous liquid. In an in vitro study, MTA Obtura showed progressive increased leakage during extended experimental periods [168]. On the other hand, another study concluded that MTA Obtura presented greater flow than the minimum recommended level in the ADA_{57} specification [19].

7.3.3.5 ProRoot Endo Sealer

ProRoot Endo Sealer (Dentsply Maillefer, Ballaigues, Switzerland) is reported to be calcium silicate based with liquid-to-powder ratio of 1:2. The liquid is composed of water and a viscous water-soluble polymer. The addition of a polymer to improve the workability had been reported previously [44]. The polymer addition does not seem to affect the biocompatibility of the material [34, 44]. Sealing property of ProRoot Endo Sealer is comparable to other tested sealers [172], and also the presence of spherical amorphous calcium phosphate-like and apatite-like phases after immersion in simulated body fluid is demonstrated [94].

Conclusion

The introduction of *mineral trioxide aggregate* (MTA) in 1993 started a new revolutionary phase in endodontic practice. However, despite solving many problems in the treatment of complicated cases, some difficulties have been reported with MTA. The loose and sandy nature and also lack of uniformity in MTA mixture have caused some difficulties for application of MTA paste into the desired space.

While some modifications have been proposed for easier application of MTA in order to overcome its disadvantages, these modifications have had a negative influence on some properties of the material.

A new generation of materials with at least similar properties to those of original ProRoot MTA have also been introduced as its suitable alternatives in complicated cases. More evidence is required to support these materials as an improved MTA or as its new alternatives.

References

1. Abbasipour F, Akheshteh V, Rastqar A, Khalilkhani H, Asgary S, Janahmadi M. Comparing the effects of mineral trioxide aggregate and calcium enriched mixture on neuronal cells using an electrophysiological approach. Iran Endod J. 2012;7(2):79–87.
2. Abdullah D, Ford TR, Papaioannou S, Nicholson J, McDonald F. An evaluation of accelerated Portland cement as a restorative material. Biomaterials. 2002; 23(19):4001–10.
3. Aguilar FG, Roberti Garcia LF, Panzeri Pires-de-Souza FC. Biocompatibility of new calcium aluminate cement (EndoBinder). J Endod. 2012;38(3): 367–71.
4. Akbari M, Rouhani A, Samiee S, Jafarzadeh H. Effect of dentin bonding agent on the prevention of tooth discoloration produced by mineral trioxide aggregate. Int J Dent. 2012;2012:563203.
5. Alanezi AZ, Jiang J, Safavi KE, Spangberg LS, Zhu Q. Cytotoxicity evaluation of endosequence root repair material. Oral Surg Oral Med Oral Pathol Oral Radiol Endod. 2010;109(3):e122–5.
6. Alanezi AZ, Zhu Q, Wang YH, Safavi KE, Jiang J. Effect of selected accelerants on setting time and biocompatibility of mineral trioxide aggregate (MTA). Oral Surg Oral Med Oral Pathol Oral Radiol Endod. 2011;111(1):122–7.
7. Amin SA, Seyam RS, El-Samman MA. The effect of prior calcium hydroxide intracanal placement on the bond strength of two calcium silicate-based and an epoxy resin-based endodontic sealer. J Endod. 2012;38(5):696–9.
8. Asgary S, Eghbal MJ. Treatment outcomes of pulpotomy in permanent molars with irreversible pulpitis using biomaterials: a multi-center randomized controlled trial. Acta Odontol Scand. 2013;71(1):130–6.
9. Asgary S, Eghbal MJ, Ghoddusi J. Two-year results of vital pulp therapy in permanent molars with irreversible pulpitis: an ongoing multicenter randomized clinical trial. Clin Oral Investig. 2014;18(2):635–41. Epub 2013 May 28.
10. Asgary S, Eghbal MJ, Ghoddusi J, Yazdani S. One-year results of vital pulp therapy in permanent molars with irreversible pulpitis: an ongoing multicenter, randomized, non-inferiority clinical trial. Clin Oral Investig. 2013;17(2):431–9.
11. Asgary S, Eghbal MJ, Parirokh M. Sealing ability of a novel endodontic cement as a root-end filling material. J Biomed Mater Res A. 2008;87(3):706–9.
12. Asgary S, Eghbal MJ, Parirokh M, Ghanavati F, Rahimi H. A comparative study of histologic response to different pulp capping materials and a novel endodontic cement. Oral Surg Oral Med Oral Pathol Oral Radiol Endod. 2008;106(4):609–14.
13. Asgary S, Eghbal MJ, Parirokh M, Ghoddusi J. Effect of two storage solutions on surface topography of two root-end fillings. Aust Endod J. 2009;35(3):147–52.
14. Asgary S, Kamrani FA. Antibacterial effects of five different root canal sealing materials. J Oral Sci. 2008;50(4):469–74.
15. Asgary S, Moosavi SH, Yadegari Z, Shahriari S. Cytotoxic effect of MTA and CEM cement in human gingival fibroblast cells. Scanning electronic microscope evaluation. N Y State Dent J. 2012;78(2):51–4.
16. Asgary S, Shahabi S, Jafarzadeh T, Amini S, Kheirieh S. The properties of a new endodontic material. J Endod. 2008;34(8):990–3.
17. Belobrov I, Parashos P. Treatment of tooth discoloration after the use of white mineral trioxide aggregate. J Endod. 2011;37(7):1017–20.
18. Ber BS, Hatton JF, Stewart GP. Chemical modification of proroot MTA to improve handling characteristics and decrease setting time. J Endod. 2007;33(10):1231–4.
19. Bernardes RA, de Amorim Campelo A, Junior DS, Pereira LO, Duarte MA, Moraes IG, et al. Evaluation of the flow rate of 3 endodontic sealers: Sealer 26, AH Plus, and MTA Obtura. Oral Surg Oral Med Oral Pathol Oral Radiol Endod. 2010;109(1):e47–9.
20. Bin CV, Valera MC, Camargo SE, Rabelo SB, Silva GO, Balducci I, et al. Cytotoxicity and genotoxicity of root canal sealers based on mineral trioxide aggregate. J Endod. 2012;38(4):495–500.
21. Bird DC, Komabayashi T, Guo L, Opperman LA, Spears R. In vitro evaluation of dentinal tubule penetration and biomineralization ability of a new root-end filling material. J Endod. 2012;38(8):1093–6.

22. Boëck-Neto RJ, Gabrielli MF, Shibli JA, Marcantonio E, Lia RC. Histomorphometric evaluation of human sinus floor augmentation healing responses to placement of calcium phosphate or Ricinus communis polymer associated with autogenous bone. Clin Implant Dent Relat Res. 2005;7(4):181–8.
23. Borges RP, Sousa-Neto MD, Versiani MA, Rached-Júnior FA, De-Deus G, Miranda CE, et al. Changes in the surface of four calcium silicate-containing endodontic materials and an epoxy resin-based sealer after a solubility test. Int Endod J. 2012;45(5): 419–28.
24. Bortoluzzi EA, Broon NJ, Bramante CM, Consolaro A, Garcia RB, de Moraes IG, et al. Mineral trioxide aggregate with or without calcium chloride in pulpotomy. J Endod. 2008;34(2):172–5.
25. Bortoluzzi EA, Broon NJ, Bramante CM, Garcia RB, de Moraes IG, Bernardineli N. Sealing ability of MTA and radiopaque Portland cement with or without calcium chloride for root-end filling. J Endod. 2006;32(9):897–900.
26. Bortoluzzi EA, Guerreiro-Tanomaru JM, Tanomaru-Filho M, Duarte MA. Radiographic effect of different radiopacifiers on a potential retrograde filling material. Oral Surg Oral Med Oral Pathol Oral Radiol Endod. 2009;108(4):628–32.
27. Boutsioukis C, Noula G, Lambrianidis T. Ex vivo study of the efficiency of two techniques for the removal of mineral trioxide aggregate used as a root canal filling material. J Endod. 2008;34(10): 1239–42.
28. Camargo SE, Camargo CH, Hiller KA, Rode SM, Schweikl H, Schmalz G. Cytotoxicity and genotoxicity of pulp capping materials in two cell lines. Int Endod J. 2009;42(3):227–37.
29. Camargo SE, Rode SEM, do Prado RF, Carvalho YR, Camargo CH. Subcutaneous tissue reaction to castor oil bean and calcium hydroxide in rats. J Appl Oral Sci. 2010;18(3):273–8.
30. Camilleri J. Hydration mechanisms of mineral trioxide aggregate. Int Endod J. 2007;40(6):462–70.
31. Camilleri J. Modification of mineral trioxide aggregate. Physical and mechanical properties. Int Endod J. 2008;41(10):843–9.
32. Camilleri J. The physical properties of accelerated Portland cement for endodontic use. Int Endod J. 2008;41(2):151–7.
33. Camilleri J. Characterization of hydration products of mineral trioxide aggregate. Int Endod J. 2008;41:408–17.
34. Camilleri J. The biocompatibility of modified experimental Portland cement with potential for use in dentistry. Int Endod J. 2008;41:1107–14.
35. Camilleri J. Hydration characteristics of calcium silicate cements with alternative radiopacifiers used as root-end filling materials. J Endod. 2010;36(3): 502–8.
36. Camilleri J. Characterization and hydration kinetics of tricalcium silicate cement for use as a dental biomaterial. Dent Mater. 2011;27(8):836–44.
37. Camilleri J. Investigation of Biodentine as dentine replacement material. J Dent. 2013;41(7):600–10.
38. Camilleri J. Colour stability of white mineral trioxide aggregate. J Endod. 2014;40(3):436–40.
39. Camilleri J, Formosa L, Damidot D. The setting characteristics of MTA Plus in different environmental conditions. Int Endod J. 2013;46(9):831–40.
40. Camilleri J, Gandolfi MG. Evaluation of the radiopacity of calcium silicate cements containing different radiopacifiers. Int Endod J. 2010;43(1):21–30.
41. Camilleri J, Grech L, Galea K, Keir D, Fenech M, Formosa L, Damidot D, Mallia B. Assessment of porosity and sealing ability of tricalcium silicate-based root-end filling materials. Clin Oral Invest. 2014;18:1437–46.
42. Camilleri J, Kralj P, Veber M, Sinagra E. Characterization and analyses of acid-extractable and leached trace elements in dental cements. Int Endod J. 2012;45(8):737–43.
43. Camilleri J, Montesin FE, Curtis RV, Ford TR. Characterization of Portland cement for use as a dental restorative material. Dent Mater. 2006;22(6): 569–75.
44. Camilleri J, Montesin FE, Di Silvio L, Pitt Ford TR. The chemical constitution and biocompatibility of accelerated Portland cement for endodontic use. Int Endod J. 2005;38(11):834–42.
45. Camilleri J, Montesin FE, Papaioannou S, McDonald F, Pitt Ford TR. Biocompatibility of two commercial forms of mineral trioxide aggregate. Int Endod J. 2004;37(10):699–704.
46. Camilleri J, Sorrentino F, Damidot D. Investigation of the hydration and bioactivity of radiopacified tricalcium silicate cement, Biodentine and MTA Angelus. Dent Mater. 2013;29:580–93.
47. Carvalho TL, Araújo CA, Teófilo JM, Brentegani LG. Histologic and histometric evaluation of rat alveolar wound healing around polyurethane resin implants. Int J Oral Maxillofac Surg. 1997;26(2):149–52.
48. Castro-Raucci LM, Oliveira IR, Teixeira LN, Rosa AL, Oliveira PT, Jacobovitz M. Effects of a novel calcium aluminate cement on the early events of the progression of osteogenic cell cultures. Braz Dent J. 2011;22(2):99–104.
49. Cutajar A, Mallia B, Abela S, Camilleri J. Replacement of radiopacifier in mineral trioxide aggregate; characterization and determination of physical properties. Dent Mater. 2011;27(9):879–91.
50. da Silva GF, Guerreiro-Tanomaru JM, Sasso-Cerri E, Tanomaru-Filho M, Cerri PS. Histological and histomorphometrical evaluation of furcation perforations filled with MTA. CPM and ZOE. Int Endod J. 2011;44(2):100–10.
51. de Martins GR, Carvalho CA, Valera MC, de Oliveira LD, Buso L, Carvalho AS. Sealing ability of castor oil polymer as a root-end filling material. J Appl Oral Sci. 2009;17(3):220–3.
52. de Morais CA, Bernardineli N, Garcia RB, Duarte MA, Guerisoli DM. Evaluation of tissue response to MTA and Portland cement with iodoform. Oral Surg

Oral Med Oral Pathol Oral Radiol Endod. 2006; 102(3):417–21.
53. De-Deus G, Canabarro A, Alves G, Linhares A, Senne MI, Granjeiro JM. Optimal cytocompatibility of a bioceramic nanoparticulate cement in primary human mesenchymal cells. J Endod. 2009;35(10):1387–90.
54. De-Deus G, de Souza MC, Sergio Fidel RA, Fidel SR, de Campos RC, Luna AS. Negligible expression of arsenic in some commercially available brands of Portland cement and mineral trioxide aggregate. J Endod. 2009;35(6):887–90.
55. De-Deus G, Reis C, Brandão C, Fidel S, Fidel RA. The ability of Portland cement, MTA, and MTA Bio to prevent through-and-through fluid movement in repaired furcal perforations. J Endod. 2007;33(11):1374–7.
56. Ding SJ, Kao CT, Shie MY, Hung C, Huang TH. The physical and cytological properties of white MTA mixed with Na_2HPO_4 as an accelerant. J Endod. 2008;34(6):748–51.
57. Duarte MA, Alves de Aguiar K, Zeferino MA, Vivan RR, Ordinola-Zapata R, Tanomaru-Filho M, et al. Evaluation of the propylene glycol association on some physical and chemical properties of mineral trioxide aggregate. Int Endod J. 2012;45(6):565–70.
58. Duarte MA, De Oliveira Demarchi AC, Yamashita JC, Kuga MC, De Fraga Campos S. Arsenic release provided by MTA and Portland cement. Oral Surg Oral Med Oral Pathol Oral Radiol Endod. 2005;99(5): 648–50.
59. El Sayed M, Saeed M. In vitro comparative study of sealing ability of Diadent BioAggregate and other root-end filling materials. J Conserv Dent. 2012;15(3):249–52.
60. Ersahan S, Aydin C. Dislocation resistance of iRoot SP, a calcium silicate-based sealer, from radicular dentine. J Endod. 2010;36(12):2000–2.
61. Ersahan S, Aydin C. Solubility and apical sealing characteristics of a new calcium silicate-based root canal sealer in comparison to calcium hydroxide-, methacrylate resin- and epoxy resin-based sealers. Acta Odontol Scand. 2013;71(3–4):857–62.
62. Estrela C, Bammann LL, Estrela CR, Silva RS, Pécora JD. Antimicrobial and chemical study of MTA, Portland cement, calcium hydroxide paste. Sealapex and Dycal. Braz Dent J. 2000;11(1):3–9.
63. Fallahinejad Ghajari M, Asgharian Jeddi T, Iri S, Asgary S. Direct pulp-capping with calcium enriched mixture in primary molar teeth: a randomized clinical trial. Iran Endod J. 2010;5(1).27–30.
64. Foley JI. Use of mineral trioxide aggregate (MTA by postgraduates in restorative dentistry in the UK. Eur J Prosthodont Restor Dent. 2011;19(4):179–83.
65. Formosa LM, Mallia B, Camilleri J. A quantitative method for determining the antiwashout characteristics of cement-based dental materials including mineral trioxide aggregate. Int Endod J. 2013;46(2):179–86.
66. Formosa LM, Mallia B, Camilleri J. The chemical properties of light- and chemical-curing composites with mineral trioxide aggregate filler. Dent Mater. 2013;29(2):e11–9.
67. Fridland M, Rosado R. Mineral trioxide aggregate (MTA) solubility and porosity with different water-to-powder ratios. J Endod. 2003;29(12):814–7.
68. Gandolfi MG, Siboni F, Prati C. Chemical-physical properties of TheraCal, a novel light-curable MTA-like material for pulp capping. Int Endod J. 2012; 45(6):571–9.
69. Gandolfi MG, Taddei P, Siboni F, Modena E, Ciapetti G, Prati C. Development of the foremost light-curable calcium-silicate MTA cement as root-end in oral surgery. Chemical-physical properties, bioactivity and biological behavior. Dent Mater. 2011;27(7): e134–57.
70. Gandolfi MG, Taddei P, Siboni F, Modena E, De Stefano ED, Prati C. Biomimetic remineralization of human dentin using promising innovative calcium-silicate hybrid "smart" materials. Dent Mater. 2011;27(11):1055–69.
71. Garcia LD, Aguilar FG, Rossetto HL, Sabino MG, Pires-de-Souza FD. Staining susceptibility of new calcium aluminate cement (EndoBinder) in teeth: a 1-year in vitro study. Dent Traumatol. 2013;29(5):383–8. Epub 2012 Oct 16.
72. Glickman GN, Koch KA. 21st-century endodontics. J Am Dent Assoc. 2000;131(Suppl):39S–46.
73. Gomes-Filho JE, de Faria MD, Bernabé PF, Nery MJ, Otoboni-Filho JA, Dezan-Júnior E, et al. Mineral trioxide aggregate but not light-cure mineral trioxide aggregate stimulated mineralization. J Endod. 2008;34(1):62–5.
74. Gomes-Filho JE, de Moraes Costa MT, Cintra LT, Lodi CS, Duarte PC, Okamoto R, et al. Evaluation of alveolar socket response to Angelus MTA and experimental light-cure MTA. Oral Surg Oral Med Oral Pathol Oral Radiol Endod. 2010;110(5):e93–7.
75. Gomes-Filho JE, Moreira JV, Watanabe S, Lodi CS, Cintra LT, Dezan Junior E, et al. Sealability of MTA and calcium hydroxide containing sealers. J Appl Oral Sci. 2012;20(3):347–51.
76. Gomes-Filho JE, Watanabe S, Bernabé PF, de Moraes Costa MT. A mineral trioxide aggregate sealer stimulated mineralization. J Endod. 2009;35(2):256–60.
77. Gomes-Filho JE, Watanabe S, Gomes AC, Faria MD, Lodi CS, Penha Oliveira SH. Evaluation of the effects of endodontic materials on fibroblast viability and cytokine production. J Endod. 2009;35(11):1577–9.
78. Gomes-Filho JE, Watanabe S, Lodi CS, Cintra LT, Nery MJ, Filho JA, et al. Rat tissue reaction to MTA FILLAPEX®. Dent Traumatol. 2012;28(6):452–6.
79. Grech L, Mallia B, Camilleri J. Characterization of set IRM, Biodentine, Bioaggregate and a prototype calcium silicate cement for use as root-end filling materials. Int Endod J. 2013;46:632–41.
80. Grech L, Mallia B, Camilleri J. Investigation of the physical properties of tricalcium silicate cement-based root-end filling materials. Dent Mater. 2013;29:e20–8.
81. Han L, Okiji T. Uptake of calcium and silicon released from calcium silicate-based endodontic materials into root canal dentine. Int Endod J. 2011;44(12):1081–7.

82. Hansen SW, Marshall JG, Sedgley CM. Comparison of intracanal EndoSequence Root Repair Material and ProRoot MTA to induce pH changes in simulated root resorption defects over 4 weeks in matched pairs of human teeth. J Endod. 2011;37(4): 502–6.
83. Hasan Zarrabi M, Javidi M, Naderinasab M, Gharechahi M. Comparative evaluation of antimicrobial activity of three cements: new endodontic cement (NEC), mineral trioxide aggregate (MTA) and Portland. J Oral Sci. 2009;51(3):437–42.
84. Hasheminia M, Loriaei Nejad S, Asgary S. Sealing Ability of MTA and CEM Cement as Root-End Fillings of Human Teeth in Dry, Saliva or Blood-Contaminated Conditions. Iran Endod J. 2010;5(4): 151–6.
85. Hebling J, Lessa FC, Nogueira I, Carvalho RM, Costa CA. Cytotoxicity of resin-based light-cured liners. Am J Dent. 2009;22(3):137–42.
86. Hernandez EP, Botero TM, Mantellini MG, McDonald NJ, Nör JE. Effect of ProRoot MTA mixed with chlorhexidine on apoptosis and cell cycle of fibroblasts and macrophages in vitro. Int Endod J. 2005; 38(2):137–43.
87. Hirschberg CS, Patel NS, Patel LM, Kadouri DE, Hartwell GR. Comparison of sealing ability of MTA and EndoSequence Bioceramic Root Repair Material: a bacterial leakage study. Quintessence Int. 2013; 44(5):e157–62.
88. Hirschman WR, Wheater MA, Bringas JS, Hoen MM. Cytotoxicity comparison of three current direct pulp-capping agents with a new bioceramic root repair putty. J Endod. 2012;38(3):385–8.
89. Holt DM, Watts JD, Beeson TJ, Kirkpatrick TC, Rutledge RE. The anti-microbial effect against Enterococcus faecalis and the compressive strength of two types of mineral trioxide aggregate mixed with sterile water or 2 % chlorhexidine liquid. J Endod. 2007;33(7):844–7.
90. Hong ST, Bae KS, Baek SH, Kum KY, Lee W. Microleakage of accelerated mineral trioxide aggregate and Portland cement in an in vitro apexification model. J Endod. 2008;34(1):56–8.
91. Hong ST, Bae KS, Baek SH, Kum KY, Shon WJ, Lee W. Effects of root canal irrigants on the push-out strength and hydration behavior of accelerated mineral trioxide aggregate in its early setting phase. J Endod. 2010;36(12):1995–9.
92. Hsieh SC, Teng NC, Lin YC, Lee PY, Ji DY, Chen CC, et al. A novel accelerator for improving the handling properties of dental filling materials. J Endod. 2009;35(9):1292–5.
93. Huang TH, Shie MY, Kao CT, Ding SJ. The effect of setting accelerator on properties of mineral trioxide aggregate. J Endod. 2008;34(5):590–3.
94. Huffman BP, Mai S, Pinna L, Weller RN, Primus CM, Gutmann JL, et al. Dislocation resistance of ProRoot Endo Sealer, a calcium silicate-based root canal sealer, from radicular dentine. Int Endod J. 2009; 42(1):34–46.
95. Húngaro Duarte MA, De Oliveira El Kadre GD, Vivan RR, Guerreiro Tanomaru JM, TanomaruFilho M, De Moraes IG. Radiopacity of portland cement associated with different radiopacifying agents. J Endod. 2009;35(5):737–40.
96. Jacobovitz M, de Lima RK. Treatment of inflammatory internal root resorption with mineral trioxide aggregate: a case report. Int Endod J. 2008;41(10): 905–12.
97. Jafarnia B, Jiang J, He J, Wang YH, Safavi KE, Zhu Q. Evaluation of cytotoxicity of MTA employing various additives. Oral Surg Oral Med Oral Pathol Oral Radiol Endod. 2009;107(5):739–44.
98. Ji DY, Wu HD, Hsieh SC, Teng NC, Chen CC, Ke ES, et al. Effects of a novel hydration accelerant on the biological and mechanical properties of white mineral trioxide aggregate. J Endod. 2011;37(6): 851–5.
99. Kang JY, Lee BN, Son HJ, Koh JT, Kang SS, Son HH, et al. Biocompatibility of mineral trioxide aggregate mixed with hydration accelerators. J Endod. 2013;39(4):497–500.
100. Kao CT, Shie MY, Huang TH, Ding SJ. Properties of an accelerated mineral trioxide aggregate-like root-end filling material. J Endod. 2009;35(2):239–42.
101. Karabucak B, Li D, Lim J, Iqbal M. Vital pulp therapy with mineral trioxide aggregate. Dent Traumatol. 2005;21(4):240–3.
102. Karimjee CK, Koka S, Rallis DM, Gound TG. Cellular toxicity of mineral trioxide aggregate mixed with an alternative delivery vehicle. Oral Surg Oral Med Oral Pathol Oral Radiol Endod. 2006;102(4): e115–20.
103. Kazem M, Eghbal MJ, Asgary S. Comparison of bacterial and dye microleakage of different root-end filling materials. Iran Endod J. 2010;5(1):17–22.
104. Khalil WA, Eid NF. Biocompatibility of BioAggregate and mineral trioxide aggregate on the liver and kidney. Int Endod J. 2013;46(8):730–7. Epub 2013 Mar 7.
105. Kim EC, Lee BC, Chang HS, Lee W, Hong CU, Min KS. Evaluation of the radiopacity and cytotoxicity of Portland cements containing bismuth oxide. Oral Surg Oral Med Oral Pathol Oral Radiol Endod. 2008;105(1):e54–7.
106. Kogan P, He J, Glickman GN, Watanabe I. The effects of various additives on setting properties of MTA. J Endod. 2006;32(6):569–72.
107. Laurent P, Camps J, About I. Biodentine(TM) induces TGF-β1 release from human pulp cells and early dental pulp mineralization. Int Endod J. 2012;45(5):439–48.
108. Leal F, De-Deus G, Brandão C, Luna AS, Fidel SR, Souza EM. Comparison of the root-end seal provided by bioceramic repair cements and White MTA. Int Endod J. 2011;44(7):662–8.
109. Lee BN, Hwang YC, Jang JH, Chang HS, Hwang IN, Yang SY, et al. Improvement of the properties of mineral trioxide aggregate by mixing with hydration accelerators. J Endod. 2011;37(10):1433–6.

110. Lee SJ, Monsef M, Torabinejad M. Sealing ability of a mineral trioxide aggregate for repair of lateral root perforations. J Endod. 1993;19(11):541–4.
111. Leiendecker AP, Qi YP, Sawyer AN, Niu LN, Agee KA, Loushine RJ, et al. Effects of calcium silicate-based materials on collagen matrix integrity of mineralized dentin. J Endod. 2012;38(6):829–33.
112. Leite FR, Ramalho LT. Bone regeneration after demineralized bone matrix and castor oil (Ricinus communis) polyurethane implantation. J Appl Oral Sci. 2008;16(2):122–6.
113. Lessa FC, Aranha AM, Hebling J, Costa CA. Cytotoxic effects of White-MTA and MTA-Bio cements on odontoblast-like cells (MDPC-23). Braz Dent J. 2010;21(1):24–31.
114. Lovato KF, Sedgley CM. Antibacterial activity of endosequence root repair material and proroot MTA against clinical isolates of Enterococcus faecalis. J Endod. 2011;37(11):1542–6.
115. Ma J, Shen Y, Stojicic S, Haapasalo M. Biocompatibility of two novel root repair materials. J Endod. 2011;37(6):793–8.
116. Malekafzali B, Shekarchi F, Asgary S. Treatment outcomes of pulpotomy in primary molars using two endodontic biomaterials. A 2-year randomised clinical trial. Eur J Paediatr Dent. 2011;12(3): 189–93.
117. Matsunaga T, Tsujimoto M, Kawashima T, Tsujimoto Y, Fujiwara M, Ookubo A, et al. Analysis of arsenic in gray and white mineral trioxide aggregates by using atomic absorption spectrometry. J Endod. 2010;36(12):1988–90.
118. McNamara RP, Henry MA, Schindler WG, Hargreaves KM. Biocompatibility of accelerated mineral trioxide aggregate in a rat model. J Endod. 2010;36(11):1851–5.
119. Min KS, Chang HS, Bae JM, Park SH, Hong CU, Kim EC. The induction of heme oxygenase-1 modulates bismuth oxide-induced cytotoxicity in human dental pulp cells. J Endod. 2007;33(11):1342–6.
120. Mittag SG, Eissner C, Zabel L, Wrbas KT, Kielbassa AM. The influence of chlorhexidine on the antibacterial effects of MTA. Quintessence Int. 2012;43(10):901–6.
121. Miyagak DC, de Carvalho EM, Robazza CR, Chavasco JK, Levorato GL. In vitro evaluation of the antimicrobial activity of endodontic sealers. Braz Oral Res. 2006;20(4):303–6.
122. Modareszadeh MR, Di Fiore PM, Tipton DA, Salamat N. Cytotoxicity and alkaline phosphatase activity evaluation of endosequence root repair material. J Endod. 2012;38(8):1101–5.
123. Monteiro Bramante C, Demarchi AC, de Moraes IG, Bernadineli N, Garcia RB, Spångberg LS, et al. Presence of arsenic in different types of MTA and white and gray Portland cement. Oral Surg Oral Med Oral Pathol Oral Radiol Endod. 2008;106(6):909–13.
124. Morgental RD, Vier-Pelisser FV, Oliveira SD, Antunes FC, Cogo DM, Kopper PM. Antibacterial activity of two MTA-based root canal sealers. Int Endod J. 2011;44(12):1128–33.
125. Mozayeni MA, Milani AS, Marvasti LA, Asgary S. Cytotoxicity of calcium enriched mixture cement compared with mineral trioxide aggregate and intermediate restorative material. Aust Endod J. 2012;38(2):70–5.
126. Nagas E, Uyanik MO, Eymirli A, Cehreli ZC, Vallittu PK, Lassila LV, et al. Dentin moisture conditions affect the adhesion of root canal sealers. J Endod. 2012;38(2):240–4.
127. Nair U, Ghattas S, Saber M, Natera M, Walker C, Pileggi R. A comparative evaluation of the sealing ability of 2 root-end filling materials: an in vitro leakage study using Enterococcus faecalis. Oral Surg Oral Med Oral Pathol Oral Radiol Endod. 2011;112(2):e74–7.
128. Nosrat A, Seifi A, Asgary S. Pulpotomy in caries-exposed immature permanent molars using calcium-enriched mixture cement or mineral trioxide aggregate: a randomized clinical trial. Int J Paediatr Dent. 2013;23(1):56–63.
129. Odabaş ME, Cinar C, Akça G, Araz I, Ulusu T, Yücel H. Short-term antimicrobial properties of mineral trioxide aggregate with incorporated silver-zeolite. Dent Traumatol. 2011;27(3):189–94.
130. Oliveira IR, Andrade TL, Jacobovitz M, Pandolfelli VC. Bioactivity of calcium aluminate endodontic cement. J Endod. 2013;39(6):774–8.
131. Oliveira IR, Pandolfelli VC, Jacobovitz M. Chemical, physical and mechanical properties of a novel calcium aluminate endodontic cement. Int Endod J. 2010;43(12):1069–76.
132. Owadally ID, Pitt Ford TR. Effect of addition of hydroxyapatite on the physical properties of IRM. Int Endod J. 1994;27(5):227–32.
133. Pandolfelli VC, Oliveira IR, Rossetto HL, Jacobovitz M. A composition based on aluminate cement for application in endodontics and the obtained cement product. Patent registration INPI 0704502-6. Assignee: Fundação Universidade Federal de São Carlos, November 29, 2007 (in Portuguese).
134. Parirokh M, Asgary S, Eghbal MJ, Kakoei S, Samiee M. A comparative study of using a combination of calcium chloride and mineral trioxide aggregate as the pulp-capping agent on dogs' teeth. J Endod. 2011;37(6):786–8.
135. Parirokh M, Asgary S, Eghbal MJ, Stowe S, Eslami B, Eskandarizade A, et al. A comparative study of white and grey mineral trioxide aggregate as pulp capping agents in dog's teeth. Dent Traumatol. 2005;21(3):150–4.
136. Parirokh M, Mirsoltani B, Raoof M, Tabrizchi H, Haghdoost AA. Comparative study of subcutaneous tissue responses to a novel root-end filling material and white and grey mineral trioxide aggregate. Int Endod J. 2011;44(4):283–9.
137. Park JW, Hong SH, Kim JH, Lee SJ, Shin SJ. X-Ray diffraction analysis of white ProRoot MTA and

Diadent BioAggregate. Oral Surg Oral Med Oral Pathol Oral Radiol Endod. 2010;109(1):155–8.
138. Parker KM, Sharp JH. Refractory calcium aluminate cements. Transact J Br Ceram Soc. 1982;81:35–42.
139. Porter ML, Bertó A, Primus CM, Watanabe I. Physical and chemical properties of new-generation endodontic materials. J Endod. 2010;36(3):524–8.
140. Primus CM. Comments on "arsenic release provided by MTA and Portland cement" by Duarte MA, et al. Oral Surg Oral Med Oral Pathol Oral Radiol Endod. 2006;101(4):416–7; author reply 417–8.
141. Profeta AC, Mannocci F, Foxton R, Watson TF, Feitosa VP, De Carlo B, Mongiorgi R, Valdré G, Sauro S. Experimental etch-and-rinse adhesives doped with bioactive calcium silicate-based micro-fillers to generate therapeutic resin-dentin interfaces. Dent Mater. 2013;29(7):729–41.
142. Rahimi S, Mokhtari H, Shahi S, Kazemi A, Asgary S, Eghbal MJ, et al. Osseous reaction to implantation of two endodontic cements: Mineral trioxide aggregate (MTA) and calcium enriched mixture (CEM). Med Oral Patol Oral Cir Bucal. 2012; 17(5):e907–11.
143. Rao AJ, Pagilla KR, Wagh AS. Stabilization and solidification of metal-laden wastes by compaction and magnesium phosphate-based binder. J Air Waste Manag Assoc. 2000;50(9):1623–31.
144. Saatchi M, Hosseini HS, Farhad AR, Narimany T. The effect of various concentrations of iodine potassium iodide on the antimicrobial properties of mineral trioxide aggregate – a pilot study. Dent Traumatol. 2012;28(6):474–7.
145. Saghiri MA, Asgar K, Lotfi M, Garcia-Godoy F. Nanomodification of mineral trioxide aggregate for enhanced physiochemical properties. Int Endod J. 2012;45(11):979–88.
146. Saghiri MA, Garcia-Godoy F, Asatourian A, Lotfi M, Banava S, Khezri-Boukani K. Effect of pH on compressive strength of some modification of mineral trioxide aggregate. Med Oral Patol Oral Cir Bucal. 2013;18(4):e714–20.
147. Saghiri MA, Garcia-Godoy F, Gutmann JL, Lotfi M, Asatorian A, Ahmadi H. Push-out bond strength of a nano-modified mineral trioxide aggregate. Dent Traumatol. 2013;29(4):323–7. Epub 2012 Aug 13.
148. Sagsen B, Ustün Y, Demirbuga S, Pala K. Push-out bond strength of two new calcium silicate-based endodontic sealers to root canal dentine. Int Endod J. 2011;44(12):1088–91.
149. Salles LP, Gomes-Cornélio AL, Guimarães FC, Herrera BS, Bao SN, Rossa-Junior C, et al. Mineral trioxide aggregate-based endodontic sealer stimulates hydroxyapatite nucleation in human osteoblast-like cell culture. J Endod. 2012;38(7):971–6.
150. Sauro S, Osorio R, Osorio E, Watson TF, Toledano M. Novel light-curable materials containing experimental bioactive micro-fillers remineralise mineral-depleted bonded-dentine interfaces. J Biomater Sci Polym Ed. 2013;24(8):940–56.
151. Sawyer AN, Nikonov SY, Pancio AK, Niu LN, Agee KA, Loushine RJ, et al. Effects of calcium silicate-based materials on the flexural properties of dentin. J Endod. 2012;38(5):680–3.
152. Shahi S, Rahimi S, Yavari HR, Shakouie S, Nezafati S, Abdolrahimi M. Sealing ability of white and gray mineral trioxide aggregate mixed with distilled water and 0.12 % chlorhexidine gluconate when used as root-end filling materials. J Endod. 2007;33(12):1429–32.
153. Shokouhinejad N, Nekoofar MH, Razmi H, Sajadi S, Davies TE, Saghiri MA, et al. Bioactivity of EndoSequence root repair material and bioaggregate. Int Endod J. 2012;45(12):1127–34.
154. Sönmez IS, Oba AA, Sönmez D, Almaz ME. In vitro evaluation of apical microleakage of a new MTA-based sealer. Eur Arch Paediatr Dent. 2012;13(5): 252–5.
155. Stowe TJ, Sedgley CM, Stowe B, Fenno JC. The effects of chlorhexidine gluconate (0.12 %) on the antimicrobial properties of tooth-colored ProRoot mineral trioxide aggregate. J Endod. 2004;30(6): 429–33.
156. Sumer M, Muglali M, Bodrumlu E, Guvenc T. Reactions of connective tissue to amalgam, intermediate restorative material, mineral trioxide aggregate, and mineral trioxide aggregate mixed with chlorhexidine. J Endod. 2006;32(11):1094–6.
157. Tabarsi B, Parirokh M, Eghbal MJ, Haghdoost AA, Torabzadeh H, Asgary S. A comparative study of dental pulp response to several pulpotomy agents. Int Endod J. 2010;43(7):565–71.
158. Tanalp J, Karapinar-Kazandag M, Ersev H, Bayirli G. The status of mineral trioxide aggregate in endodontics education in dental schools in Turkey. J Dent Educ. 2012;76(6):752–8.
159. Tanomaru JM, Tanomaru-Filho M, Hotta J, Watanabe E, Ito IY. Antimicrobial activity of endodontic sealers based on calcium hydroxide and MTA. Acta Odontol Latinoam. 2008;21(2):147–51.
160. Tanomaru-Filho M, Chaves Faleiros FB, Saçaki JN, Hungaro Duarte MA, Guerreiro-Tanomaru JM. Evaluation of pH and calcium ion release of root-end filling materials containing calcium hydroxide or mineral trioxide aggregate. J Endod. 2009;35(10): 1418–21.
161. Tay KC, Loushine BA, Oxford C, Kapur R, Primus CM, Gutmann JL, et al. In vitro evaluation of a Ceramicrete-based root-end filling material. J Endod. 2007;33(12):1438–43.
162. Torabinejad M, Hong CU, McDonald F, Pitt Ford TR. Physical and chemical properties of a new root-end filling material. J Endod. 1995;21(7):349–53.
163. Torabinejad M, Hong CU, Pitt Ford TR, Kettering JD. Antibacterial effects of some root end filling materials. J Endod. 1995;21(8):403–6.
164. Tuna EB, Dinçol ME, Gençay K, Aktören O. Fracture resistance of immature teeth filled with BioAggregate, mineral trioxide aggregate and calcium hydroxide. Dent Traumatol. 2011;27(3):174–8.

165. Valera MC, Maekawa LE, Chung A, de Oliveira LD, Carvalho CA, Koga-Ito CY, et al. Effectiveness of castor oil extract on Escherichia coli and its endotoxins in root canals. Gen Dent. 2012;60(4):e204–9.
166. Vallés M, Mercadé M, Duran-Sindreu F, Bourdelande JL, Roig M. Color stability of white mineral trioxide aggregate. Clin Oral Investig. 2013;17(4):1155–9.
167. Vallés M, Mercadé M, Duran-Sindreu F, Bourdelande JL, Roig M. Influence of light and oxygen on the color stability of five calcium silicate-based materials. J Endod. 2013;39(4):525–8.
168. Vasconcelos BC, Bernardes RA, Duarte MA, Bramante CM, Moraes IG. Apical sealing of root canal fillings performed with five different endodontic sealers: analysis by fluid filtration. J Appl Oral Sci. 2011;19(4):324–8.
169. Vivan RR, Zapata RO, Zeferino MA, Bramante CM, Bernardineli N, Garcia RB, et al. Evaluation of the physical and chemical properties of two commercial and three experimental root-end filling materials. Oral Surg Oral Med Oral Pathol Oral Radiol Endod. 2010;110(2):250–6.
170. Washington JT, Schneiderman E, Spears R, Fernandez CR, He J, Opperman LA. Biocompatibility and osteogenic potential of new generation endodontic materials established by using primary osteoblasts. J Endod. 2011;37(8):1166–70.
171. Wei W, Qi YP, Nikonov SY, Niu LN, Messer RL, Mao J, et al. Effects of an experimental calcium aluminosilicate cement on the viability of murine odontoblast-like cells. J Endod. 2012;38(7):936–42.
172. Weller RN, Tay KC, Garrett LV, Mai S, Primus CM, Gutmann JL, et al. Microscopic appearance and apical seal of root canals filled with gutta-percha and ProRoot Endo Sealer after immersion in a phosphate-containing fluid. Int Endod J. 2008;41(11):977–86.
173. Wiltbank KB, Schwartz SA, Schindler WG. Effect of selected accelerants on the physical properties of mineral trioxide aggregate and Portland cement. J Endod. 2007;33(10):1235–8.
174. Yan P, Peng B, Fan B, Fan M, Bian Z. The effects of sodium hypochlorite (5.25 %), Chlorhexidine (2 %), and Glyde File Prep on the bond strength of MTA-dentin. J Endod. 2006;32(1):58–60.
175. Yan P, Yuan Z, Jiang H, Peng B, Bian Z. Effect of bioaggregate on differentiation of human periodontal ligament fibroblasts. Int Endod J. 2010; 43(12):1116–21.
176. Yasuda Y, Kamaguchi A, Saito T. In vitro evaluation of the antimicrobial activity of a new resin-based endodontic sealer against endodontic pathogens. J Oral Sci. 2008;50(3):309–13.
177. Yuan Z, Peng B, Jiang H, Bian Z, Yan P. Effect of bioaggregate on mineral-associated gene expression in osteoblast cells. J Endod. 2010;36(7):1145–8.
178. Zhang W, Li Z, Peng B. Assessment of a new root canal sealer's apical sealing ability. Oral Surg Oral Med Oral Pathol Oral Radiol Endod. 2009;107(6): e79–82.
179. Zhang W, Li Z, Peng B. Ex vivo cytotoxicity of a new calcium silicate-based canal filling material. Int Endod J. 2010;43(9):769–74.
180. Zhang H, Pappen FG, Haapasalo M. Dentin enhances the antibacterial effect of mineral trioxide aggregate and bioaggregate. J Endod. 2009;35(2):221–4.
181. Zhang H, Shen Y, Ruse ND, Haapasalo M. Antibacterial activity of endodontic sealers by modified direct contact test against Enterococcus faecalis. J Endod. 2009;35(7):1051–5.
182. Zhang S, Yang X, Fan M. BioAggregate and iRoot BP Plus optimize the proliferation and mineralization ability of human dental pulp cells. Int Endod J. 2013;46(10):962–70. Epub 2013 Mar 11.

8 Products and Distinctions

Carolyn M. Primus

8.1 Introduction

This chapter describes the dental products that contain or are based on tri- or dicalcium silicates. Resin-based products that contain these powders are included. For simplicity, these products are denoted at MTA-type materials because they rely on the hydration reactions in Eqs. 8.1 and 8.2.

Tricalcium silicate:

$$2Ca_3SiO_5 + 7H_2O = 3CaO_2SiO_2 \cdot 4H_2O + 3Ca(OH)_2 \quad (8.1)$$

Dicalcium silicate:

$$2Ca_2SiO_4 + 5H_2O = 3CaO \cdot 2SiO_2 \cdot 4H_2O + Ca(OH)_2 \quad (8.2)$$

Secondary or lesser hydration reactions occur involving the minor phases, but the strength and the release of calcium hydroxide for bioactivity arise from these two reactions. The key to the bioactivity of MTA-type products is the precipitation of hydroxyapatite when the calcium hydroxide reacts with phosphate ions in body fluids, as shown in Eq. 8.3.

$$7Ca(OH)_2 + 3Ca(H_2PO_4)_2 \rightarrow Ca_{10}(PO_4)6(OH)_2 + 12H_2O \quad (8.3)$$

Calcium silicate, $CaSiO_3$ (wollastonite), is not part of this discussion because this compound does not react with water and hydrate. However, this distinction is not always clear in the literature. Calcium silicate was used in another experimental magnesium phosphate dental product [32, 79, 93]. The calcium silicate was not a hydraulic phase but a phase that reacted in situ contributing to bioactivity.

8.2 Commercial Products

From 1993 to 1998, Dr. Torabinejad of Loma Linda University (Loma Linda, CA, USA) distributed experimental samples of MTA from his laboratory to endodontists. Commercial introduction of MTA products began in 1998 by the Tulsa Dental Specialties division of Dentsply International with ProRoot® MTA. This product was introduced after two applications to the US Food and Drug Administration (FDA) for clearance of these indications: repair of pulpal exposures, apexification, root perforation, root-end filling, and management of internal resorption. A picture of this gray MTA product is shown in Fig. 8.1a. In 2008, the US FDA cleared additional indications of cavity liner, pulpotomies, obturation, and root canal sealer, for MTA-type products from Dentsply. In Korea, MTA-type products are used for replantation [36, 72], transplantation, file separation, and vertical

C.M. Primus, PhD
Primus Consulting, 7046 Owl's Nest Terrace, Bradenton, FL 34203, USA
e-mail: cprimus@me.com

J. Camilleri (ed.), *Mineral Trioxide Aggregate in Dentistry*,
DOI 10.1007/978-3-642-55157-4_8, © Springer-Verlag Berlin Heidelberg 2014

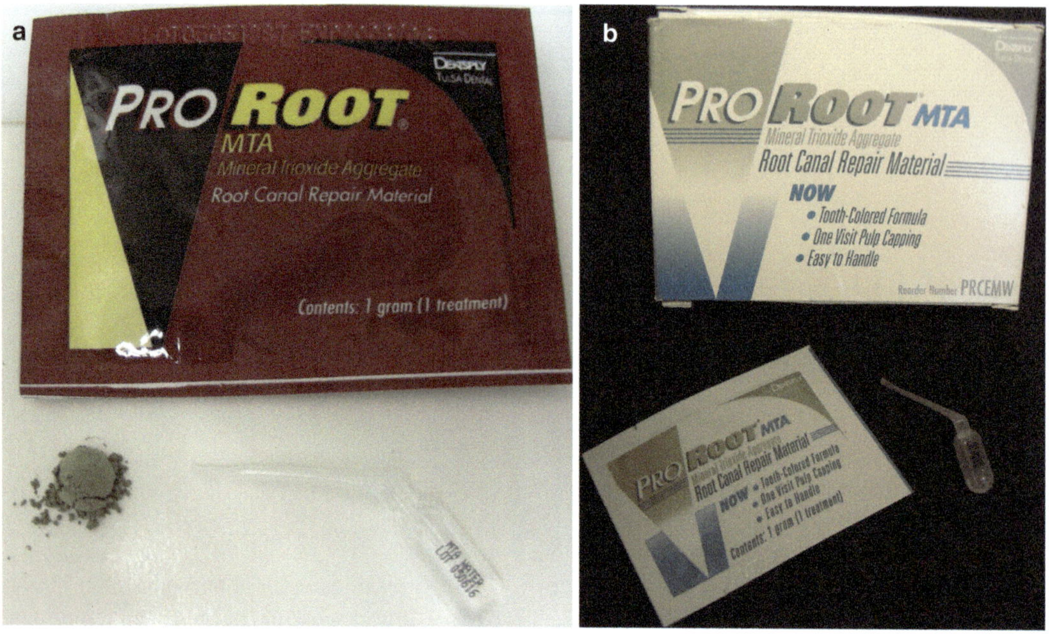

Fig. 8.1 (**a**) Packet of ProRoot MTA powder, ampoule of water and powder, introduced in 1998. (**b**) Packet of tooth-colored (*white*) ProRoot MTA powder, ampoule of water and powder, introduced in 2002

cracks. MTA-type products are generally suitable for dental procedures that contact with pulpal or periapical tissues, as described in this chapter and others. The performance and the convenience of products for a procedure have varied, as can be gleaned in the following discussion.

Since the introduction of ProRoot MTA, a shorter setting time has been desired, so that the clinician can feel confident that the product has set before the procedure is finished, as is conventional for dental materials. Several products and many researchers have sought to achieve this goal, often by the addition of calcium chloride, a known accelerant for Portland cement setting even though calcium chloride is not necessarily the most effective salt for accelerating the set. The elimination of calcium sulfate is known to reduce setting time for Portland cement [68], and this approach has also been used by several manufacturers. Calcium sulfate is necessary in construction concrete pouring to avoid flash or "false" setting, as described in Chap. 1. In dentistry, flash setting is unimportant and may be beneficial as noted below.

Researchers and clinicians have reported that the ProRoot MTA product had poor handling characteristics and "looses consistency in the presence of excess liquid, even at the proportion recommended by the manufacturer," creating a low viscosity, "soupy mix" [62]. Since 1998, many investigators and companies have developed alternatives that were less "sandy", faster setting and less expensive.

The key characteristics for comparisons of MTA products are crystalline phases, particle-size distribution, setting time, handling adjuvants, radiopacifier, and resistance to washout. All of these characteristics contribute to the clinician's ability to satisfactorily prepare and mix the material. Washout resistance is important for stable placement of the material, particularly for the products that have a long setting time. The evolution of the available products and supporting research is described here.

The first patented MTA was a blend of a particular Portland cement composition, which included about 5 % iron oxide, and was believed to be unique in its ability to "work" (private communication about US Patents 5,415,547 and 5,769,638). Dentsply fabricated the patented cement formula under controlled environmental conditions and created a finer powder than the original samples, with better bismuth oxide distribution. This product became ProRoot MTA. The color of the powder was dark gray, as shown in Fig. 8.1a. The powder was packaged in foil pouches and supplied with ampoules of water in the kit (Fig. 8.1a). In 2002, a "tooth-colored" (white) ProRoot MTA (US Patent 7,892,342) product superseded the gray ProRoot MTA. This product was very similar but contained less than 0.5 % iron, so that the cement was yellowish white in color. The bismuth oxide contributed the yellow cast. In many articles, the tooth-colored ProRoot MTA product is denoted as white ProRoot MTA (Fig. 8.1b). Market demand required the original gray-colored ProRoot MTA to be reintroduced, and it has been sporadically available since then. Some papers have proposed greater biocompatibility for the gray version [37, 78].

The Angelus company in Londrina, Brazil, founded by Dr. Roberto Q. M. Alcântara, commercialized a more affordable MTA product in 2001. This product was available in Brazil and now is available through Henry Schein distributors. The format of their gray and white Angelus products is bottles of powder and water in a vial, different from ProRoot MTA powder in 1 g pouches with water ampoules. Originally, commercial Portland cement was used to create MTA Angelus, a gray-colored powder with bismuth oxide, which was followed by MTA Bianco, a white Portland cement with bismuth oxide.

When evaluating products, researchers have often repeated the term "sandy" feel of MTA [64] Coarse particles give this sensation and scratchy sound when a powder is mixed with water on a glass slab. Therefore, the particle-size distributions have been compared for several powders. The particle-size distribution of the experimental samples of MTA from Loma Linda University is shown in Fig. 8.2a, and this powder has a significant portion of particles coarser than 40 μm, hence the "sandy feel." The material was coarser than ProRoot MTA [65] and had incompletely dispersed bismuth oxide which appeared as bright spots in radiographs. The particle-size distributions in Fig. 8.2b, c are for the Angelus company's white and gray MTA powders. The median particle sizes are below 10 μm, but each powder contains many particles which are coarser than 40 μm, up to 100 μm. The line at 20 μm allows a comparison of the number of particles that are coarse. Figure 8.2d–f show the distributions of particle sizes in ProRoot (gray and white) and DiaRoot powders (DiaDent Group International, Burnaby, British Columbia, Canada), which have significantly fewer coarse particles than the original MTA or the Angelus materials. Figure 8.3 has particle-size distributions for three newer materials, which are remarkably finer: Biodentine, EndoSequence sealer, and RetroMTA powders. None of these powders is "nano-sized." Nano-sized particles are 1/1,000 of a micron and none of these materials is even submicron (1/10 of a micron).

Nano-sized particles are of interest because of the high surface-to-volume ratio versus micron-sized particles. The surface-to-volume ratio changes from less than 10 % for micron-sized particles to more than 50 % for nanoparticles, which is important because a higher surface-to-volume ratio can dramatically increase reactivity, such as hydration. Fumed or colloidal silica are nano-sized particles that are commonly added to many dental products. Such silica products may be a minor addition to some MTA products; however, no MTA product has been identified that is primarily composed of nanoparticles.

Calcium sulfate is used in construction uses of Portland cement to delay setting. Without calcium sulfate, the calcium aluminate phase of Portland cement quickly hydrates and causes initial setting by stiffening the cement, which is undesirable for bulk pouring of concrete. For MTA indications, faster setting is desired. The Angelus company has integrated the manufacture of the tricalcium silicate powders into their operations so that their MTA products are now made with fewer trace metal oxides and without calcium sulfate (private communication, 2013). The initial setting time of their products is reported to be only 10 min, by allowing the tricalcium aluminate phase to quickly hydrate [54]. Later, the Angelus Corporation developed a sealer containing MTA powder (MTA Fillapex®), which is described in the ensuing sealer section.

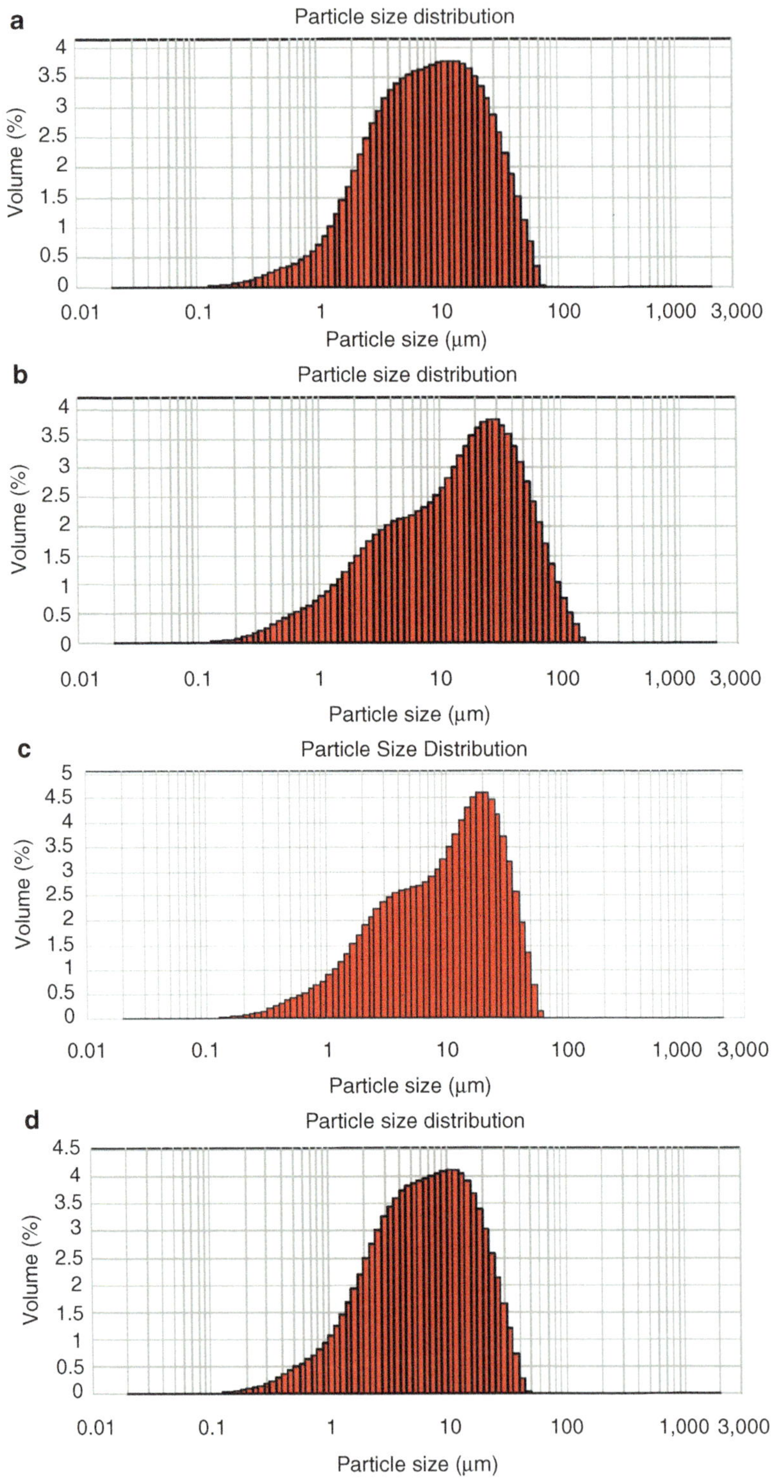

Fig. 8.2 (**a**) Original, pre-commercial MTA powder particle-size distribution. (**b**) MTA Bianco from Angelus Corporation powder particle-size distribution. (**c**) MTA Angelus (*gray*) from Angelus Corporation powder particle-size distribution. (**d**) Early version of (*gray*) ProRoot MTA powder particle-size distribution. (**e**) Tooth-colored (*white*) ProRoot MTA powder particle-size distribution. (**f**) DiaRoot powder particle-size distribution

Fig. 8.2 (continued)

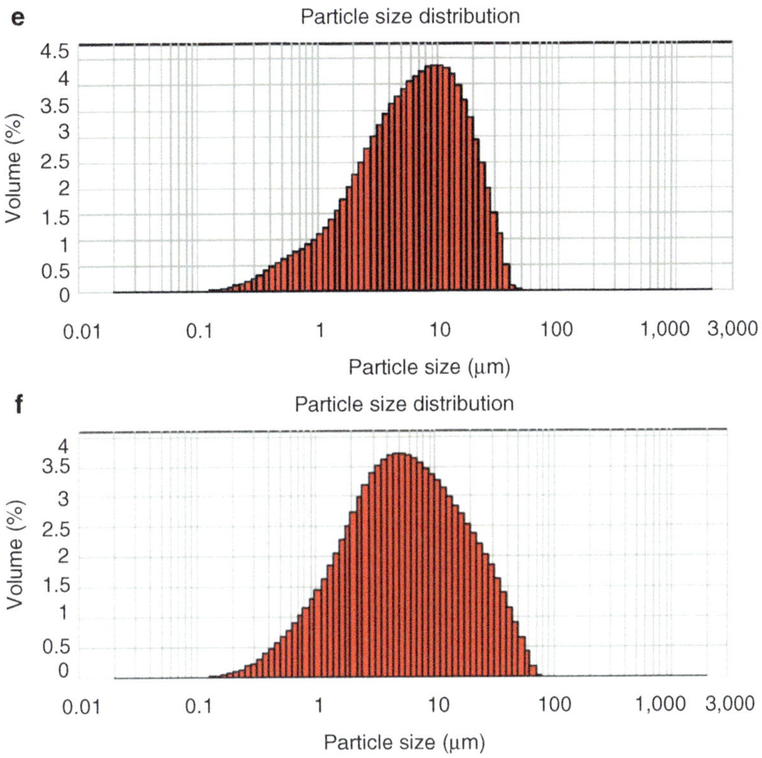

DiaRoot® from DiaDent® was introduced by 2007, and this material was manufactured without tricalcium aluminate; therefore, no calcium sulfate phase is needed to control the rapid hydration of the tricalcium silicate. Tantalite (Ta_2O_5) is used as the radiopaque powder, making this material very white, by comparisons to gray ProRoot MTA or tooth-colored (white) ProRoot MTA that contain bismuth oxide. DiaRoot was advertised as containing calcium phosphate monobasic, but no phosphate phase was detected with XRD (Table 8.1), indicating that the phosphate was either amorphous or was present at less than 1 %. The format of this product is very similar to ProRoot MTA with one gm sachets of powder and water ampoules shown in Fig. 8.4. Currently, this product is sold through Verio Dental Co. (Vancouver, Canada) from Innovative BioCeramix Inc. (IBC) (Vancouver, Canada).

The Brasseler Co. (Savannah, GA, USA) offers MTA-type products, under the trade name EndoSequence BC or Bioceramic. These products appear to be related to the DiaRoot and iRoot products, and IBC is believed to be the supplier/manufacturer. The Brasseler products are based on fine tricalcium silicate powders that do not contain alumina. The products are offered in four formats: powder for mixing with water, a paste, a putty, and a sealer (Fig. 8.5). The EndoSequence BC putty, paste, and sealer have the powder mixed with various carrier liquids that do not cause setting; hence, the liquid must be anhydrous. These paste/putty forms of the EndoSequence BC material do not require mixing before placement and they allow a clinician to choose a viscosity suitable for the indication or case. When placed, water must diffuse from the tissues into the paste, putty, or sealer to displace the carrier liquid and cause hydration/setting of the tricalcium silicate powder. The percentage of the ceramic powder in any of the products is not known, but is estimated as 60–80 % MTA-type powder. The fine powders and convenience as putty or paste are solutions to the criticisms of MTA being coarse and hard to place. The time for diffusion of water to cause setting will vary with the indication and location. Brasseler EndoSequence putty sets more slowly than ProRoot MTA [28], but the setting times

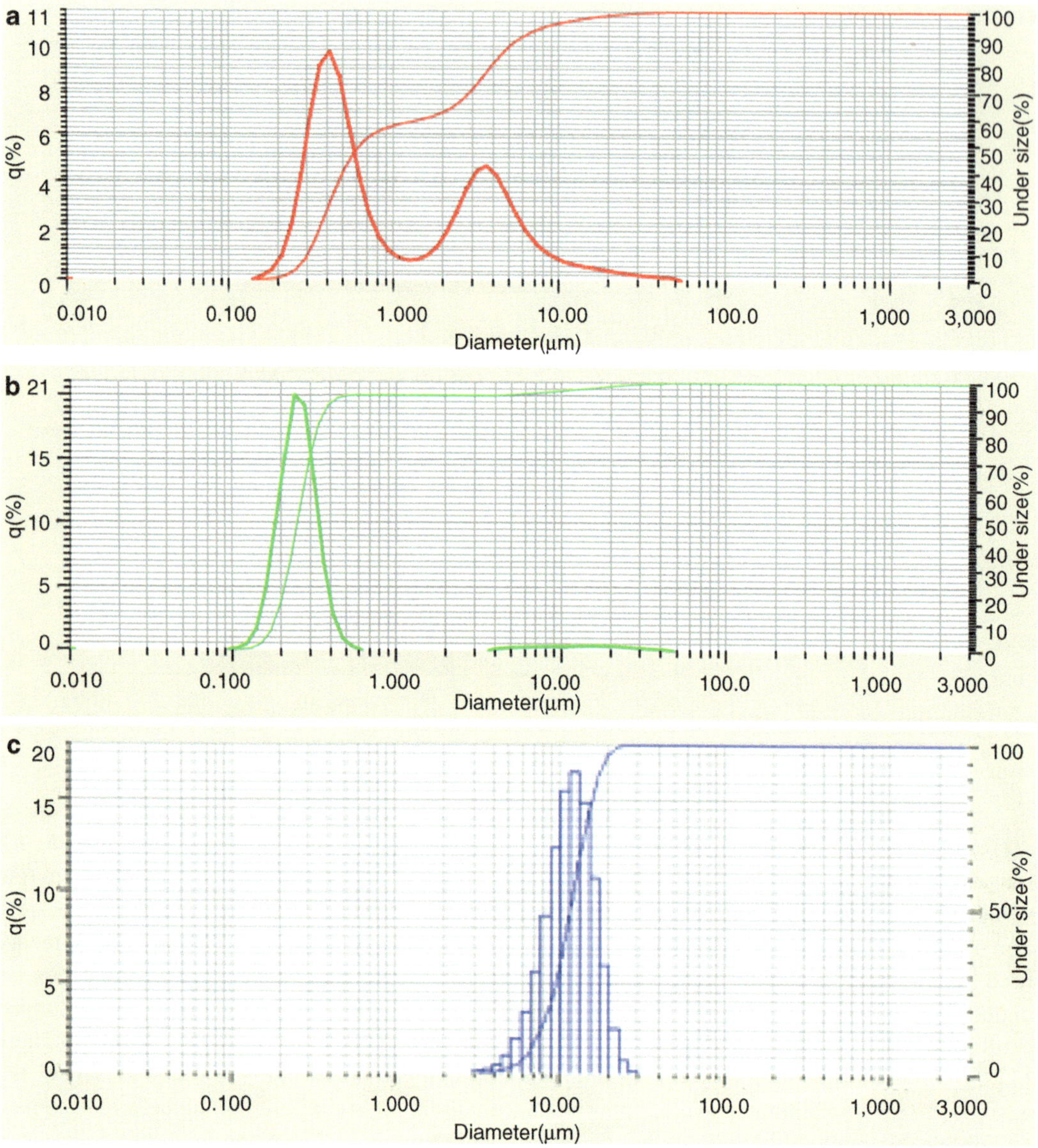

Fig. 8.3 (**a**) Biodentine powder particle-size distribution. (**b**)EndoSequence sealer powder particle-size distribution. (**c**) RetroMTA powder particle-size distribution

for these materials are more than 24 h, therefore irrelevant for the procedure. In vitro testing shows that setting of the sealer takes more than 1 week [71]. However, the ability to place the putty and complete the procedure may outweigh other concerns.

Brasseler and IBC companies use the terms bioaggregate and bioceramic for their products. Bioaggregate has no technical meaning, but does imply the bioactivity that occurs when tri- and dicalcium silicates are placed in contact with tissue fluid. Bioceramic is a term used to refer any ceramic (nonmetallic and inorganic) material, including glass, in the body of suitable biocompatibility. Bioceramics are not limited to the Brasseler products, but include resorbable ceramics and inert ceramics such as alumina or zirconia used in dentistry and other medical devices.

Table 8.1 X-ray diffraction results for some MTA products (weight percent)

Phase detected by XRD	(White) ProRoot MTA	DiaRoot	Biodentine	RetroMTA	Endocem	MTA+ (Cerkamed)	MTA Plus	MTA Caps	CPM Endo-XRD analysis
Tricalcium silicate	57.8	61.2	82.7	43.8		62.7	59.3	20.7	62.6
Dicalcium silicate	18.5	26.7		18.6	36.2	2.8	17.7	17.7	15.0
Tricalcium aluminate				3.2				9.8	
Calcium sulfate	1.7						1.5		3.3
Calcium carbonate			13.7		42.0		0.7	18.3	11.5
Tetracalcium aluminoferrite	0.09						0.6		
Calcium hydroxide	1.9	3.2			1.7				
Bismuth oxide	20.0				15.2	9.3	20.0		3.7
Calcium tungstate								30.8	
Zirconium oxide			3.6	25.4		9.2			
Barium sulfate									3.2
Tantalite		6.7							
Calcium phosphate (various)					1.7				
Magnesium oxide					1.1				
Calcium chloride hydrate								2.3	
Silica-crystalline					2.0		0.1	0.4	/7
Amorphous (silica)				9.0		14.0			
Tetracalcium monocarboaluminate $Ca_4Al_2(OH)_{12}(CO_3)(H_2O)_5$						2.0			0.7

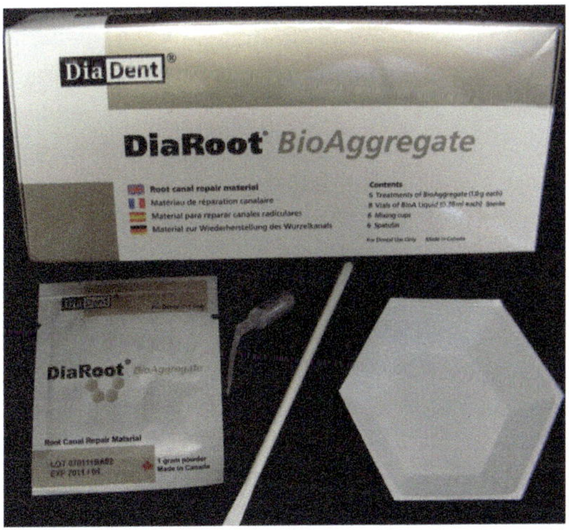

Fig. 8.4 DiaRoot BioAggregate product showing powder sachet, water ampoule, and mixing tools

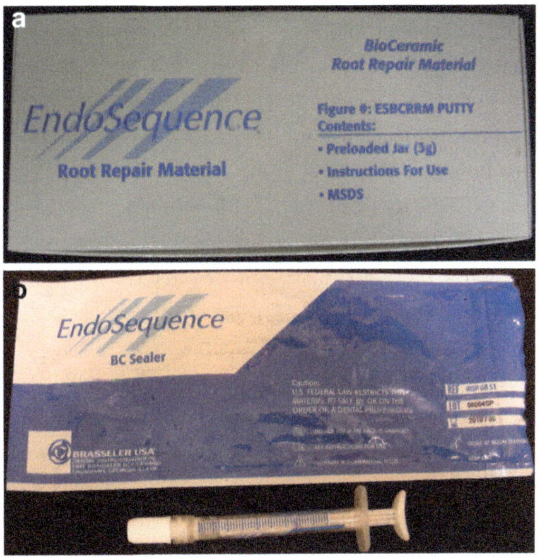

Fig. 8.5 Two of Brasseler's EndoSequence products, putty (**a**) and sealer (**b**), are shown

Brasseler also manufactures EndoSequence BC gutta-percha points that contain the same tricalcium silicate powder used in their other tricalcium silicate products. This product is their approach to bonding the sealer to the gutta-percha and the dentin as a "monoblock" [94]. The use of MTA powder in gutta-percha has been patented (US 7,838,573).

Biodentine® (Septodont, Saint-Maur-des-Fossés, France) is a fast-setting tricalcium silicate product, which has the same indications as ProRoot MTA. The company has emphasized using the material to replace dentine lost to caries. Its use as a dentine replacement may not prevent leakage [22]. A composite resin should be placed over the Biodentine as the material will not be sufficiently stable when exposed to the oral cavity. Biodentine powder is packaged in unit doses of 0.75 g, more than is usually used for endodontic or vital pulp therapy indications (Fig. 8.6). The user manually adds the liquid to the powder's capsule and the mixture is triturated. The water-based liquid, supplied in ampoules, contains a "plasticizer" (polycarboxylate) and calcium chloride to enhance the properties and speed the setting. Although advertised as "dentin in a capsule," the Biodentine powder contains mostly tricalcium silicate (83 %) with 14 % calcium carbonate and 4 % zirconia (Table 8.1) and does not contain hydroxyapatite and collagen. Biodentine does not contain dentine and should not be confused with bone grafting material, which is hydroxyapatite. However, its fine powder and faster setting are improvements over the original MTA. The low amount of zirconia in Biodentine makes the material only as radiopaque as dentin. High radiopaque contrast is desired for dental materials, such as composite resins, which are also dentin replacements, for X-ray visibility. However, this product was stable to discoloration [95], unlike ProRoot MTA [9, 12, 59, 67, 70].

TheraCal™ LC (Bisco Inc. Schaumburg, IL, USA) is the only commercial light-curing version of MTA to date and is indicated for pulpal tissue contact. This material contains less than 20 % MTA powder, a radiopacifier of barium zirconate ($BaZrO_3$), and dimethacrylate resins. The

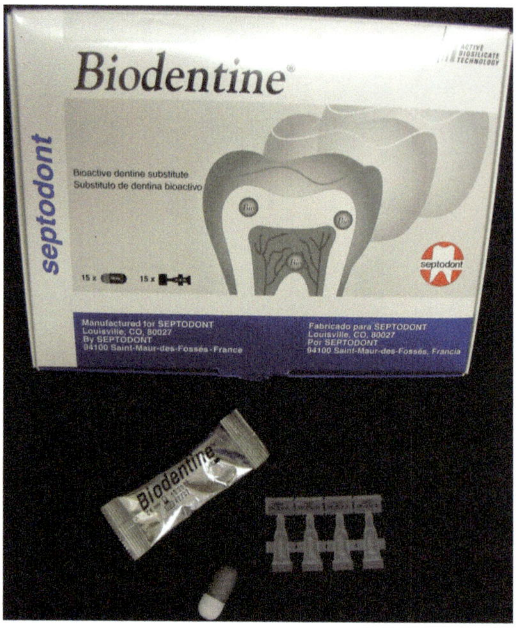

Fig. 8.6 Biodentine by Septodont, showing the triturator capsule and its foil packaging, liquid for addition to the capsule

product literature describes the MTA component as Type III Portland cement, which denotes a finer powder than Type I Portland cement. The particle size is less important for a premixed material that needs no spatulation prior to light curing. TheraCal has been tested and shown to release more calcium ions than Dycal® (Dentsply International, York, Pennsylvania, USA), a calcium hydroxide-based pulp-capping material [44]. Also the TheraCal product has higher radiopacity, lower solubility, and better bonding than Dycal, the current "gold standard" for pulp capping. TheraCal is not indicated for the endodontic indications for which MTA has become known and may not be suitable for such indications based on cytotoxicity studies [55].

New endodontic cement (NEC, AKA calcium-enriched mixture or CEM) has been introduced (BioniqueDent, Tehran, Iran) and contains calcium compounds not found in ProRoot MTA. The NEC material contains more calcia than MTA does by the addition of [8] calcium oxide, calcium phosphate, calcium carbonate, calcium silicate, calcium sulfate, calcium hydroxide, and calcium chloride. Over time, calcium oxide powder will form hydroxide and then carbonate in the container, to create more calcium carbonate. Asgary has not disclosed the presence of tri- or dicalcium silicates, nor a radiopaque agent in the literature; however, the material's similar performance to MTA makes this material likely to be based on the familiar MTA phases of tri- and dicalcium silicate phases. NEC has been reported to be bioactive and have good handling and sealing [6] as a root-end filling material. Its film thickness was lower than ProRoot MTA's and its flow was higher, indicative of a finer particle size than the ProRoot MTA, which has the same indications. A study with pulp capping in canines has shown equivalent results of MTA and NEC, and NEC's superiority to calcium hydroxide-based IRM® [91]. A root-end filling study in canines was successful (after 60 days) versus MTA when apical lesions were induced [5]. Pulpotomies in humans showed similar success (about 75 %) for NEC and MTA [76] for apical development for as long as a 1-year follow-up. A second study in humans compared conventional root canal therapy to pulpotomies (with NEC) for postoperative pain and 6-month radiographic outcome. Significantly less pain occured in the first 7 days for pain and radiographic superiority [4].

Two manufacturers from Korea have introduced MTA products to the USA and elsewhere: OrthoMTA and RetroMTA (BioMTA, Daejeon, Korea), and Endocem MTA (Maruchi, Gangwon-do, Korea) shown in Fig. 8.7. OrthoMTA and RetroMTA products are fine powders, advertised as having an average particle size of 2.6 μm, although independent testing has shown that the powders have a median particle size of about 10 μm (Fig. 8.3c). The indications for OrthoMTA and RetroMTA overlap, although RetroMTA has more vital pulp indications.

OrthoMTA is sold in (centrifuge vials) containing 0.2 g of powder. The user adds his/her own water to the powder in the vial and places the vial in a battery-powered centrifuge to spin for 20 s. Then the excess water is decanted and the retained powder is considered hydrated for dispensing. Special instruments are used for dispensing. Initial setting time is 3 min. and the final setting is about 6 h. The phases present are said to include tri- and dicalcium silicate, tricalcium aluminate, tetracalcium aluminoferrite, less than 1 % free calcia, and 3 % of amorphous phase. Its radiopaque component is bismuth oxide. The material is indicated for orthograde use.

RetroMTA has a different format from OrthoMTA. Sachets of 0.3 g of powder are packaged in a flat plastic container disk with separate ampoules of water, which are manually mixed by the user. This light gray tri- and dicalcium silicate powder has about 25 % zirconia, some tricalcium aluminate phase, calcium chloride, and silica (Table 8.1). It is advertised as containing calcium aluminozirconate for radiopacity, but this was not detected by X-ray diffraction. The RetroMTA brochure lists "lack of discoloration" as an attribute; discoloration has been attributed to bismuth oxide [23]. RetroMTA does not contain bismuth oxide, so the discoloration claim seems valid. The initial setting time of RetroMTA is said to be 1.5 min, which is likely caused by the calcium chloride.

Endocem MTA shown in Fig. 8.7c is advertised as setting in 3:15 min. Like the OrthoMTA, the powder is sold in a flip-top vial of the kind that is often used in centrifuging biological samples. The Endocem product literature states that zirconia is present, but bismuth oxide was identified in X-ray diffraction (Table 8.1). Endocem was the only product tested that contained only dicalcium silicate, with no tricalcium silicate for the hydraulic reaction. The setting was not tested independently; however, dicalcium silicate is slower setting than tricalcium silicate. About 40 % calcium carbonate was also identified, with minor amounts of calcium phosphate, crystalline silica, and magnesia. This excess calcium carbonate indicates that the material is pozzolanic.

Cerkamed PPH (Wojciech Pawlowski, Nisko, Poland) has introduced an MTA+ product (Fig. 8.8), which is distinct from the product MTA Plus® described below. The MTA+ product is distributed in small polymer bottles containing 0.3 g of powder with a separate vial of water. This white powder contained primarily tricalcium

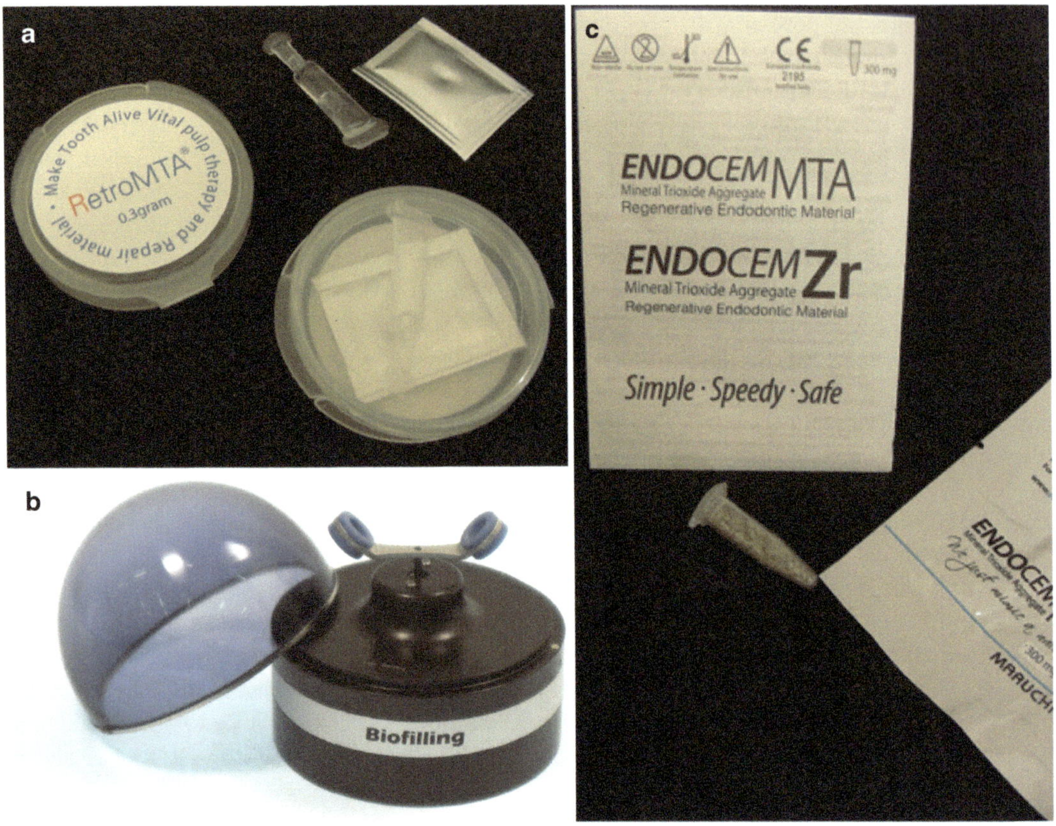

Fig. 8.7 (**a**) RetroMTA shown in sachet, packaged with water ampoule. (**b**) OrthoMTA shown in vial placed in centrifuge (Image courtesy of Dr. Yoojin Shin, BioMTA.) (**c**) Endocem shown in vial, having a *gray* color

silicate (63 %) with silica, and about 9 % each of bismuth oxide and zirconia, and a small amount of an aluminate phase (Table 8.1) in X-ray diffraction.

Medcem GmbH (Weinfelden, CH) offers a Portland cement powder for use instead of formocresol [83]. However, this powder has no radiopaque material; therefore, its radiopacity is similar to dentin.

Two MTA Plus® products are available and both are tri/dicalcium silicate powders with bismuth oxide. The white version is sold outside the USA, and is manufactured by Prevest Denpro (Jammu, India); its phase composition is substantially identical to that of tooth-colored ProRoot MTA (Table 8.1). Grey MTA Plus is manufactured in the USA by Avalon Biomed Inc. (Bradenton, FL, USA). Both products include a powder and gel for mixing.

Both MTA Plus products are indicated for pulp and periapical tissue contact. This is the only MTA product that is indicated for the additional indication of a root canal sealer. The variety of indications from pulp-capping to root-end filling can be satisfied by varying the ratio of powder to gel to the desired consistency for the procedure. The benefit of the gel is the washout resistance, versus other MTA products mixed with water. The MTA Plus powders are finer than ProRoot MTA powder, as can be seen in the scanning electron micrographs of Fig. 8.9. The coarse particles of ProRoot MTA create the "sandy" feeling when mixing with water. The MTA Plus powder is packaged in a desiccant-lined bottle, which is more protective and convenient than sachets of other manufacturers against water absorption by the cement, and permits the clinician to use any amount of powder without

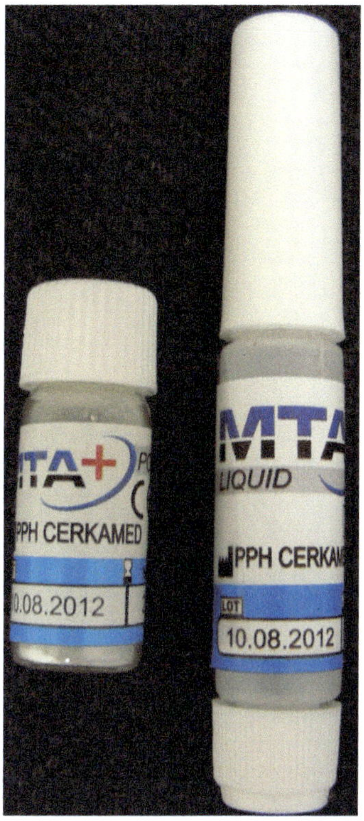

Fig. 8.8 MTA+material from Cerkamed, shown in vial, having a white color

waste. Several articles have been written about the properties of MTA Plus including remineralization, anti-washout, and use as a root canal sealer [25, 40, 69, 75, 84]. A product similar in appearance to the white-version of MTA Plus is marketed by Dentonics (Charlotte, NC, USA) as Masterdent® MTA.

In 2013, several European companies introduced MTA products that have 0.3 g "unit doses" in triturator capsules containing powder. When the capsules are squeezed to activate (like an amalgam capsule), a separate compartment with water is opened and the powder and water are triturated. Harvard Dental International's (Hoppegarten, Germany) MTA, Micro-Mega (Besancon, France) MM-MTA™, S&C Polymer Silicon's (Elmshorn, Schleswig-Holstein, Germany) MTA cement, and MTA Caps by Acteon (Merignac, France) all have unit-dose triturator capsules (Fig. 8.10). These capsules are sold in foil pouches, to protect the powder in the capsule from humidity. Ironically, the capsules also contain water for mixing. The water must be sufficiently segregated to avoid harming the powder during storage, or the shelf life will be impaired.

The MTA Caps powder was analyzed (Table 8.1) and found to contain tricalcium and dicalcium silicate, tricalcium aluminate, about 18 % calcium carbonate, and 31 % calcium tungstate (for radiopacity). A small amount of silica and calcium chloride hydrate is included, which presumably enhance handling and accelerate initial setting. MM-MTA is also said to have a "faster set time" (20 min), achieved by the addition of calcium carbonate.

Other products are close to marketing such as Trioxident (VladMiVa, Belgorod, Russia)'s NEX MTA (Tokyo, Japan) cement or Endo–Eze MTA by Ultradent (South Jordan, UT, USA). The Trioxident product is a powder–water system, with the powder sold in sachets. The powder has some coarse particle but appears to be a conventional MTA formula with bismuth oxide. The NEX MTA is a powder–liquid system and the powder is provided in sachets. The format of the Endo–Eze MTA is unknown.

The spectrum of formulas, packaging, properties, and colors is widening. Undoubtedly, more calcium silicate products will enter the marketplace in the coming years.

8.3 Experimental Products

In 2005–2010, experimental products from Dentsply were described in the literature: ProRoot MTA Advanced [79, 97] and ProRoot MTA sealer (AKA Generex A and B, respectively). The former had the usual periapical and pulpal contact indications; the latter was indicated only for root canal sealing. Although the results were favorable for sealing [57, 99] and bioactivity [99], these powder/gel products have not been commercially introduced. The experimental Dentsply products were disclosed as being more radiopaque and having improved handling compared to ProRoot MTA. Each product had a unique liquid for use for its indications.

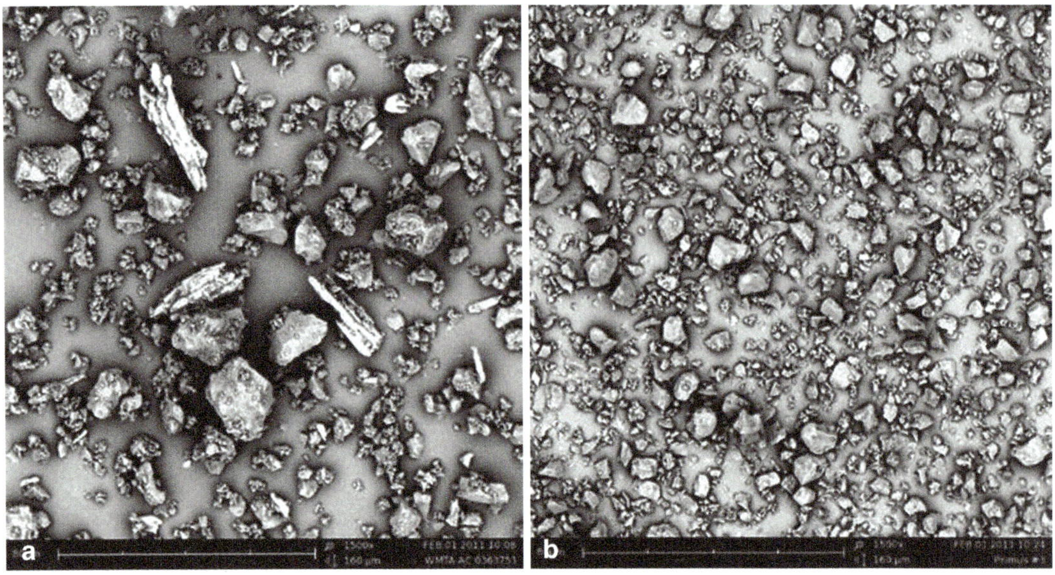

Fig. 8.9 Particle-size comparison of ProRoot MTA (**a**) versus MTA Plus with (**b**)

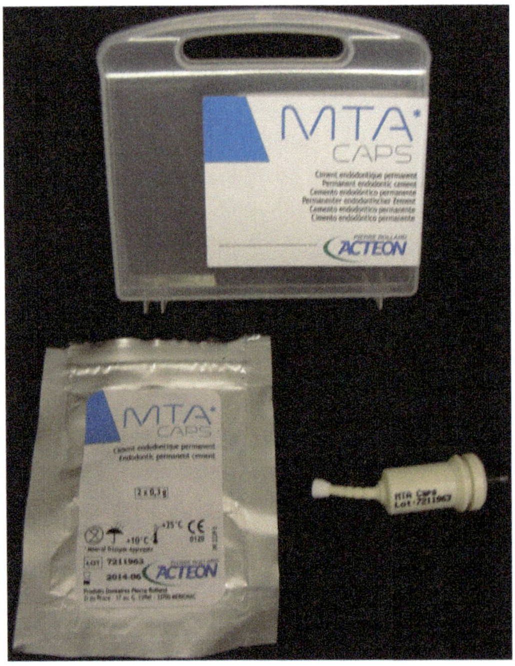

Fig. 8.10 MTA Caps by Acteon showing the triturator capsule and foil pouch

Another experimental product was Viscosity Enhanced Root Repair Material (VERRM) [30] which contained Portland cement, bismuth oxide, and "other compounds" such as polyvinyl alcohol, polyethylene oxide, natural gums, cellulose, or clay dispersions to improve the handling versus MTA. Cellulose and calcium chloride have also been tested by others [10] for mixing with MTA products.

Camilleri has been a forerunner in experimental materials by testing gray and white Portland cements, with the addition of an industrial plasticizer. The plasticizer improved the handling (workability) and did not reduce biocompatibility [26]. The absence of calcium sulfate in a tricalcium silicate accelerated setting [18]. She did pioneering work [19] in investigating the suitability of MTA products for use as a sealer, when MTA-type materials were mixed with Glenium® (Degussa, Manchester, UK), a polycarboxylic ether polymer, to attempt to meet the requirements of ISO 6876 for root canal sealers.

Ding has researched sol–gel–processed dicalcium silicate cement for endodontics and possibly bone cement. He used mixtures of the cement with sodium phosphate dibasic (Na_2HPO_4) as an accelerant [34]. Recently he reported on ß-Ca_2SiO_4 powder, combined with gelatin and chitosan oligosaccharide (COS) solution in a liquid phase [29]. Research has also been performed by his group regarding incorporating zinc oxide, magnesia, and iron oxide additions to tricalcium silicate powders [63] for improved properties.

Gandolfi and Prati have tested Portland cement-based materials (denoted as TC materials) using variations that include montmorillonite (a type of inorganic clay that is a layered phyllosilicate), calcium chloride, and fluoride, sometimes mixed with Articaine®. Their MTA formulas were as biocompatible as the ProRoot MTA product and more biocompatible than AH Plus® (Dentsply, Konstanz, Germany) root canal sealer [42]. Other experimental formulas, also denoted as TC, used another white Portland cement and showed the bioactivity of the experimental materials [48], although the pushout strengths of their experimental formulas were not as high as for ProRoot MTA [61]. A promising light-curable formula has also been reported [47].

An experimental material containing barium sulfate, Portland cement, and undisclosed emulsifiers has been investigated. Like other Portland cement products, implantation was equal to MTA (Angelus) [51].

Asgary, the inventor of NEC, mentioned other materials that were being developed for MTA-type applications, but information on these experimental materials was not available: Root MTA (Salamifar in Iran) ([41]), Abyek cement (Abyek company in Iran), Melcann cement or Melcann white cement (Melcann cement in Australia), and Saveh white cement (Saveh company in Iran) [7]. However, the latter three cements seem to reference cement brands, not dental companies or brands.

An experimental root canal sealer has been reported in the literature, MTAS [96], having a composition of 80 % white Portland cement with zirconia for radiopacity. Its liquid contains water, calcium chloride, and a "resinous vehicle" [81].

Many studies have used commercial Portland cements as a substitute for MTA products on the market and as the basis for experimental products [3, 7, 13, 14, 24, 31, 33, 35, 43, 45, 50, 58, 60–62, 65, 66, 74, 82, 86–88, 90, 92, 100]. Often, the focus has been on biocompatibility of the Portland cements, usually cell culture studies, versus ProRoot MTA. Other studies have measured the arsenic or other trace metal oxides in Portland cements versus commercial products. The total arsenic oxide content of the noncommercial preproduction MTA powder was 5 ppm (unpublished data, 2007), determined by inductively coupled plasma technique (ICP), although the leachable content would be less. Researchers disagree on methods for arsenic determinations and the reports of the amounts in commercial cements or MTA products have varied, ranging from <1 ppm to over 50 ppm. The potential arsenic content has been discussed [80], as a possible contaminant in commercial Portland cements designed for construction, versus medical devices. The International Standards Organization (ISO) 9917 document limits the leachable arsenic content to 2 ppm for water-based dental cements. No researcher has reported a commercial construction grade Portland cement that meets all the important attributes of sealing, fine particle size, freedom from lead and arsenic, and conformance to ISO 6876 standards such as insolubility and radiopacity.

8.4 Alternative Formulas

Portland (calcium silicate) cement has been combined with calcium aluminate cement for some tests as a dental material. Monocalcium aluminate cements should not be confused with the tricalcium aluminate phase of Portland cements. The monocalcium aluminates, hereafter referred to as calcium aluminate cement, are commercially used for high-temperature linings of furnaces and as a coating in some sewer systems. The calcium aluminate cements have the advantages of higher early strength and greater resistance to acid than calcium silicate (Portland-type) cements; however, the calcium aluminate cements undergo "conversion," a reversible hydration reaction at environmental temperatures, making them unsound for massive construction. The main setting reaction calcium aluminate cements at body temperature is given in Eq. 8.4, which is a dissolution–precipitation reaction.

$$6(CaO \cdot Al_2O_3) + 24H_2O \rightarrow 2(CaO) \cdot Al_2O_3 \cdot 6H_2O + 4Al(OH)_3 \quad (8.4)$$

Calcium aluminate cements have higher strength than the minor phase of tricalcium aluminate, present in most Portland cements as described earlier. Furthermore, some reactivity of the monocalcium aluminate occurs with silica, which seems to contribute to the Quick-Set material described below.

Capasio, now known as Quick-Set, is an experimental material that has been investigated as an MTA improvement. The Quick-Set system includes a fine calcium aluminosilicate powder and a water-based gel. This material is quick-setting, washout resistant, and acid resistant [97]. Quick-Set is chemically distinct from MTA because it does not contain tri- or dicalcium silicate. This fine aluminosilicate powder has been shown to penetrate dentinal tubules [11] and to biocompatible [38, 98]. EndoBinder material (Binderware, São Carlos, SP, Brazil) is a calcium aluminate product, which does not contain silica but is a water-setting hydraulic material. EndoBinder has less MMP-2 activity than other hydraulic dental materials [89]. Other properties of Endobinder have been shown to be favorable [1, 2, 49]. The monocalcium aluminate in EndoBinder and in Quick-Set powders is known to be more acid resistant, which is beneficial for placing the cement in infected conditions or for the placement of a composite, which requires acid etching, over the cement.

Camilleri also tested combinations of calcium aluminate, calcium silicate cements, and fluoride-containing silicate cements with calcium sulfate additions reporting adequate in vitro properties [15, 17], acceptable biocompatibility [16], and successful reduction of the initial and final setting times. While some companies have removed calcium sulfate, Camilleri added about 8 % $CaSO_4$ and a plasticizer to achieve desirable test results. Dye leakage was noted with these experimental materials [20], but bacteria may be killed by the high pH of the interstitial liquid in the cement, preventing harm from leakage. Attack by acid on these predominantly tricalcium silicate materials did occur [21].

8.5 Root Canal Sealers

MTA-based root canal sealers are intriguing because of the biocompatibility of MTA and its osteogenic potential for accidental extrusion beyond the apex. The American Dental Association (ADA) 57 and ISO 6876 requirements for root canal sealers are useful for evaluating such root canal sealer products. These two documents' requirements and methods are identical with two exceptions. The ISO 6876 standard uses a flow and working time sample of 0.05 ml versus 0.5 ml for the ADA 57 standard. The second difference is the ISO 6876 version has no requirement regarding dimensional stability, whereas the ADA 57 standard requires the linear dimensional stability over 30 days to be less than 1 % shrinkage and less than 0.1 % expansion ($1\ \% < \Delta L < +0.1\ \%$.). Data from the literature have been gathered in Table 8.2 for several materials discussed above. The requirements provide a basis for comparisons; however, the standards are not designed to compare clinical handling, sealing of the canal, or clinical efficacy. The following discussion of MTA-containing sealers refers to the methods of these standards.

The EndoSequence BC sealer of Brasseler is a single paste sealer that contains a very fine tricalcium silicate powder and an unidentified liquid medium. The fill percentage of powder is also undisclosed. Within the tooth, water must interact with the powder, displace the medium, and cause hydration and setting of the tricalcium silicate around the gutta-percha. The sealer has been reported to meet the ISO 6876 requirements [27, 101], as shown in Table 8.2. When used with EndoSequence BC gutta-percha, some hydration and bonding of the tricalcium silicate in the gutta-percha can be expected with the sealer. However, the benefits of this interaction have not been published, such as, evidence that hydration does bond the sealer to the gutta-percha. The EndoSequence BC sealer's setting time is quite long (>24 h), depending on the testing methodology, but zinc oxide eugenol (ZOE) sealers also have a long setting time.

MTA Plus products are indicated for use as a root canal sealer. The MTA Plus powders are very similar in composition to the original MTA, but the powder is finer and a gel is included, not water. The finer powder and gel allows the small film thickness to be achieved (<50 μm is required) for a root canal sealer, which was not possible with ProRoot MTA (Table 8.2), or in

Table 8.2 Properties tested per ADA 57, ISO 6876, and ISO 9917 tests (From Asgary et al. [8], Candeiro et al. [27] and Zhou et al. [101]; Otherwise measured by the author)

Test	Criteria for conformance or desired value, if none stated	ProRoot MTA (mixed at 3:1 w/water)	OrthoMTA/ RetroMTA	MTA Plus® material w/gel		EndoSequence BC sealer [101]	MTA Fillapex [101]	NEC (Asgary et al. [7, 8]
				Gray	White			
Radiopacity (mm equivalent of Al)	Exceed 3 mm of equivalent Al	5	**5**	**5.5**	**4.9**	**3.8** [27]		
Working time (min)	Preferably 10–20 min	5 [8], 70		**12** at **P:L = 3:1** **20** at **P:L = 1:1**		**>1440/24 h**	**45 ± 15**	**5 ± 0.8**
Setting time (hours)	Preferably less than 20 min, but may be longer if the clinical use is satisfactory with a short working time and high washout resistance	1:10 [8], ~5 h	**3/3**	**1:15** at **P:L = 3:1** **10** at **P:L = 1:1**		**2.7 ± 0.3**	**2.5 ± 0.3**	**0.8 ± 0:1**
Solubility in water (weight %)	Must be less than 3 % by weight after setting, ideally after 24 h, but definitely after the final set time	1.3		**1.2** at **3:1 & 2:1**; **1.9** at **1:1, after 3 days of setting**		**2.9 ± 0.5**	**1.1 ± 0.2**	
Dimensional stability (linear %)	Shall be less than 1 % shrinkage and less than 0.1 % expansion after 30 days	0.3 0.085 [8]		**0.04, 0.07**		**0.09 ± 0.04**	**−0.7 ± 0.01**	**0.08 ± 0.03**
Film thickness measurement (μm)	Must be less than 50 μm for sealers, but acceptable >50 μm for other indications	470, 452 [8]		**470** at **P:L = 3:1** **180** at **P:L = 2:1** **47–69** at **P:L = 1:1**		**22 ± 5**	**24 ± 7**	**175 ± 25**
Flow (mm)	Flow should be more 20 mm for sealer. (Less than 20 mm is needed for other indications)	2 10		**29-31 at P:L=1:1** **8** at **P:L = 3:1**		**23.1±0.7**	**24.9 ± 0.5**	**10 ± 0.8**
Leachable As and Pb	<2 ppm As, <100 ppm Pb in acid leaching test	Meets standard		**1.3 ppm TOTAL As; no detectable Pb**				
Compressive strength (MPa)	More than 50 MPa	55		**42** at **2:1** **80** at **3:1**				

general, for construction grade Portland cements. Setting time is less than 10 h in vivo, using the ISO 6876 test method, when mixed to the consistency needed for a sealer.

MTA Fillapex (Angelus, Londrina, Brazil) is a two-paste root canal sealer that contains MTA powder in a salicylate resin (Fig. 8.11). The 1,2 butylene glycol disalicylate resin creates a 35 min working time and a 2:10 h setting time; however, the sealer contains only 13.2 % MTA powder. Studies are needed to find out if the MTA will hydrate within the resin and if bioactivity occurs in this format. If not, then the sealer's resin carrier is more similar to the pulp-capping material called Dycal, without the calcium hydroxide. Studies have shown Fillapex to be antibacterial but also to be more soluble than AH Plus sealer [39].

Retreatability has been an issue regarding MTA-based sealers, because of the challenge of removing the old sealer before retreatment. Two studies have shown that complete removal of the EndoSequence sealer, Fillapex, and MTA Plus sealers is not possible [56, 75]. No study has shown that retreatment will be more or less important for these sealers.

Endoseal by Maruchi is an MTA powder that is mixed with water for use with gutta-percha cones. This material is provided in a plastic vial within a foil pouch for unit doses of 0.3 g. The material is said to contain zirconia and no heavy metals.

Endo CPM material (EGEO SRL, Buenos Aires, Argentina), shown in Fig. 8.12, is a powder–liquid system for use as a root canal sealer. The composition is reported to be 50 % MTA (SiO_2, K_2O, Al_2O_3, SO_3, CaO), 7 % SiO_2, 10 % $CaCO_3$, 10 % Bi_2O_3, and 10 % $BaSO_4$, with a liquid containing 1 % propylene glycol alginate, 1 % propylene glycol, 1 % sodium citrate, and 10 % calcium chloride in water [52]. Small differences from the stated formula were found by X-ray diffraction as presented in Table 8.2. Bacterial leakage for this sealer was reported to be worse [77] and antibacterial action was less than AH 26 sealer (Dentsply International, Konstanz, Germany) [73]. However, implantation studies show equivalence to MTA and superiority to AH Plus [85] and bioactivity [52].

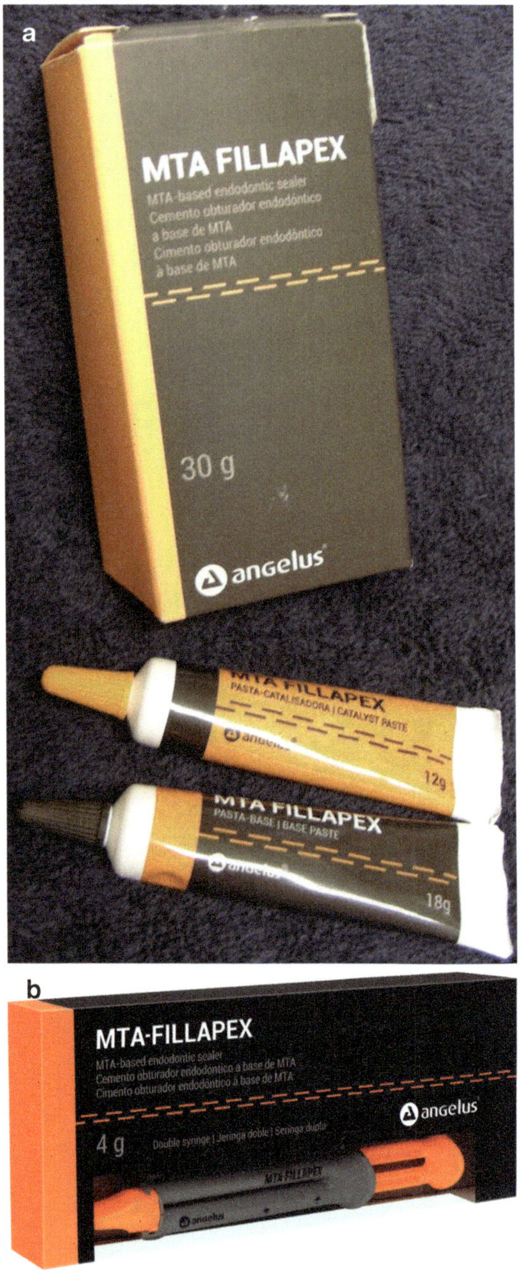

Fig. 8.11 MTA Fillapex shown in its 2-tube format (**a**) and auto-mixing tip format (**b**)

Tech Biosealer products from Isasan SRL (Rovello Porro (CO; Italy)) seem to be based on the compositions of Gandolfi et al. [46, 53], where a phyllosilicate is added to improve handling of the tricalcium silicate powder. The powder is a mixture of white CEM (presumably

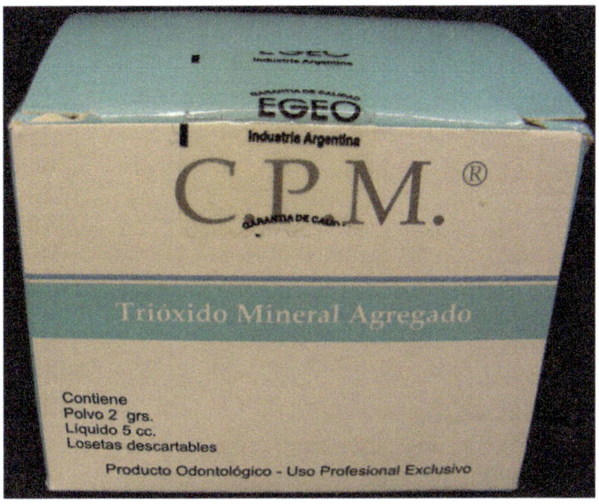

Fig. 8.12 CPM root canal sealer kit by EGEO, containing a powder and a "physiological" liquid

Portland cement), $CaSO_4$, $CaCl_2$, Bi_2O_3, "water-swelling silicate" (montmorillonite), and NaF. The liquid contains Dulbecco's phosphate-buffered saline (DPBS). The cement is milled and heat-treated before packaging into kits with capsules containing 0.27 g of powder, with one vial of liquid containing 5 cm^3 of DPBS. The product is offered in three formats: root-end, pulp capping, endodontic, and apexification. The four product differentiations could not be discerned as to which was best for root canal sealing.

8.6 Summary

A wide variety of commercial MTA-type materials are now available for pulp-capping, endodontic treatment, and root canal sealing, many having improved characteristics and wider indications that the original MTA products. Several products have finer particles, less "sandy" handling, and faster initial or final setting. Adjuvants are incorporated in some products for faster setting achieved by the addition of fluoride, the elimination of calcium sulfate, or an increase in tricalcium aluminate phase. Additions to the mixing liquid to speed setting include calcium chloride, polycarboxylate, or various organic resins. Several new products have enhanced calcium content compared to the original MTA, although the biological benefits of excess calcium oxide or carbonate have not been substantiated. A gel system has been developed (MTA Plus) to reduce washout resistance and speed setting. Even a light-cured MTA-containing material is marketed. Depending on the product, the radiopacity and the radiopacity agent may vary. The product formats include bulk powder/liquid containers (1–8 g), unit doses as small as 0.27 g in triturator capsules, or unit doses in centrifuge tubes. All-purpose materials, for use for all endodontic and pulpal indications, including root canal sealer, are also available.

No studies have shown superior biocompatibility over the original MTA formula. Portland cements normally used for construction have not been shown to be biologically inferior, despite their slow setting, impurities, low radiopacity, and coarseness. The bioactivity of tri- and dicalcium silicate powders, by the release of calcium hydroxide during setting, dominate the biological response. The resulting layer of HA masks the underlying cement, reducing the opportunity for leaching of any impurity into the tissues.

Major advances have been made to create more convenient MTA products that have good handling, faster setting, good radiopacity, washout resistance, and resistance to discoloration. However, no product has definitively improved on the biocompatibility or bioactivity of the original formula.

Key Terms/Definitions

Alumina Aluminum oxide Al_2O_3.
Amorphous Lacking a crystalline structure identifiable by x-ray diffraction.
Ceramic Inorganic, nonmetallic material, usually an oxide, but includes other compounds such as sulfates, carbonates, sulfides, or carbides.
Bioceramic Any ceramic material that is used in the body; includes all MTA products.
Calcia Calcium oxide, usually created by calcining (heating) calcium carbonate ($CaCO_3$) to release carbon dioxide.
Calcium aluminate cement A high-temperature (refractory) cement based on hydration of $CaO{\cdot}Al_2O_3$

Calcium hydroxide Portlandite, a reaction phase of hydrating tri- or dicalcium silicates; $Ca(OH)_2$ or CH in cement notation.
Calcium silicate $CaSiO_3$, AKA wollastonite, a non-hydraulic compound of calcium oxide and silica.
Calcium sulfate $CaSO_4$, which may be present as anhydrous, hemihydrate, and dihydrate.
Cement notation Abbreviations used for the phases of Portland cement for brevity and convenience.
Clinker The cement product, usually a particle larger than 1 cm, that exits from a rotary kiln.
Component (1) The materials that are used before firing a ceramic. For example, calcium carbonate is used to make Portland cement; or (2) the compound in a phase diagram to show the interrelations of several components usually over a range of temperatures.
Dicalcium silicate Belite, the second most common phase in Portland cement. Ca_2SiO_4, also written as $2CaO{\cdot}SiO_2$ or C_2S in cement chemist notation.
Ettringite A hydrated calcium aluminum sulfate mineral with formula $(CaO)_6(Al_2O_3)(SO_3)_3{\cdot}32H_2O$ or $(CaO)_3(Al_2O_3)(CaSO_4)_3{\cdot}32H_2O$, formed by reaction of tricalcium aluminate with calcium sulfate.
Ferrite Tetracalcium aluminoferrite; $4CaO{\cdot}Al_2O_3{\cdot}Fe_2O_3$, also shown in cement notation as C_4AF.
Glass An amorphous (noncrystalline) ceramic, usually based on silica but can also be based on boron oxide or phosphorous oxide as the main components.
Hydraulic material A powdered ceramic material that hardens (sets) when mixed with water.
Hydroxyapatite The mineral component of the bone having the formula $Ca_{10}(PO_4)_6(OH)_2$. Carbonated calcium-deficient hydroxyapatite is the main mineral of dental enamel and dentin.
Kiln/rotary kiln A furnace capable for high temperature (higher than 1,200 °C) for firing materials such as Portland cement. A rotary kiln rotates the feedstock (usually balls of 1–3 in. in diameter) to economically, uniformly, and continuously fire (react and sinter) Portland cement.
Minerals Compounds that are mined which may vary in purity depending on the source. Some deposits of minerals are one nearly pure phase, or they may be a combination of phases or purities. For instance, calcium carbonate sources can be very pure, white calcium carbonate, with less than 1 % or any other carbonate, such as strontium carbonate or magnesium carbonate. Other mines may have calcium carbonate mineral interspersed with iron oxide; such raw material sources will create a gray-colored Portland cement by the presence of iron.
Mineral trioxide aggregate (MTA) An inorganic powder composed primarily of tricalcium and dicalcium silicates, usually with a radiopacifier and other minor ceramic phases.
Nano-sized Particles that are close to a nanometer (nm) in size, which is 1/1,000 of a micron (μm).
Phase A chemical compound that is present in a material, uniquely identifiable by X-ray diffraction.
Pozzolan, pozzolanic (1) A Portland cement that has free silica added which reacts with calcium hydroxide released from the Portland cement during the hydration of its calcium silicate phases, or (2) Roman-era cement that relied on the reaction of calcium oxide, made by heating calcium carbonate, with silica to form calcium silicate hydrates, via the reaction below, which differs from the Portland cement hydration (Eq. 8.5):

$$Ca(OH)_2 + H_4SiO_4 \rightarrow Ca^{2+} + H_2SiO_4{}^{2-} + 2H_2O \rightarrow CaH_2SiO_4 \cdot 2H_2O \quad (8.5)$$

Portland cement A range of compositions based on reacting calcia, silica, and alumina to form powders containing tricalcium silicate and dicalcium silicate, usually with some minor phases. Calcium sulfate is commonly added to the silicate powders to control and slow the setting time for use in large scale constructions. Type I and Type III are the common categories for construction uses of Portland cement. The properties are similar, but the Type III product is a finer powder.
Silica Silicon dioxide, SiO_2, usually amorphous, but the quartz form is crystalline.

Sintering A heating process for powders that reduces the overall surface area by various atomic movements, to cause a powder to form a solid mass, and usually reduces porosity. For Portland cement, the sintering process is concomitant with the reaction process to create the calcium silicate phases from the raw materials in the kiln.

Tricalcium aluminate $Ca_3Al_2O_6$, also written as $3CaO{\cdot}Al_2O_3$, or C_3A in cement notation. A minor phase in most Portland cements.

Tricalcium silicate Ca_3SiO_5, also written as $3CaO{\cdot}SiO_2$ or as C_3S in cement chemist notation. The main component of Portland cement.

Zirconia Zirconium oxide, ZrO_2.

Ziron Zirconium silicate, $ZrSiO_3$

Zirconates Compounds that combine another oxide with zirconia into a unique compound such as $CaZrO_3$.

Tungstate Compounds that combine another oxide with tungsten into a unique compound such as $CaWO_4$, which is commonly used for radiopacity in dental materials.

References

1. Aguilar FG, Garcia Lda F, Rossetto HL, Pardini LC, Pires-de-Souza Fde C. Radiopacity evaluation of calcium aluminate cement containing different radiopacifying agents. J Endod. 2011;37(1):67–71.
2. Aguilar FG, Roberti Garcia LF, Panzeri Pires-de-Souza FC. Biocompatibility of new calcium aluminate cement (EndoBinder). J Endod. 2012;38(3):367–71.
3. Appelbaum KS, Stewart JT, Hartwell GR. Effect of sodium fluorosilicate on the properties of portland cement. J Endod. 2012;38(7):1001–3.
4. Asgary S, Eghbal MJ. A clinical trial of pulpotomy vs. root canal therapy of mature molars. J Dent Res. 2010;89(10):1080–5.
5. Asgary S, Eghbal MJ, Ehsani S. Periradicular regeneration after endodontic surgery with calcium-enriched mixture cement in dogs. J Endod. 2010;36(5):837–41.
6. Asgary S, Eghbal MJ, Parirokh M. Sealing ability of a novel endodontic cement as a root-end filling material. J Biomed Mater Res A. 2008;87(3):706–9.
7. Asgary S, Eghbal MJ, Parirokh M, Ghoddusi J, Kheirieh S, Brink F. Comparison of mineral trioxide aggregate's composition with Portland cements and a new endodontic cement. J Endod. 2009;35(2):243–50.
8. Asgary S, Shahabi S, Jafarzadeh T, Amini S, Kheirieh S. The properties of a new endodontic material. J Endod. 2008;34(8):990–3.
9. Belobrov I, Parashos P. Treatment of tooth discoloration after the use of white mineral trioxide aggregate. J Endod. 2011;37(7):1017–20.
10. Ber B, Hatton J, Stewart G. Chemical modification of ProRoot MTA to improve handling characteristics and decrease setting time. J Endod. 2007;33(10):1231–4.
11. Bird DC, Komabayashi T, Guo L, Opperman LA, Spears R. In vitro evaluation of dentinal tubule penetration and biomineralization ability of a new root-end filling material. J Endod. 2012;38(8):1093–6.
12. Bortoluzzi EA, Araujo GS, Guerreiro Tanomaru JM, Tanomaru-Filho M. Marginal gingiva discoloration by gray MTA: a case report. J Endod. 2007;33(3):325–7.
13. Bortoluzzi EA, Broon NJ, Bramante CM, Felippe WT, Tanomaru Filho M, Esberard RM. The influence of calcium chloride on the setting time, solubility, disintegration, and pH of mineral trioxide aggregate and white Portland cement with a radiopacifier. J Endod. 2009;35(4):550–4.
14. Bortoluzzi EA, Broon NJ, Bramante CM, Garcia RB, de Moraes IG, Bernardineli N. Sealing ability of MTA and radiopaque Portland cement with or without calcium chloride for root-end filling. J Endod. 2006; 32(9):897–900.
15. Camilleri J. Characterization and chemical activity of Portland cement and two experimental cements with potential for use in dentistry. Int Endod J. 2008;41(9): 791–9.
16. Camilleri J. The biocompatibility of modified experimental Portland cement with potential for use in dentistry. Int Endod J. 2008;41:1107–14.
17. Camilleri J. Modification of MTA. Physical and mechanical properties. Int Endod J. 2008;41:843–9.
18. Camilleri J. The physical properties of accelerated Portland cement for endodontic use. Int Endod J. 2008;41(2):151–7.
19. Camilleri J. Evaluation of selected properties of mineral trioxide aggregate sealer cement. J Endod. 2009;35(10):1412–7.
20. Camilleri J. The sealing ability of modified experimental Portland cements with potential use in dentistry. Adv Cement Res. 2010;22:115–21.
21. Camilleri J. Characterization of modified calcium-silicate cements exposed to acidic environment. Mater Charact. 2011;62(1):70–5.
22. Camilleri J. Investigation of Biodentine as dentine replacement material. J Dent. 2013;41(7):600–10.
23. Camilleri J. Color stability of white mineral trioxide aggregate in contact with hypochlorite solution. J Endod. 2014;40(3):436–40.
24. Camilleri J, Cutajar A, Mallia B. Hydration characteristics of zirconium oxide replaced Portland cement for use as a root-end filling material. Dent Mater. 2011;27(8):845–54.
25. Camilleri J, Formosa L, Damidot D. The setting characteristics of MTA Plus in different environmental conditions. Int Endod J. 2013;46(9):831–40.
26. Camilleri J, Montesin FE, Di Silvio L, Pitt Ford TR. The constitution and biocompatibility of accelerated Portland cement for endodontic use. Int Endod J. 2005;38:834–42.

27. Candeiro GT, Correia FC, Duarte MA, Ribeiro-Siqueira DC, Gavini G. Evaluation of radiopacity, pH, release of calcium ions, and flow of a bioceramic root canal sealer. J Endod. 2012;38(6):842–5.
28. Charland T, Hartwell GR, Hirschberg C, Patel R. An evaluation of setting time of mineral trioxide aggregate and EndoSequence root repair material in the presence of human blood and minimal essential media. J Endod. 2013;39(8):1071–2.
29. Chen CC, Wang WC, Ding SJ. In vitro physiochemical properties of a biomimetic gelatin/chitosan oligosaccharide/calcium silicate cement. J Biomed Mater Res B Appl Biomater. 2010;95(2):456–65.
30. Chng H, Islam I, Yap A, Tong Y, Koh E. Properties of a new root-end filling material. J Endod. 2005;31(9): 665–8.
31. Coomaraswamy K, Lumley P, Hofmann M. Effect of bismuth oxide radioopacifier content on the material properties of an endodontic Portland cement–based (MTA-like) system. J Endod. 2007;33(3):295–8.
32. De Souza ET, Nunes Tameirao MD, Roter JM, De Assis JT, De Almeida Neves A, De-Deus GA. Tridimensional quantitative porosity characterization of three set calcium silicate-based repair cements for endodontic use. Microsc Res Tech. 2013;76(10):1093–8.
33. De-Deus G, de Souza MCB, Sergio Fidel RA, Fidel SR, de Campos RC, Luna AS. Negligible expression of arsenic in some commercially available brands of Portland cement and mineral trioxide aggregate. J Endod. 2009;35(6):887–90.
34. Ding SJ, Kao CT, Shie MY, Hung Jr C, Huang TH. The physical and cytological properties of white MTA mixed with Na_2HPO_4 as an accelerant. J Endod. 2008;34(6):748–51.
35. Dreger LA, Felippe WT, Reyes-Carmona JF, Felippe GS, Bortoluzzi EA, Felippe MC. Mineral trioxide aggregate and Portland cement promote biomineralization in vivo. J Endod. 2012;38(3):324–9.
36. Dyanne de Souza Gomes W. MTA and calcium hydroxide as root canal filling materials in delayed replantation of monkey's teeth. Proceedings from the 17th World Congress on Dental Traumatology: 19–22 Sept 2012, Rio de Janeiro. Braz J Dent Traumatol. 2012;(Special issue), p 110.
37. Eid AA, Gosier JL, Primus CM, Hammond BD, Susin LF, Pashley DH, et al. In vitro biocompatibility and oxidative stress profiles of different hydraulic calcium silicate cements. J Endod. 2014;40(2):255–60. Epub 2013 Aug 31.
38. Eid AA, Niu LN, Primus CM, Opperman LA, Pashley DH, Watanabe I, et al. In vitro osteogenic/dentinogenic potential of an experimental calcium aluminosilicate cement. J Endod. 2013;39(9):1161–6.
39. Faria-Junior NB, Tanomaru-Filho M, Berbert FL, Guerreiro-Tanomaru JM. Antibiofilm activity, pH and solubility of endodontic sealers. Int Endod J. 2013; 46(8):755–62.
40. Formosa LM, Mallia B, Camilleri J. The chemical properties of light- and chemical-curing composites with mineral trioxide aggregate filler. Dent Mater. 2013;29(2):e11–9.
41. Froughreyhani M, Milani AS, Barakatein B, Shiezadeh V. Treatment of strip perforation using Root MTA: a case report. Iran Endod J. 2013;8(2): 80–3.
42. Gandolfi MG, Pagani S, Perut F, Ciapetti G, Baldini N, Mongiorgi R, et al. Innovative silicate-based cements for endodontics: a study of osteoblast-like cell response. J Biomed Mater Res A. 2008;87(2): 477–86.
43. Gandolfi M, Perut F, Ciapetti G, Mongiorgi R, Prati C. New Portland cement–based materials for endodontics mixed with Articaine solution: a study of cellular response. J Endod. 2008;34(1):39–44.
44. Gandolfi MG, Siboni F, Prati C. Chemical-physical properties of TheraCal, a novel light-curable MTA-like material for pulp capping. Int Endod J. 2012;45(6): 571–9.
45. Gandolfi M, Silvia F, Pashley David H, Gasparotto G, Carlo P. Calcium silicate coating derived from Portland cement as treatment for hypersensitive dentine. J Dent. 2008;36(8):565–78.
46. Gandolfi MG, Taddei P, Modena E, Siboni F, Prati C. Biointeractivity-related versus chemi/physisorption-related apatite precursor-forming ability of current root end filling materials. J Biomed Mater Res B Appl Biomater. 2013;101(7):1107–23.
47. Gandolfi MG, Taddei P, Siboni F, Modena E, Ciapetti G, Prati C. Development of the foremost light-curable calcium-silicate MTA cement as root-end in oral surgery. Chemical-physical properties, bioactivity and biological behavior. Dent Mater. 2011;27(7): e134–57.
48. Gandolfi MG, Van Landuyt K, Taddei P, Modena E, Van Meerbeek B, Prati C. Environmental scanning electron microscopy connected with energy dispersive x-ray analysis and Raman techniques to study ProRoot mineral trioxide aggregate and calcium silicate cements in wet conditions and in real time. J Endod. 2010;36(5):851–7.
49. Garcia LD, Aguilar FG, Rossetto HL, Sabino MG, Pires-de-Souza FD. Staining susceptibility of new calcium aluminate cement (EndoBinder) in teeth: a 1-year in vitro study. Dent Traumatol. 2013;29(5): 383–8. Epub 2012 Oct 16.
50. Gomes Cornelio AL, Salles LP, Campos da Paz M, Cirelli JA, Guerreiro-Tanomaru JM, Tanomaru Filho M. Cytotoxicity of Portland cement with different radiopacifying agents: a cell death study. J Endod. 2011;37(2):203–10.
51. Gomes-Filho JE, Rodrigues G, Watanabe S, Estrada Bernabe PF, Lodi CS, Gomes AC, et al. Evaluation of the tissue reaction to fast endodontic cement (CER) and Angelus MTA. J Endod. 2009;35(10):1377–80.
52. Gomes-Filho JE, Watanabe S, Bernabe PF, de Moraes Costa MT. A mineral trioxide aggregate sealer stimulated mineralization. J Endod. 2009;35(2):256–60.
53. Hakki SS, Bozkurt BS, Ozcopur B, Gandolfi MG, Prati C, Belli S. The response of cementoblasts to calcium phosphate resin-based and calcium silicate-based commercial sealers. Int Endod J. 2013;46(3): 242–52.

54. Hashem AA, Hassanien EE. ProRoot MTA, MTA-Angelus and IRM used to repair large furcation perforations: sealability study. J Endod. 2008;34(1):59–61.
55. Hebling J, Lessa FC, Nogueira I, Carvalho RM, Costa CA. Cytotoxicity of resin-based light-cured liners. Am J Dent. 2009;22(3):137–42.
56. Hess D, Solomon E, Spears R, He J. Retreatability of a bioceramic root canal sealing material. J Endod. 2011;37(11):1547–9.
57. Huffman BP, Mai S, Pinna L, Weller RN, Primus CM, Gutmann JL, et al. Dislocation resistance of ProRoot Endo Sealer, a calcium silicate-based root canal sealer, from radicular dentine. Int Endod J. 2009;42(1):34–46.
58. Hungaro Duarte MA, Minotti PG, Rodrigues CT, Zapata RO, Bramante CM, Tanomaru Filho M, et al. Effect of different radiopacifying agents on the physicochemical properties of white Portland cement and white mineral trioxide aggregate. J Endod. 2012;38(3):394–7.
59. Hutcheson C, Seale NS, McWhorter A, Kerins C, Wright J. Multi-surface composite vs stainless steel crown restorations after mineral trioxide aggregate pulpotomy: a randomized controlled trial. Pediatr Dent. 2012;34(7):460–7.
60. Hwang Y-C, Kim D-H, Hwang I-N, Song S-J, Park Y-J, Koh J-T, et al. Chemical constitution, physical properties, and biocompatibility of experimentally manufactured Portland cement. J Endod. 2011;37(1):58–62.
61. Iacono F, Gandolfi MG, Huffman B, Sword J, Agee K, Siboni F, et al. Push-out strength of modified Portland cements and resins. Am J Dent. 2010;23(1):43–6.
62. Islam I, Chng HK, Yap AU. Comparison of the physical and mechanical properties of MTA and Portland cement. J Endod. 2006;32(3):193–7.
63. Kao C, Shie M, Huang T, Ding S. Properties of an accelerated mineral trioxide aggregate–like root-end filling material. J Endod. 2009;35(2):239–42.
64. Kogan P, He J, Glickman G, Watanabe I. The effects of various additives on setting properties of MTA. J Endod. 2006;32(6):569–72.
65. Komabayashi T, Spangberg L. Comparative analysis of the particle size and shape of commercially available mineral trioxide aggregates and Portland cement: a study with a flow particle image analyzer. J Endod. 2008;34(1):94–8.
66. Komabayashi T, Spangberg L. Particle size and shape analysis of MTA finer fractions using Portland cement. J Endod. 2008;34(6):709–11.
67. Krastl G, Allgayer N, Lenherr P, Filippi A, Taneja P, Weiger R. Tooth discoloration induced by endodontic materials: a literature review. Dent Traumatol. 2013; 29(1):2–7.
68. Lea FM, Hewlett PC. Lea's chemistry of cement and concrete. 4th ed. London/New York: Arnold; 1998; Copublished in North, Central, and South America by J. Wiley.
69. Leiendecker AP, Qi YP, Sawyer AN, Niu LN, Agee KA, Loushine RJ, et al. Effects of calcium silicate-based materials on collagen matrix integrity of mineralized dentin. J Endod. 2012;38(6):829–33.
70. Lenherr P, Allgayer N, Weiger R, Filippi A, Attin T, Krastl G. Tooth discoloration induced by endodontic materials: a laboratory study. Int Endod J. 2012; 45(10):942–9.
71. Loushine BA, Bryan TE, Looney SW, Gillen BM, Loushine RJ, Weller RN, et al. Setting properties and cytotoxicity evaluation of a premixed bioceramic root canal sealer. J Endod. 2011;37(5):673–7.
72. Luvizuto ER. Periapical tissue reactions to MTA after external root resorption in delayed tooth replantation. Proceedings from the 17th World Congress on Dental Traumatology: 19–22 Sept 2012, Rio de Janeiro. Braz J Dent Traumatol. 2012;(Special issue). p. 63.
73. Mohammadi Z, Giardino L, Palazzi F, Shalavi S. Antibacterial activity of a new mineral trioxide aggregate-based root canal sealer. Int Dent J. 2012; 62(2):70–3.
74. Monteiro Bramante C, Demarchi AC, de Moraes IG, Bernadineli N, Garcia RB, Spangberg LS, et al. Presence of arsenic in different types of MTA and white and gray Portland cement. Oral Surg Oral Med Oral Pathol Oral Radiol Endod. 2008;106(6):909–13.
75. Neelakantan P, Grotra D, Sharma S. Retreatability of 2 mineral trioxide aggregate-based root canal sealers: a cone-beam computed tomography analysis. J Endod. 2013;39(7):893–6.
76. Nosrat A, Seifi A, Asgary S. Pulpotomy in caries-exposed immature permanent molars using calcium-enriched mixture cement or mineral trioxide aggregate: a randomized clinical trial. Int J Paediatr Dent. 2013;23(1):56–63.
77. Oliveira AC, Tanomaru JM, Faria-Junior N, Tanomaru-Filho M. Bacterial leakage in root canals filled with conventional and MTA-based sealers. Int Endod J. 2011;44(4):370–5.
78. Perez AL, Spears R, Gutmann JL, Opperman LA. Osteoblasts and MG-63 osteosarcoma cells behave differently when in contact with ProRoot MTA and White MTA. Int Endod J. 2003;36(8):564–70.
79. Porter ML, Berto A, Primus CM, Watanabe I. Physical and chemical properties of new-generation endodontic materials. J Endod. 2010;36(3):524–8.
80. Primus CM. Comments on "arsenic release provided by MTA and Portland cement" by Duarte MA, et al. Oral Surg Oral Med Oral Pathol Oral Radiol Endod. 2006;101(4):416–7; author reply 417–418.
81. Rawtiya M, Verma K, Singh S, Munuga S, Khan S MTA-based root canal sealers. J Orofac Res. 2013;3(1):16–21. doi:10.5005/jp-journals-10026-1057.
82. Reyes-Carmona JF, Felippe MS, Felippe WT. The biomineralization ability of mineral trioxide aggregate and Portland cement on dentin enhances the push-out strength. J Endod. 2010;36(2):286–91.
83. Richard Steffen D, Hubertus van Waes CM. Regenerative endodontie. Endod J. 2011;10(2):6–12.
84. Sawyer AN, Nikonov SY, Pancio AK, L-n N, Agee KA, Loushine RJ, et al. Effects of calcium silicate–based materials on the flexural properties of dentin. J Endod. 2012;38(5):680–3.
85. Scarparo RK, Haddad D, Acasigua GA, Fossati AC, Fachin EV, Grecca FS. Mineral trioxide aggregate-based sealer: analysis of tissue reactions to a new endodontic material. J Endod. 2010;36(7):1174–8.

86. Schembri M, Peplow G, Camilleri J. Analyses of heavy metals in mineral trioxide aggregate and Portland cement. J Endod. 2010;36(7):1210–5.
87. Seong K-P, Jeon S-Y, Singh B, Hwang J-H, Song S-J. Comparative study of an experimental Portland cement and ProRoot MTA by electrochemical impedance spectroscopy. Ceram Int. 2014;40(1 Part B): 1741–6.
88. Shahi S, Rahimi S, Yavari HR, Mokhtari H, Roshangar L, Abasi MM, et al. Effect of mineral trioxide aggregates and Portland cements on inflammatory cells. J Endod. 2010;36(5): 899–903.
89. Silva EJ, Herrera DR, Almeida JF, Ferraz CC, Gomes BP, Zaia AA. Evaluation of cytotoxicity and up-regulation of gelatinases in fibroblast cells by three root repair materials. Int Endod J. 2012;45(9): 815–20.
90. Storm B, Eichmiller F, Tordik P, Goodell G. Setting expansion of gray and white mineral trioxide aggregate and Portland cement. J Endod. 2008;34(1): 80–2.
91. Tabarsi B, Parirokh M, Eghbal MJ, Haghdoost AA, Torabzadeh H, Asgary S. A comparative study of dental pulp response to several pulpotomy agents. Int Endod J. 2010;43(7):565–71.
92. Tanomaru-Filho M, Tanomaru JM, Barros DB, Watanabe E, Ito IY. In vitro antimicrobial activity of endodontic sealers, MTA-based cements and Portland cement. J Oral Sci. 2007;49(1):41–5.
93. Tay KC, Loushine BA, Oxford C, Kapur R, Primus CM, Gutmann JL, et al. In vitro evaluation of a Ceramicrete-based root-end filling material. J Endod. 2007;33(12):1438–43.
94. Tay FR, Pashley DH. Monoblocks in root canals: a hypothetical or a tangible goal. J Endod. 2007;33(4): 391–8.
95. Valles M, Mercade M, Duran-Sindreu F, Bourdelande JL, Roig M. Influence of light and oxygen on the color stability of five calcium silicate-based materials. J Endod. 2013;39(4):525–8.
96. Viola NV, Guerreiro-Tanomaru JM, da Silva GF, Sasso-Cerri E, Tanomaru-Filho M, Cerri PS. Biocompatibility of an experimental MTA sealer implanted in the rat subcutaneous: quantitative and immunohistochemical evaluation. J Biomed Mater Res B Appl Biomater. 2012;100(7):1773–81.
97. Washington JT, Schneiderman E, Spears R, Fernandez CR, He J, Opperman LA. Biocompatibility and osteogenic potential of New generation endodontic materials by using primary osteoblasts. J Endod. 2011;37(8):1166–70.
98. Wei W, Qi YP, Nikonov SY, Niu LN, Messer RL, Mao J, et al. Effects of an experimental calcium aluminosilicate cement on the viability of murine odontoblast-like cells. J Endod. 2012;38(7):936–42.
99. Weller RN, Tay KC, Garrett LV, Mai S, Primus CM, Gutmann JL, et al. Microscopic appearance and apical seal of root canals filled with gutta-percha and ProRoot Endo Sealer after immersion in a phosphate-containing fluid. Int Endod J. 2008;41(11):977–86.
100. Wongkornchaowalit N, Lertchirakarn V. Setting time and flowability of accelerated Portland cement mixed with polycarboxylate superplasticizer. J Endod. 2011;37(3):387–9.
101. Zhou H-M, Shen Y, Zheng W, Li L, Zheng Y-F, Haapasalo M. Physical properties of five root canal sealers. J Endod. 2013;39(10):1281–6.

Mineral Trioxide Aggregate and Evidence-Based Practice

9

Saeed Asgary

9.1 Introduction

This new millennium has seen a huge 'information explosion'; each day produces vast amounts of data and knowledge in all branches of science. Knowledge doubling studies indicate that the trend of human data production has gradually increased over time. Within the recent decades, growth has become exponential, with significant amounts of data being added regularly to the pool.

It has been estimated that the doubling time of medical knowledge in 1950 was 50 years, in 2010 it was as little as 3.5 years, and in 2020, if this trend continues, it will be a staggering 73 days [37]. It means that students who began medical school in 2010 will experience roughly three doubling of knowledge before graduation, whilst students who graduate in the year 2020 will experience at least four doubling of medical knowledge throughout the course. Incredibly, medical knowledge till the beginning of the third millennium is likely to be less than 2 % of what will be known by 2020.

This exponential growth in medical/dental knowledge has created new and complex problems when clinicians wish to retrieve suitable information. Numerous new scientific articles and journals are added to various databases each day. PubMed at present is the most popular medical database covering 5,500 journals and more than 24 million citations, nearly 1 % of which are dental publications. In the presence of this huge amount of data, the question posed is: Are dental practitioners accessing and utilising the correct information? Clearly, keeping up to date is an overwhelming task.

Such a task can only be efficiently carried out by utilising the principles and methods of *evidence-based practice*. EBP involves scientific ranking of studies, selection of beneficial data and summarisation of results from the selected studies. Ultimately, these steps lead to a wealth of information into a simple and coherent statement: the *clinical bottom line*.

9.2 What Is 'Evidence-Based Practice'?

Aim
To define evidence-based practice (EBP) and to introduce the steps of EBP.

The first and most important question is 'what is *evidence-based practice*?' The term 'evidence-based' was first described by Gordon Guyatt in Canada in the early 1990s; now it is a very established term in medical and dental glossaries.

Based on the book entitled *Evidence-Based Medicine: How to Practice and Teach EBM*, by Sackett et al. [95], EBP is a way of thinking and working. It can be defined as a systematic approach

S. Asgary, DDS, MS
Department of Endodontics, Iranian Center for Endodontic Research, Shahid Beheshti Dental School, Shahid Beheshti University of Medical Sciences, Velenjak, Daneshjoo Blv., Tehran, 1983963113, Iran
e-mail: saasgary@yahoo.com

J. Camilleri (ed.), *Mineral Trioxide Aggregate in Dentistry*,
DOI 10.1007/978-3-642-55157-4_9, © Springer-Verlag Berlin Heidelberg 2014

to clinical problem solving which allows integration of (1) the best current/available evidence with (2) our clinical knowledge/skills and (3) our patient's value/preferences. When these three elements are integrated, clinicians and patients form a diagnostic and therapeutic alliance, which optimises clinical outcomes and quality of life [95]. In addition, EBP is not a static state of information but rather represents a continuously developing state of knowledge. In this systematic approach, employment of the best valid evidence invalidates or further elaborates previously accepted treatments and replaces or strengthens their evidence with proven successful and safe interventions.

To accomplish EBP, the following five steps are essential: (1) constructing an answerable, relevant and foreground clinical question; (2) finding/collecting the best available evidence to answer the question; (3) appraising critically the evidence for its results/validity/relevance; (4) pragmatic integration of the best current evidence with the practitioner's knowledge/skills and the patient's value/preferences; and (5) self-evaluating and audit of the effectiveness/efficiency of previous steps with a view to improvement.

The main objective of EBP using these five steps is the application of the best current evidence in forming clinical decisions/actions to improve the quality of the patient's management and life. Dental clinicians need to be familiar with the concept of *levels of evidence* (LoE), have knowledge of correct appraisal of evidence and identify the *grades of recommendation* (GoR). These significant skills are discussed in detail in this chapter, alongside with the aforementioned steps 1–3 entitled 'endodontic practice with mineral trioxide aggregate'. The application of the final two steps will be the clinicians' responsibility.

9.3 Levels of Evidence and Grades of Recommendation

Aim

To learn the different schemes of levels of evidence and grades of recommendation available when making clinical decisions.

Table 9.1 Levels of evidence according to study design

Level of evidence	Study design
LoE1	High-quality meta-analyses and systematic reviews of randomised controlled trials (RCTs), or
	RCTs with a very low risk of bias (high-quality RCTs)
LoE2	High-quality semi-experimental studies, or
	High-quality systematic reviews of cohort studies, or
	High-quality cohort studies with a very low risk of confounding or bias and a high probability that the relationship is causal, or
	High-quality systematic reviews of semi-experimental studies, or
	RCTs with a moderate-high risk of bias (low-quality RCTs)
LoE3	High-quality systematic reviews of case-control studies, or
	High-quality case-control studies with a low risk of confounding or bias and a moderate probability that the relationship is causal, or
	Low-quality semi-experimental studies
LoE4	Case series, or
	Case-control or cohort studies with a high risk of confounding or bias and a significant risk that the relationship is not causal
LoE5	Case reports, or
	Narrative reviews, or
	Expert opinion

As a component of EBP, there are a range of ranking systems that are used to sort published studies into their respective *levels of evidence* (LoE). These systems are designed as guidance and can be very useful in acquiring a quick overview of the desirable LoE.

LoE is classified in many different ways; the Oxford Centre for Evidence-Based Medicine and the Scottish Intercollegiate Guidelines Network (SIGN) are two of the best-known ranking systems worldwide. Using these two systems, a new modified ranking system was developed in the Knowledge Management Unit (KMU) of the Iranian Center for Endodontic Research (Table 9.1). In this ranking system, the strength of published studies is determined in accordance to their study designs and quality ranking.

High-quality systematic reviews and prospective randomised clinical trials (RCTs) with a very low risk of bias (well-designed methodology) are designated the highest rank (LoE1), followed by high-quality semi-experimental studies or low-quality randomised controlled trials (LoE2), high-quality systematic reviews of case-control studies (LoE3), case series (LoE4) and finally case reports as well as an expert opinion (LoE5). Notably, high-quality studies require stronger research methodology, are more difficult to carry out and consequently are rarer. Also, in vitro and animal studies are not considered valid evidence as the effects of materials/techniques in laboratory (in vitro) situations are not essentially the same as in the human body; the intervention outcomes are often dissimilar in animals and humans and likely to be dissimilar within various mammals.

When biomaterials like MTA become available to the dental market, they are usually subjected to a number of studies conducted in vitro or ex vivo assessment of their biological/chemical/physical properties. However, these usually have no meaningful correlation with in situ clinical situations; the results of a limited number of review articles in the field of dental materials have revealed that there are poor correlations between laboratory test values and clinical performance [20, 21, 50]. Further reports have shown a lack of consistency between the results of two bacterial and dye microleakage methods for sealing ability of the same root-end filling materials [57]. Therefore, as the results of these methodologies do not have clinical significance, the results of in vitro and animal studies are not considered as valid evidence. As a final note, diagnosis, prognosis and treatment topics require different LoE for clinical application/decision.

Finding the appropriate evidence via searching scientific databases is a difficult task due to the large pool of *individual* studies available. This usually requires clinicians to access and critically appraise studies in order to classify the LoE and assess the clinical application of the best evidence. In contrast, *summaries* (systematic reviews) assess and present evidences from primary individual studies and tend to alleviate the need for accessing and appraising individual studies, thus greatly facilitating evidenced-based clinical decision-making.

In addition to individual original studies and systematic reviews, there are also two other categories of clinical information resources named *synopses* and *systems*. Synopses are summaries of research evidence that usually include guidance/advice regarding specific clinical application by qualified experts. This form of guidance externally assesses the evidence and provides strengths and weaknesses for each study; there are a limited number of synopses in dental literature. Systems are defined as textbook-like resources that summarise clinical evidence with other types of information directed at clinical practice decisions; this type of evidence is also limited but provides clear answers leading to appropriate clinical action/care, i.e. 'health technology assessment (HTA)' and 'evidence-based practice guideline (EBPG)'. HTA is used for the evaluation and determination of safety and effectiveness of a new technology; for example, new biotechnology of 'MTA pulpotomy of mature molars with irreversible pulpitis' can be evaluated in terms of effectiveness as well as safety-related factors and social implications, i.e. affordability, availability, accessibility and acceptability. These studies usually evaluate the ethical, social and economic implications of a new technology on health status and health-related quality of life for the general populations. Like a bridge between the world of research and decision-making, HTA studies help health policymakers adopt appropriate decisions and subsequently propagate, popularise and establish the new technology.

Based on unbiased analysis of the best available evidence, numerous EBPGs have been developed by medical associations or governmental bodies as national/international recommendations to guide high-quality patient care. Typically, EBPGs can provide recommendations for prevention and treatment of diseases; they generally contain a simple summarised consensus statement on best practice in health care. A health-care provider is required to know the EBPG of his/her profession and has to decide whether or not to practise the recommendations for that individual patient.

Table 9.2 Grades of recommendation according to study design

Grades of recommendation	Study design
GoR-A	LoE1 documents, directly applicable to the target population
GoR-B	LoE2 documents, directly applicable to the target population, or LoE1 documents, indirectly[a] applicable to the target population
GoR-C	LoE3 documents, directly applicable to the target population, or LoE2 documents, indirectly applicable to the target population
GoR-D	LoE4 documents, directly applicable to the target population, or LoE3 documents, indirectly applicable to the target population
GoR-E	LoE5 documents, directly applicable to the target population, or LoE4 documents, indirectly applicable to the target population

[a]Selected population, major intervention and/or main outcomes of the study are somewhat different to the present clinical situation

Grades of recommendation (GoR) defined as the strength of evidence for a recommendation is determined by searching/reviewing all the related literature on that subject. The number and quality of available related literature should be used as the basis for ranking the recommendation. Most of the multiple grading schemes are based on LoE. The definitions of GoR used in this chapter are modification of those used in the classification system proposed by the Scottish Intercollegiate Guidelines Network (SIGN). Grades of recommendation are usually stated with letters. In this modified GoR, constructed in the Knowledge Management Unit (KMU) of the Iranian Center for Endodontic Research, grades A to E stand for good- to poor-quality evidence for recommending intervention (Table 9.2).

9.4 Framing a Foreground Question (Using PICO)

Aim

To present the process of formulating an accurate and effective foreground Population, Intervention, Comparison and Outcome (PICO) question.

> A good question is half the science. (Hasan-ibn Ali Alayhis-salam)

In current clinical practice, answering to relevant questions requires special types of data/information. An imprecise question results in an imprecise answer; the more specifically we can formulate the question, the greater our chance of getting a decent answer in dental literature. Formulating a high-quality and answerable question is the preliminary step of EBP.

Sackett et al. identified two types of questions: background and foreground [95]. *Background questions* are general knowledge questions and are usually answered by original articles (primary resource), review articles (secondary resource) and textbooks (tertiary resource); review articles are the best source as they condense and summarise evidence derived from original studies. These articles cover a broad topic, are rich sources of background information, are usually readily available and provide numerous references. Background questions typically have two parts: a question root, 'i.e. what, why, when, where, who and how?' and 'the name of a disease/treatment'. For example, 'What is irreversible pulpitis?' or 'How do I perform primary molar formocresol pulpotomy?' Dental students and junior residents most frequently ask background questions.

Foreground questions concentrate on specific information required for clinical decision/actions and include questions of diagnosis, treatment or prognosis of a disease, e.g. *Can irreversible pulpitis be accurately diagnosed clinically?* and *Is root canal therapy the only treatment available?* These questions are best answered by searching the high-LoE published articles, not by textbooks; foreground questions are the most frequent type of questions generated by senior residents and clinicians. Generally, the question must be phrased in a way that directs the subsequent search to relevant and precise answers. Finding an accurate answer in scientific literature can be attained by subdividing the foreground question into four parts: (P) Patient(s)/Problem, (I) Intervention, (C) Comparison and (O) Outcomes; the acronym PICO helps to remember the key components of a clear and well-focused question. The question needs to identify the main problem of the patient, the main intervention/treatment considering the patient's problem, the standard management, and the effectiveness/outcome(s) of interest. A PICO feature is also accessible on PubMed (http://pubmedhh.nlm.nih.gov).

PICO formulating method provides a conceptual framework for more effective searching. An example for a single, well-focused and clearly identified foreground question is: 'In children with asymptomatic pulp exposure (P) how does MTA pulpotomy (I) compare with conventional formocresol pulpotomy (C) for the successful clinical and radiographic outcomes (O)?'

9.5 Finding the Evidence

Aim

To develop a research strategy in order to locate and find published high-level evidences in that field of dentistry.

After framing a PICO question, the next step is good literature search for evidence with the highest LoE. Searching for evidence is a difficult and time-consuming task, particularly with the rapid growth of knowledge in peer-reviewed published literature. To identify relevant studies, the search strategy may include hand searching of hard copies or electronic searching of databases and search engines; however, hand searching is a difficult job for clinicians and even researchers.

Question type (i.e. aetiology, diagnosis, treatment and prognosis) can play a significant role to determine the best source of evidence. For example, a PICO *treatment question* regarding 'outcome comparison of current best practice with a new therapy' needs to find LoE1 studies from the Cochrane Library, Medline (PubMed) and evidence-based websites (i.e. The Dental Elf); however, for a *prognosis question*, searching Medline (PubMed) alone for cohort studies suffices.

The *Cochrane Library* is the best source of summarised high-quality systematic reviews of randomised controlled trials, named *Cochrane Reviews*. Cochrane researchers usually perform hand searching as well as searches of Medline (PubMed) and Embase databases to identify studies that are relevant to the question they are trying to answer. Then, the quality of studies found is carefully assessed using valid quality scales such as Delphi or van Tulder Lists. They apply statistical analysis to compare the data of the clinical trials and to create a systematic review which usually gives the best current word on the effectiveness/efficacy of an intervention. The reviews are available at http://www.thecochranelibrary.com.

If there are no Cochrane reviews that can answer the PICO question, the next step is search *PubMed*. PubMed is a free search service of the US National Library of Medicine (NLM) that collects >22,500,000 citations from 5,500 indexed journal on life sciences and biomedical topics; 13,326 million articles are recorded with their abstracts, and 14,369 million articles have links to full text; there are 3,916 million free full-text articles. A staggering 700,000 new articles were added to the database in year 2012. This useful and easy-to-use bibliographic database contains titles, citations, keywords and abstracts for most of the peer-reviewed scientific biomedical literature dating back to the 1950s. PubMed is part of the Entrez information retrieval system accessing primarily the *Medline* database and was first released in January 1996.

Simple search strategies on PubMed can be a mix of controlled vocabulary such as Medical Subject Headings (*MeSH*) terms and free text or keywords related to a PICO question which enter into search window (http://www.ncbi.nlm.nih.gov/pubmed/). PubMed automatically translates the term/words and adds field names, relevant *MeSH* terms and synonyms, which greatly enhances the search formulation; i.e. 'causes pulpitis' is translated as ("etiology"[Subheading] OR "etiology"[All Fields] OR "causes"[All Fields] OR "causality"[MeSH Terms] OR "causality"[All Fields]) AND ("pulpitis"[MeSH Terms] OR "pulpitis"[All Fields]). This simple broad search is likely to find most of the relevant articles; however, it may also retrieve many irrelevant citations. The appropriate use of Boolean operators AND, OR and NOT is a reliable way to control searches and retrieves a good degree of relevant citations. In addition, applying limits such as human versus animal research, age groups, year of publication, language and more importantly *publication types* reduces the number of irrelevant hits and usually uncovers the highest level of evidence.

Clinical Queries filter is a unique feature of PubMed tools and provides a quick/simple way to search 'Clinical Study Categories', as well as 'Systematic Reviews' subjects. The *Category* and *Scope* methodological filters can retrieve clinically relevant studies with significant precision. It was shown that 'systematic reviews can be retrieved from Medline with close to perfect sensitivity or specificity, or with high precision, by using empirical search strategies' [67].

Assessing the evidence-based synopses such as *The Dental ELF* or critically appraised topic such as *UTHSCSA Dental School CAT Library* are another options for finding the required evidence. These databases show CATs or synopses of individual studies that have been critically appraised and include evidence-based journal reviews, critically appraised topics and clinical evidence.

There are a few useful evidence-based dentistry resources on the Internet including 'Journal of Evidence-Based Dental Practice' and 'Evidence-Based Dentistry' journals as well as websites such as 'The Centre for Evidence-Based Dentistry'. The two journals report on high-quality clinical studies that can impact dental practice. In addition, *ClinicalTrials.gov* as a service of the US National Institutes of Health is a registry site and searchable database of clinical trials in progress which are being conducted around the world. Even then the clinician is required to use his/her own critical appraisal.

Locating and exploiting print and electronic resources has normally been the role of the librarian; therefore, assistance of an expert familiar with various electronic resources, search terms and search strategies is always valuable.

9.6 Interpreting the Best Evidence (Critical Appraisal)

Aim

To focus on the skills necessary to critically evaluate and weigh information concerning the effectiveness of a new intervention.

Many clinicians believe that a wide range of study types can be brought to bear on answering clinical questions; undoubtedly, that is an accepted initial concept [94]. However, for an 'A' grade evidence-based clinical recommendation (GoR-A) regarding a *treatment* topic, the best level of evidence includes results from high-quality meta-analyses/systematic reviews of randomised controlled trials or high-quality randomised controlled trials. This chapter focuses on such evidences, as the next level of the recommendation (GoR-B) might be from low-quality conducted meta-analyses/systematic reviews of good trials or high-quality conducted of fair studies (Table 9.2), which are both insufficiently powered.

Development of critical appraisal skills is essential for clinicians to have an evidence-based approach to practice; the individual practitioner should be able to review and rate the evidence. However, time can be saved by looking for sources of summarised LoE1; the first port of call and the easiest is searching the Cochrane Library for *Cochrane Reviews*. If a suitable paper is not found, we would recommend searching Medline via PubMed for systematic reviews and randomised controlled trials.

There is a general consensus that systematic reviews provide the highest evidence; however, they are not equally reliable and successful in minimising bias. A number of techniques are available to assess the methodological quality of systematic reviews; amongst which is AMSTAR (*a* *meas*urement *t*ool to *a*ssess *s*ystematic *r*eviews), a reliable and valid measurement tool that has been widely accepted and utilised [101].

It consists of eleven items with good face and content validity (available at http://www.amstar.ca/Amstar_Checklist.php); when all the checklist items have been fully addressed, a well-done systematic review is established.

Published randomised controlled trials in peer-reviewed journals also have different quality and level of evidence. The LoE provided by a randomised controlled trial depends on the ability of the study design to minimise the possibility of bias. To assess the risk of bias, the methodological quality of randomised controlled trials is commonly evaluated using various quality scales. It was reported that there are more than 20 scales and associated modifications to assess the quality of randomised controlled trails [81]. Most of these scales have not been adequately developed for assessing the internal and external validity of trails.

Internal validity is the degree to which research results are likely to be correct and free of bias. It usually reflects the extent to which the trial meets the criteria of random allocation, concealment, baseline comparability, blinding of patients/therapist(s)/assessor(s), withdrawal/dropout rate/reasons and statistical analysis. Internal validity is a prerequisite for external validity. *External validity* refers to the ability to generalise the results of a trial to other settings/populations outside the experimental situation; this is also called generalisability.

There are usually five main items in the various quality assessment scales; these consist of patient selection, blinding, interventions, outcomes and statistics. *Jadad scale* is the most common tool for 'pain' research assessment; however, it contains very few items ($n=5$). On the other hand, *Nguyen scale*, which is based on generally accepted methodological criteria for evaluation of 'dental injury' trials, contains too many items ($n=100$). The 9-item *Delphi List*, as a generic criteria list, was developed by international consensus and introduced in 1998 [119]. It was reported that this list is the original source for most of the quality scales. The Cochrane Collaboration Review Groups (CCRG) also used the Delphi List for their analysis in more than 2000 reviews before 2003. More recently, CCRG adopted the *van Tulder List* with 11 items as the latest modification of the Delphi List for many of its systematic reviews [118]. This criteria list has been adequately developed and tested for face and content validity and reliability. A modified *van Tulder* comprehensive list was adapted by our KMU, which consists of the following items:

1. *Patient selection* (i) randomisation, (ii) allocation concealment and (iii) groups' similarity at baseline
2. *Blinding* (iv) of outcome assessor(s), (v) care provider(s) and (vi) patient(s) and also calibration (vii) of outcome assessor(s)
3. *Interventions*: (viii) avoidance of co-interventions, (ix) adequate follow-up period, (x) description of withdrawal and dropouts, (xi) comparison of the outcome assessment timing in all groups, (xii) relevant outcomes, (xiii) adequate sample size and (xiv) using of objective outcome measures
4. *Statistics* (xv) intention-to-treat analysis (Table 9.3)

These criteria can be scored as yes (+1), or no/don't know (0). The quality score of randomised controlled trials is computed by counting the number of positive scores. A published study reporting a randomised controlled trial could therefore receive a modified *van Tulder* score of between 0 and 15 (strongest evidence).

9.7 MTA in Clinical Practice

9.7.1 Background

A recent study that conducted a keyword search 'mineral trioxide aggregate' in PubMed found 1,024 published articles from 1993 till August 2012 [17]. Only ~5 % were classified as LoE1; Iran, Brazil and the UK ranked highest for providing LoE1 MTA articles. MTA was first introduced for repair of lateral root perforations as well as root-end fillings in 1993 [58, 115]. After FDA approval of the material in 1998, Prof. Torabinejad, the inventor of this novel biomaterial, described the clinical procedures for four applications of grey-coloured ProRoot MTA based on 19 published in vitro and animal studies; these include direct pulp capping

Table 9.3 Modified van Tulder List

		Yes/no/don't know
(i)	Was an appropriate method of randomisation performed?	
(ii)	Treatment allocation: Was the treatment allocation concealed?	
(iii)	Were the groups similar at baseline regarding the most important prognostic indicators?	
(iv)	Was the outcome assessor(s) blinded?	
(v)	Was the care provider(s) blinded?	
(vi)	Was the patient(s) blinded?	
(vii)	Was the outcome assessor(s) calibrated?	
(viii)	Were the co-interventions avoided?	
(ix)	Was the follow-up period adequate?	
(x)	Were withdrawal and dropout rates described and acceptable? (>85 %)WCA	
(xi)	Was the timing of the outcome assessment comparable in all groups?	
(xii)	Were relevant outcomes used?	
(xiii)	Was the sample size adequate?	
(xiv)	Were the outcome measures objective?	
(xv)	Did the analysis include an intention-to-treat analysis?	

(permanent teeth with reversible pulpitis), apexification, repair of root perforations and root-end fillings [112].

To overcome the potential discolouration of tooth structure with grey MTA in aesthetically sensitive areas, a new type of MTA with a tooth-coloured formula was introduced. However, there are few reports which discuss the new white ProRoot MTA discolouration effect.

The introduction of MTA as an excellent sealant of the pathways of the pulp (inner and outer dental surfaces) has made a great worldwide impact in endodontic and general dental practice. The new millennium has seen the introduction of numerous brands of MTA and MTA-like materials worldwide as well as additional uses and applications of this biomaterial which are described in detail in this book. Many published studies showed favourable outcomes for additional clinical applications for different types of MTA including vital pulp therapies in primary teeth as well as permanent teeth with established irreversible pulpitis, revascularisation treatments, management of internal and external root resorption and root canal obturations. The various clinical applications of MTA are discussed in detail in Chap. 6.

A Cochrane Library search up to April 2013 amongst ~7,800 records revealed less than 200 reviews published in the field of dentistry/endodontics and just two reviews that only mentioned the name of MTA: 'Pulp management for caries in adults: maintaining pulp vitality' and 'Pulp treatment for extensive decay in primary teeth' [66, 70].

In the first review, however, the results revealed that there is no definitive conclusion as 'the most effective method of pulp treatment of asymptomatic carious teeth'; the authors stated that there has been a recent move towards using alternative materials and methods such as the direct/indirect placement of bonding agents and mineral trioxide aggregate for the management of the pulp in extensively decayed teeth. They concluded that 'further well-designed randomized controlled trials are needed to investigate the potential of contemporary materials which may be suitable when used in the management of carious teeth'. In the second review, the authors also stated that more evidence of effectiveness is required for mineral trioxide aggregate pulp treatment technique.

It is disappointing that after 20 years of introducing MTA in the dental world there are no high-quality Cochrane reviews discussing its clinical applications. However, we hope that in the near future such reviews will be formulated. Accordingly, data locating, finding and collection in this chapter will be based on electronic searches of the PubMed (Medline; 1966 to April 2013), The Dental ELF, UTHSCSA Dental School CAT Library, *Journal of Evidence-Based Dental Practice* as well as *Evidence-Based Dentistry* and ClinicalTrials.gov.

9.7.2 Mineral Trioxide Aggregate for Root-End Fillings

PICO Question

When endodontic surgery is indicated, how does MTA compare to other root-end filling materials in terms of clinical and radiographic outcomes?

9.7.2.1 Definition

Surgical endodontics is an important treatment option for teeth with persistent apical periodontitis (AP). It usually includes pathological tissue removal, root-end resection, root-end cavity preparation and finally insertion of a root-end filling material; the filling material seals the root canal contents and thus prevents exit of microorganisms and their by-product into the periradicular tissues.

MTA was first introduced as a root-end filling material, and it has shown good sealing property compared to traditional filling materials in vitro and favourable biocompatibility ex vivo as well as in animal studies [113]; it stimulates hard tissue healing in surrounding tissues particularly cementogenesis in animal models [12, 114]. There are many case reports and clinical studies that show positive outcomes; however, there are a few randomised controlled trials as discussed below.

Apical/periradicular periodontitis (AP) is a type of periodontal disease usually with an endodontic origin. The disease presents itself as a low-grade inflammation of the periodontium in the area around the main entrances of the root canal system at the root apex or various levels along the root surface of a tooth and is usually asymptomatic (chronic form). The inflammation is generally accompanied by bone destruction which allows radiographic detection of AP. Appearance of symptoms such as pain, swelling and impaired function is an indicator for acute form of AP. It is generally agreed that either newly developed or persistent AP in radiographic examination is a sign of failed endodontic treatment.

9.7.2.2 Incidence/Prevalence

A systematic review of epidemiological studies in 2012 on more than 300,000 teeth from 33 studies mostly performed in developed countries demonstrated that the prevalence of endodontically treated teeth is very high, broadly equivalent to two treatments per patient with 36 % failure rate (persistent AP) [83].

9.7.2.3 Aetiology

Persistent AP after endodontic treatment is an indication of inflammation of periodontal ligament which is usually due to microbial invasion. There is a dynamic process at the interface of root canal system (the source of microbial invasion in necrotic teeth) and host defence in periodontal tissues. This leads to breakdown of both soft and hard periapical tissues. However, in a vital tooth, the inflammation of the periodontal ligament is usually caused by immunological mediators.

9.7.2.4 Prognosis

When AP persists after endodontic treatment, a more complex therapeutic situation arises than in untreated teeth with AP [72]. Hence, the prognosis of AP after surgical endodontic treatment is related to a number of factors, including age [odds ratio (OR), 2.5; confidence interval (CI), 1.01–6.00], preoperative root-filling length (OR, 3.4; CI, 1.34–8.76) and size of the surgical crypt (OR, 1.9; CI, 1.19–3.16) [19], as well as interproximal bone levels at the treated tooth (OR, 5.10; CI, 1.67–16.21), the type of root-end filling material used (OR, 7.65; CI, 2.60–25.27) [120] and the position of treated teeth (OR, 3.52; CI, 1.78–6.96) [103]. According to the results of these three prognostic studies, treatment outcome was superior in subjects older than 45 years, in anterior teeth, tooth with inadequate (versus adequate) root canal fillings, surgical crypt smaller or equal to 1 cm, bone level from the cementoenamel junction more than 3 mm and root-end fillings with ProRoot MTA.

9.7.2.5 Aim of Treatment

The main aims of endodontic surgery are the eradication of microbial factors and prevention

Table 9.4 Results of four ranked randomised controlled trials using MTA as root-end filling material

Study (year)	Teeth (no.)	Intervention (no. of teeth)	Control (no. of teeth)	Follow-up (month)	Radiographic results (success)	Significance
Christiansen et al. [32]	52	MTA (n=26)	gutta-percha (n=26)	12	MTA (85 %); gutta-percha (28 %)	Yes (P <0.001)
Chong et al. [31]	122	MTA (n=64)	IRM (n=58)	12 and 24	MTA (84 %, 92 %); IRM (76 %, 87 %)	No
Song and Kim [104]	260	MTA (n=130)	Super EBA (n=130)	12	MTA (95.6 %); Super EBA (93.1 %)	No
Lindeboom et al. [60]	100	MTA (n=50)	IRM (n=50)	12	MTA (92 %); IRM (86 %)	No

of reinfection by establishing a hermetic apical seal with an ideal root-end filling material. Historically, root-end filling materials such as silver amalgam, Cavit, gold foil, polycarboxylate cement and zinc phosphate cement were suggested, as well as glass ionomer, composite resin, reinforced zinc oxide eugenol cements [intermediate restorative material (IRM), super ethoxybenzoic acid (EBA)], calcium-enriched mixture (CEM) cement and mineral trioxide aggregate biomaterials.

9.7.2.6 Outcomes

The desired outcomes of an intervention are the absence of clinical signs/symptoms of inflammation/infection as well as radiographic resolution of a persistent AP in the long term. Clinical success rates are usually higher than success rates from radiographic evaluation because AP may be asymptomatic clinically; accordingly, the outcome should be mainly extrapolated from the radiographic evaluation.

The radiographic appearance of the periapical area will reflect the gradual stages of AP healing. A common scoring system for radiographic assessment of apical periodontitis, the periapical index (PAI), was introduced by Ørstavik in 1986 [82]. However, several recent studies have shown that cone-beam computed tomography (CBCT) is more sensitive in detecting AP compared to conventional radiography [35]. In other words, conventional radiography is more likely to miss AP; however, CBCT is not recommended as routine diagnostic tool due to its high cost and patient exposure.

9.7.2.7 Methods of Search and Appraisal

Studies dating back to 1966 were located by searching PubMed (Medline). The main search terms were systematic review(s) or randomised controlled trial(s) or clinical trial(s), mineral trioxide aggregate and surgery. We also searched The Dental ELF, UTHSCSA Dental School CAT Library, *Journal of Evidence-Based Dental Practice* as well as *Evidence-Based Dentistry* and ClinicalTrials.gov for the keywords 'mineral trioxide aggregate'. Only English-language trials were assessed. Using modified van Tulder List and AMSTAR checklist, randomised controlled trials and systematic reviews of randomised controlled trials were scored, respectively.

9.7.2.8 Efficacy

Our search found four randomised controlled trials [31, 32, 60, 104] (Table 9.4) and one systematic review [111]. The only systematic review found in this field, collected and analysed quasi-controlled trials as well as randomised controlled trials; therefore, the review was classified as LoE2. Four randomised controlled trials provided evidence that MTA significantly increases the radiographic success rate in comparison to no root-end cavity preparation and filling control (gutta-percha smoothed); however, such outcomes are similar with IRM and Super EBA. There are no randomised controlled trials to compare MTA with many other root-end fillings such as amalgam and CEM cement as yet.

9.7.2.9 Drawbacks

Long setting time of MTA is a known drawback of the material for root-end filling [84].

9.7.2.10 Comments

A recent study reported that the 5-year prognosis of post-endodontic surgery to be 8 % poorer than the 1-year prognosis [120], showing that recall time can influence analysis of treatment outcomes. In addition, the similarity between the treatment outcomes in the intervention and control groups in three randomised controlled trials [31, 60, 104] reveals that 'expected power of study' was dissimilar to 'observed power' at the end of the trials. Furthermore, there are limitations in small clinical trials versus large multicentre trials that are often better representatives of a population [87]. Therefore, a greater body of evidence is required to reach definitive conclusions regarding MTA as a gold standard root-end filling material in routine clinical practice. There is still a need for prospective, multicentre, long-term and large-scale randomised controlled trials for making evidence-based decisions.

Clinical Bottom Line

To answer the PICO question, randomised controlled trials that have *LoE1* and *GoR-A* demonstrate that in surgical endodontics:

1. MTA as root-end filling has better radiographic success rates than heat smoothing of the orthograde gutta-percha (no root-end filling).
2. MTA as root-end filling has similar radiographic success rates with IRM in single-rooted teeth.
3. MTA as root-end filling has similar radiographic success rates with Super EBA after endodontic microsurgery.

9.7.3 Mineral Trioxide Aggregate for Vital Pulp Therapy of Primary Teeth

PICO Question

In case of pulp exposures in primary teeth, how does MTA pulp cover compare with other pulp covering agents in terms of treatment outcome?

9.7.3.1 Definition

Vital pulp therapy (VPT) techniques consist of six definite treatments. From the least to most invasive are non-invasive stepwise excavation [62], indirect pulp capping (IPC), direct pulp capping (DPC), miniature pulpotomy (MP) [9], partial or Cvek pulpotomy (PP) [33] and full/coronal pulpotomy (FP). Clinicians can employ these techniques in either primary or permanent teeth.

The surgical removal of the entire coronal pulp, i.e. full pulpotomy, is a common treatment modality to maintain functionality of primary molar teeth with carious/traumatic pulp exposures which would otherwise be extracted.

Treatment approaches for the pulpotomy of primary teeth consist of devitalisation, preservation or regeneration using various materials including formocresol, ferric sulphate, calcium hydroxide, calcium-enriched mixture (CEM) cement, Portland cement (PC) and MTA. Currently, formocresol pulpotomy is the most common treatment approach worldwide; however, in recent years, clinicians and researchers have voiced their concerns about the safety of formocresol use in paediatric dentistry (i.e. mutagenicity, carcinogenicity and immune sensitisation). It seems that modern pedodontics/endodontics has recently shifted the objective of pulpotomy from devitalisation to revitalisation/vitalisation: infected/inflamed coronal pulp is amputated, and the radicular pulp is covered with biomaterials to induce a favourable biological response. In other words, regeneration of dentinal bridges over uninflamed remaining pulp recreating an effective biological seal [64].

Direct pulp capping (DPC) is a less invasive treatment than pulpotomy; though, due to reported unwanted treatment outcomes of CH pulp capping (i.e. internal resorption, pulp calcification, etc.), this treatment modality is rarely employed in primary teeth. However, recent evidence demonstrates that this treatment option can be effective if good coronal seal is provided.

9.7.3.2 Incidence/Prevalence

The prevalence of dental caries in the primary dentition for children aged 2–5 years increased from 24 % in 1988–1994 to 28 % in 1999–2004, according to the most recent data released by the US Department of Health and Human Services (www.cdc.gov/nchs/data/series/sr_11/sr11_248.pdf). A recent Cochrane review stated that the overall mean incidence of pulp exposure after complete caries removal is 34.7 % for the management of dentinal caries in previously unrestored primary and permanent teeth [92].

9.7.3.3 Aetiology

Vital pulp therapies (VPT) of primary teeth are most often necessitated by progression of caries into/close to the pulp and are usually indicated due to removal of all caries/soft demineralised dentine by the dentist as well as traumatic injuries to the teeth.

9.7.3.4 Prognosis

It was reported that pulpotomy success rate for teeth restored with a stainless steel crown was higher than for those restored with amalgam [105].

9.7.3.5 Aim of Treatment (Intervention)

The objective of VPT in primary dentition is pulp dressing to relieve sensitivity/pain and also to prevent the supporting periodontal tissues from breaking down up to exfoliation time.

9.7.3.6 Outcomes

The main outcome measure for determining clinical success is the absence of spontaneous pain, abscess, sinus tract or pathologic mobility; radiographic success is determined according to the absence of furcation/periapical lesion, internal or pathologic external resorption and root canal obliteration as well as the presence of a normal periodontal ligament.

Note: Many researchers have reported cases of canal obliteration as success.

9.7.3.7 Methods of Search and Appraisal

Studies dating back to 1966 were located by searching PubMed (Medline). The main search terms were [systematic review(s) or randomized controlled trial(s) or clinical trial(s)] and [mineral trioxide aggregate] and [pulpotomy or vital pulp therapy or primary molar/teeth]. We also searched The Dental ELF, UTHSCSA Dental School CAT Library, *Journal of Evidence-Based Dental Practice* as well as *Evidence-Based Dentistry* and ClinicalTrials.gov for the key term 'mineral trioxide aggregate'. Only English-language trials were assessed. Using modified van Tulder List and AMSTAR checklist, RCTs and systematic reviews of RCTs were scored respectively.

9.7.3.8 Efficacy

MTA Versus Formocresol Pulpotomy

The only Cochrane review assessing pulp therapy for extensive decay in primary teeth concluded that based on the randomised controlled trials available, there is 'no reliable evidence' supporting the superiority of one type of treatment/material over the other for pulpally involved primary molars and that 'high quality randomized controlled trials, with appropriate unit of randomization and analysis are needed' [70]. As this review was published in 2003 and several systematic reviews as well as randomised controlled trials have been published thereafter, more recent research should be analysed.

The result of our search reveals that three systematic reviews [74, 85, 102] as well as 19 randomised controlled trials [2, 3, 5, 8, 40, 43, 47, 49, 51, 52, 54, 69, 71, 75, 106, 107, 109, 110, 125] (Table 9.5) compared the success rates of MTA alone with formocresol pulpotomies. One of systematic reviews collected and analysed clinical trials as well as randomised controlled trials [74]; therefore, the review was classified as LoE2. Based on the date of publication and selection criteria, six randomised controlled trials were included in each of two remaining reviews. Four of these RCTs are the same, and totally eight randomised controlled trials were included in the two reviews (Table 9.6) [2, 3, 40, 47, 51, 54, 71, 75]. The results of the two systematic reviews are identical, and the meta-analysis [85] indicated that 'clinical and radiographic finding show that MTA is superior to formocresol in primary molars pulpotomy resulting in a lower failure rate, with the relative risk being 0.32 (CI, 0.11–0.90) and 0.31 (CI, 0.13–0.74), respectively'; in addition, MTA has less undesirable sequelae.

Table 9.5 Results of nineteen ranked randomised controlled trials comparing MTA and formocresol pulpotomy agents in primary teeth

Study (year)	Teeth no. (dropout)	MTA no. of teeth (dropout)	Formocresol no. of teeth (dropout)	Follow-up (month)	Final clinical results (success %)	Final radiographic results (success %)
Srinivasan and Jayanthi [107]	100 (7)	50 (3)	50 (4)	3, 6, 9, 12	MTA = 100; FC = 91.3[€]	MTA = 95.74; FC = 78.26[£]
Jabbarifar et al. [54]	64 (0)	32 (0)	32 (0)	6, 12	MTA = 93.75; FC = 90.6	
Holan et al. [51]	64 (2)	33 (0)	31 (2)	4–74	MTA = 97; FC = 83	
Moretti et al. [69]	30 (1)	15 (1)	15 (0)	3, 6, 12, 18, 24	MTA = 100; FC = 100	
Naik and Hegde [71]	50 (3)	25 (1)	25 (2)	24 h, 1, 3, 6	MTA = 100; FC = 100[#]	
Sonmez et al. [106]	40 (12)	20 (5)	20 (7)	6, 12, 18, 24	MTA = 66.6; FC = 76.9	
Subramaniam et al. [109]	40 (0)	20 (0)	20 (0)	1, 6, 12, 24	MTA = 100; FC = 100	MTA = 95; FC = 85
Zealand et al. [125]	252 (49)	119 (19)	DFC:133 (30)	6	GMTA = 100; DFC = 97	GMTA = 95; DFC = 86[≠]
Erdem et al. [43]	50 (0)	25 (0)	25 (0)	6, 12, 24	MTA = 96; FC = 88	
Sushynski et al. [110]	252 (121)	119 (54)	DFC: 133 (67)	6–24	GMTA = 100; DFC = 98	GMTA = 95; DFC = 76[≠]
Airen et al. [5]	70 (0)	35	35	6, 12, 24	MTA = 97.9; FC = 83[≠]	MTA = 88.6; FC = 54.3[≠]
Eidelman et al. [40]	45 (13)	23 (6)	22 (7)	6–12, 13–18, 19–24, >24	MTA = 100; FC = 93	
Agamy et al. [3]	72 (60)	Grey = 24 (4); White = 24 (4)	24 (4)	1, 3, 6, 12	MTA = (G:100,W:80); FC = 90	
Farsi et al. [47]	120 (46)	60 (22)	60 (24)	18, 24	MTA = 100; FC = 98.6	MTA = 100; FC = 86.8[≠]
Aeinehchi et al. [2]	126 (26)	51 (8)	75 (18)	3, 6	MTA = 100; FC = 100	MTA = 100; FC = 82.5[¥]
Noorollahian [75]	60 (24)	30 (12)	30 (12)	6, 12, 24	MTA = 100; FC = 100	MTA = 94.4; FC = 100
Hugar and Deshpande [52]	60 (0)	30 (0)	30 (0)	6, 12, 18, 24, 30, 36	MTA = 100; FC = 100	MTA = 100; FC = 96.67
Ansari and Ranjpour [8]	40 (10)	20 (5)	20 (5)	1, 6, 12, 24	MTA = 100; FC = 80	MTA = 95; FC = 90
Godhi et al. [49]	50 (0)	25 (0)	25 (0)	1, 3, 6, 12	MTA = 100; FC = 100	MTA = 96; FC = 88

MTA mineral trioxide aggregate, *DFC* diluted formocresol, significant difference for [€](mobility), [£](periodontal ligament widening and inter-radicular radiolucency), [#](discolouration), [≠](primary outcomes), [¥](root resorption)

Eleven randomised controlled trials [5, 8, 43, 49, 52, 69, 106, 107, 109, 110, 125] were published after the publication of these two systematic reviews (Table 9.5); therefore, to make comprehensive conclusions, we performed meta-analyses using the Mantel-Haenszel model and calculation of pooled relative risk (RR). We only included studies with 24-month follow-up. The results clearly showed that MTA is significantly superior to formocresol in primary molar pulpotomy in terms of treatment outcomes (Fig. 9.1).

MTA Versus Other Pulpotomy Agents

Eleven studies compared MTA with various pulpotomy agents other than formocresol (Table 9.7); five of these studies compared MTA with calcium hydroxide [61, 69, 80, 86, 106], four studies compared MTA to ferric sulphate [38, 43, 79, 106], two studies compared MTA with Portland cement [80, 96], one study compared MTA with calcium-enriched mixture (CEM) cement [63], and one study compared white with grey MTA [28].

Table 9.6 Two AMSTAR ranked systematic reviews comparing MTA and formocresol as pulpotomy agent for primary teeth

Systematic reviews RCTs	Peng et al. (Jadad scale) [85]	Simancas-Pallares et al. (no scale) [102]
Eidelman et al. [40]	×(5)	–
Agamy et al. [3]	×(4)	×
Jabbarifar et al. [54]	×(4)	–
Holan et al. [51]	×(5)	×
Farsi et al. [47]	×(2)	×
Naik and Hegde [71]	×(2)	×
Aeinehchi et al. [2]	–	×
Noorollahian [75]	–	×

The results of various randomised controlled trials comparing MTA with calcium hydroxide or ferric sulphate are mixed; some report significant and others insignificant differences between the pulpotomy agents. Due to the controversy, two separate meta-analyses with the Mantel-Haenszel model with calculation of pooled relative risk (RR) were performed. Our results clearly showed that MTA is superior to calcium hydroxide as well as ferric sulphate in primary molar pulpotomy at a 24-month follow-up (Figs. 9.2 and 9.3).

MTA Versus Other DPC Materials

Two randomised controlled trials compared MTA with calcium hydroxide and calcium-enriched mixture (CEM) cement for DPC of primary molars [45, 46, 117] (Table 9.8); there were no significant differences found for all the treatment outcomes assessed.

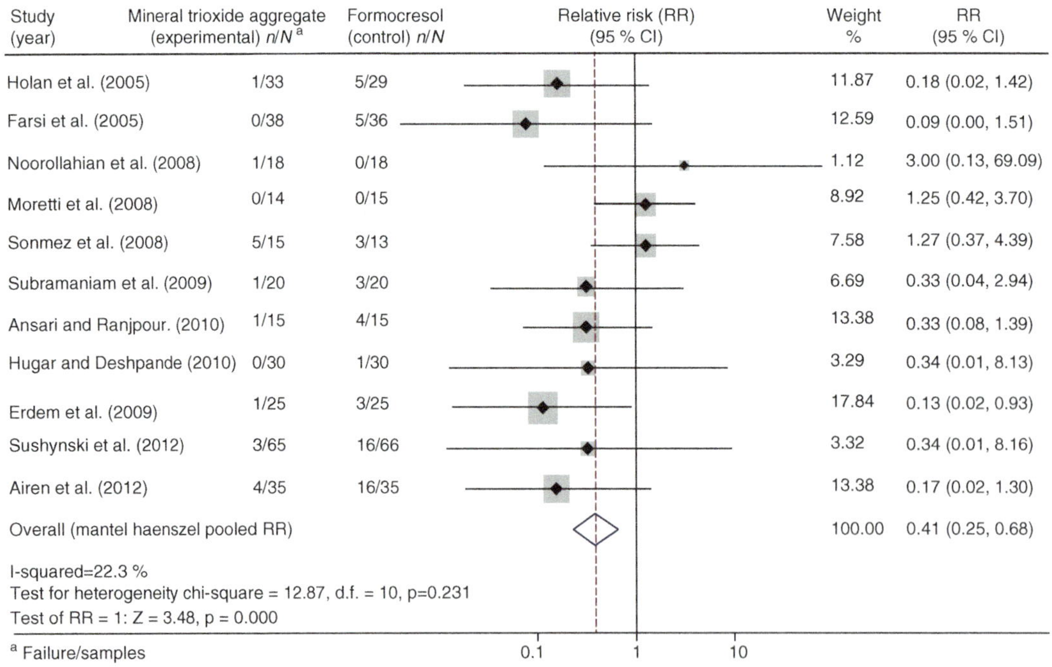

Fig. 9.1 Meta-analysis of 11 randomised clinical trials with 24-month follow-up, studying the success of mineral trioxide aggregate versus formocresol pulpotomy in primary molars

Table 9.7 Results of 11 ranked randomised controlled trials comparing MTA with other pulpotomy agents in primary teeth

Study (year)	Teeth no. (dropout)	MTA no. (dropout)	Control no. (dropout)	Follow-up (month)	Final clinical results (success%)	Final radiographic results (success%)
Moretti et al. (2008) [69]	45 (2)	15 (1)	CH = 15 (1)	3, 6, 12, 18, 24	MTA = 100; CH = 42[¥]	
Sakai et al. (2009) [96]	30 (0)	15 (0)	PC = 15 (0)	6, 12, 18, 24	MTA = 100; PC = 100	MTA = 100; PC = 100
Oliveira et al. (2013) [80]	45 (0)	15 (0)	CH = 15 (0); PC = 15 (0)	6, 12, 24	MTA = 100; CH = 38; PC = 100[£]	
Doyle et al. (2010) [38]	270 (43)	57 (10)	FS = 58 (12); EF/FS = 78 (14); FS/MTA = 77 (7)	12–38	MTA = 89; FS = 54; EF/FS = 43; FS/MTA = 73[¤]	
Percinoto et al. (2006) [86]	90 (0)	45 (0)	CH = 45 (0)	3, 6, 12	MTA = 96.56; CH = 86.67	
Malekafzali et al. (2011) [63]	80 (8)	40 (4)	40 (4)	6, 12, 24	MTA = 80; CEM = 85	
Sonmez et al. (2008) [106]	80 (24)	20 (5)	FS = 20 (5); FC = 20 (7); CH = 20 (7)	6, 12, 18, 24	MTA = 66.6; FS = 73.3; FC = 76.9; CH = 46.15	
Erdem et al. (2011) [43]	100 (0)	25 (0)	FS = 25 (0); FC = 25 (0); ZOE = 25 (0)	6, 12, 24	MTA = 96; FS = 88; FC = 88; ZOE = 68[Ⱡ]	
Cardoso-Silva et al. (2011) [28]	233 (23)	G = 74 (22)	W = 136 (1)	6–84	GMTA = 100; WMTA = 98.52	
Odabaş et al. (2012) [79]	93 (9)	42 (4)	FS = 51 (5)	1, 3, 6, 9, 12	MTA = 94.7; FS = 84.7	MTA = 92.1; FS = 78.2
Liu et al. (2011) [61]	40 (6)	20 (3)	CH = 20 (3)	10–56	MTA = 94.1; CH = 64.7[£]	

MTA mineral trioxide aggregate (*W* white, *G* grey), *CH* calcium hydroxide, *PC* Portland cement, *FS* ferric sulphate, *EF* eugenol-free, *ZOE* zinc oxide eugenol, [¥](significant difference), [£](significance not reported), [¤](MTA versus FS or EF/FS: significant difference), [Ⱡ](MTA versus ZOE: significant difference)

9.7.3.9 Drawbacks

It was reported that crown discolouration is common after ProRoot MTA pulpotomy in primary teeth [61, 71]. High price and long setting time are two other main drawbacks of MTA [84].

9.7.3.10 Comments

It appears that there are adequate randomised controlled trials and systematic reviews comparing MTA pulpotomy of primary teeth to formocresol, ferric sulphate and calcium hydroxide. The results are clear; however, we need to take into account the effects of MTA pulpotomy on the oral health-related quality of life as well as health technology assessments.

Note: MTA originated from Portland cement; however, according to FDA and CE regulations, materials that are manufactured outside of the dental industries, i.e. Portland cement, should not be used in the dental clinics [90].

Clinical Bottom Line

To answer the PICO question, systematic reviews as well as recent *LoE1* randomised controlled trials with *GoR-A* showed that in vital pulp therapy of primary teeth:

1. MTA as pulpotomy agent has superior success rates when compared to formocresol, calcium hydroxide and ferric sulphate in primary molar pulpotomies.

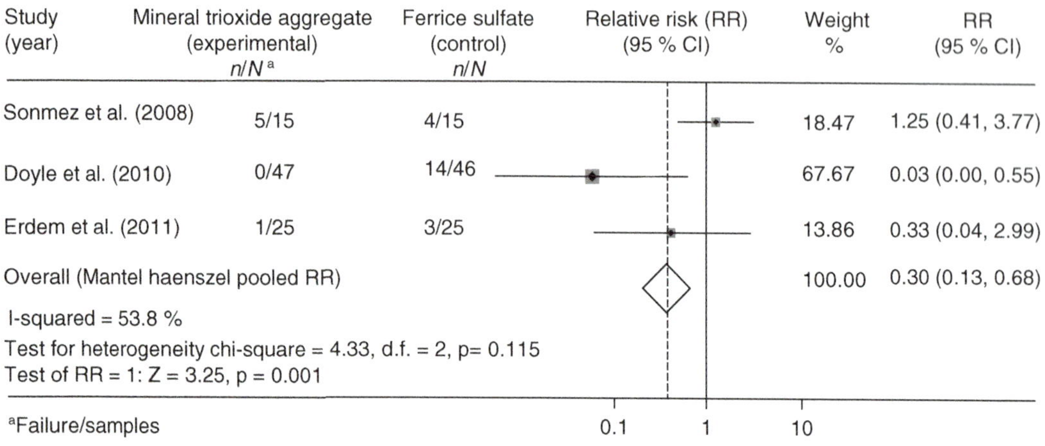

Fig. 9.2 Meta-analysis of three randomised clinical trials with 24-month follow-up studying the effect of mineral trioxide aggregate versus ferric sulphate pulpotomy in primary molars

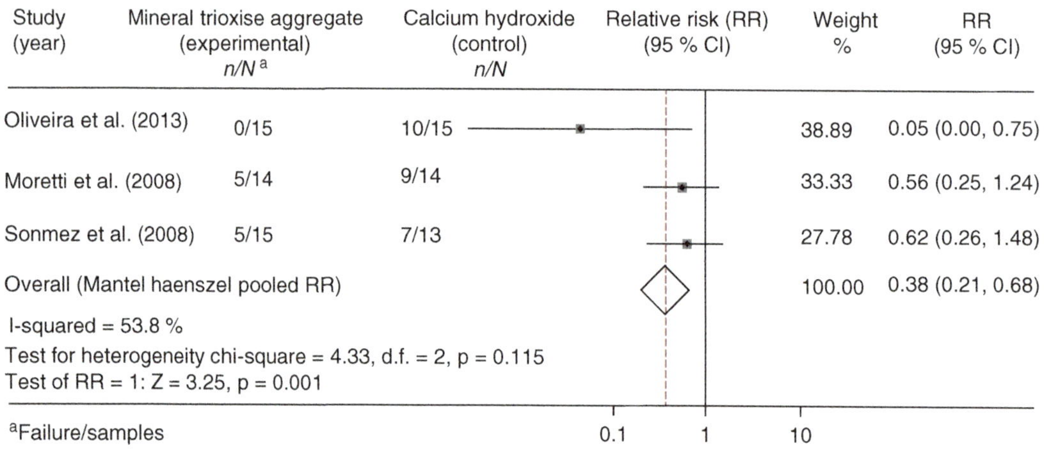

Fig. 9.3 Meta-analysis of three randomised clinical trials with 24-month follow-up studying the effect of mineral trioxide aggregate versus calcium hydroxide pulpotomy in primary molars

Table 9.8 Results of randomised controlled trials comparing MTA with calcium hydroxide (CH) or CEM cement for DPC in primary teeth

Study (year)	Teeth no. (dropout)	MTA no. of teeth (dropout)	Control no. of teeth (dropout)	Follow-up (month)	Final results (success %)
Tuna and Olmez (2008) [117]	50 (6)	25 (3)	CH = 25 (3)	3, 6, 12, 18, 24	MTA = 100; CH = 100
Fallahinejad Ghajari et al. (2010, 2013) [45, 46]	42 (4)	21 (2)	CEM = 21 (2)	6, 20	MTA = 95; CEM = 89

2. MTA as pulpotomy agent has similar success rates when compared to calcium-enriched mixture cement in primary molar pulpotomies.
3. Grey and white MTAs have similar treatment effects in primary molar pulpotomies.
4. MTA as pulp capping agent has similar success rates when compared to calcium hydroxide in primary molar direct pulp capping.
5. MTA as pulp capping agent has similar success rates when compared to calcium-enriched mixture cement in primary molar direct pulp capping.

9.7.4 Mineral Trioxide Aggregate for Management of Immature Permanent Teeth

PICO Question

In endodontic management of immature permanent teeth, how does MTA compare with other materials in terms of treatment outcomes?

9.7.4.1 Definition

When endodontic treatment is indicated for an immature open apex tooth, apexogenesis is the best treatment option. Continued root development, dentin formation and apex closure usually lead to longer and stronger roots and consequently higher survival rate for the treated vital tooth. If the immature tooth is nonvital, clinicians may choose calcium hydroxide apexification, apical plug apexification using biomaterials or revitalisation (revascularisation) technique. In the first traditional procedure, necrotic tissue is removed, and calcium hydroxide is applied in several visits to induce apical closure by stimulating the formation of a calcified barrier; the extended treatment time increases brittleness of root dentin and risk of fracture.

MTA apical plug can be also used to create an artificial apical barrier in usually one or maximum two steps; this alternative treatment reduces the treatment time as well as the required visits to the dental office. The newly introduced treatment modality, i.e. revascularisation, applies a triple antibiotic which medicates the root canal(s), providing an intra-canal clot scaffold into which blastic cells can grow. The coronal access is then sealed with a bioactive material. This procedure typically leads to formation of a vascularised tissue and subnormal development of the entire root in anterior as well as posterior teeth [18, 77].

9.7.4.2 Incidence/Prevalence

There is no comprehensive study to report the incidence/prevalence of pulp exposure of vital/nonvital immature open apex teeth after caries removal and trauma; despite the common nature of this condition in children and adolescents. It must be noted that untreated nonvital immature teeth are sometimes found in adults.

9.7.4.3 Aetiology

Pulp therapy of vital permanent immature teeth (apexogenesis) is usually indicated after iatrogenic or carious pulp exposure as well as accidental traumatic injuries to the teeth. In the case of no/inadequate treatment for such teeth, the dental pulp becomes nonvital, and apexification, apical plug or revascularisation techniques may be indicated.

9.7.4.4 Prognosis

Loss of vitality before complete root development leaves a short, thin and weak root which is more prone to fracture and has poorer crown/root ratio. It was reported that 32 % of teeth with apexification ended up with root fracture mainly subsequent to another minor trauma episode [6].

9.7.4.5 Aim of Treatment (Intervention)

As a general rule, the clinicians must always try to avoid apexification if apexogenesis is possible. In vital immature teeth with open apices, every

Table 9.9 Results of three randomised controlled trials comparing MTA with CH, ZOE or CEM cement for apexogenesis

Study (year)	Teeth (roots) (no.)	MTA no. of teeth (roots)	Control no. of teeth (roots)	Follow-up (month)	Final results (success %)
El-Meligy and Avery (2006) [41]	30	15	CH=15	3, 6, 12	MTA=100; CH=87
Ghoddusi et al. (2012) [48]	(28)	(15)	ZOE=(13)	3, 6, 12	MTA=91.7; ZOE=100
Nosrat et al. (2013) [78]	51 (102)	26 (59)	CEM=25 (59)	6, 12	MTA=100; CEM=100

attempt must be made to maintain pulp vitality until root development is complete. Simulation of apexogenesis via revascularisation is also the desired treatment. If apexogenesis cannot be achieved, then artificial apical closure and apexification must be utilised.

9.7.4.6 Outcomes

Root development and apical closure are two main treatment outcomes. Also, the absence of clinical/radiographic signs and/or symptoms of inflammation or infection is interpreted as success.

9.7.4.7 Methods of Search and Appraisal

Studies dating back to 1966 were located by searching PubMed (Medline). The main search terms were [systematic review(s) or randomized controlled trial(s) or clinical trial(s)] and [mineral trioxide aggregate] and [pulp cap or pulpotomy or vital pulp therapy or apexogenesis or apexification or apical plug or artificial apical closure or revascularization or revitalization]. We also searched The Dental ELF, UTHSCSA Dental School CAT Library, *Journal of Evidence-Based Dental Practice* as well as *Evidence-Based Dentistry* and ClinicalTrials.gov for the keywords 'mineral trioxide aggregate'. Only English-language trials were assessed. Using modified van Tulder List and AMSTAR checklist, randomised controlled trials and systematic reviews of randomised controlled trials were scored, respectively.

9.7.4.8 Efficacy

MTA Apexogenesis

The result of our search revealed that three randomised controlled trials compared the success rates of MTA apexogenesis with calcium hydroxide [41], zinc oxide eugenol [48] and calcium-enriched mixture cement [78] (Table 9.9). In comparison with calcium hydroxide, zinc oxide eugenol or CEM cement, MTA showed nonsignificant clinical and radiographic success to induce apical closure in vital immature permanent teeth.

MTA Apical Plug Versus Calcium Hydroxide Apexification

Two randomised clinical trials compared MTA with calcium hydroxide for apexification of necrotic immature permanent teeth between 1993 and 2011 [42, 88]; one was a systematic review, and the other was a meta-analysis [29]. They analysed the randomised controlled trials using Jadad scale; results of the meta-analysis showed comparable radiographic success and apical barrier formation with both calcium hydroxide and mineral trioxide aggregate in immature teeth.

Two randomised controlled trials were also published after the publication of the systematic review with similar results and without significant differences (Table 9.10); one study compared two commercial types of MTA (ProRoot vs. Angelus) [68], and the second compared MTA with calcium hydroxide [34]. In addition, there is a registered clinical trial which is completed [25]; however, the results have not been reported yet.

Table 9.10 Results of four randomised controlled trials regarding MTA apexification

Study (year)	Teeth no. (dropout)	MTA no. of teeth (dropout)	Control no. of teeth (dropout)	Follow-up (month)	Final results (success %)
El-Meligy and Avery (2006) [41]	50 (0)	25 (0)	CH=25 (0)	3, 6, 12	MTA=100; CH=86.66
Pradhan et al. (2006) [88]	20 (0)	10 (0)	CH=10 (0)	11	MTA=100; CH=100
Moore et al. (2011) [68]	22	ProRoot=11	Angelus=11	3 months and every 6 months	ProRoot=81.8; Angelus=100
Damle et al. (2012) [34]	30 (0)	15 (0)	CH=15 (0)	3, 6, 9, 12	MTA=100; CH=93.33

MTA for Regenerative Endodontic Procedures

There is a lack of randomised controlled trials for MTA.

9.7.4.9 Drawbacks

The use of MTA promotes a mild grey discolouration in the crown after apexification [55]; it was reported that coronal discolouration was observed in 22.7 % of teeth following white MTA placement in immature open apex teeth [68]. Severe discolouration after grey MTA pulpotomy in immature permanent teeth was also reported [108]. It was also reported that the roots of two maxillary central incisors were not developed after regenerative endodontic treatment using MTA [76]. High price and long setting time are two other main drawbacks of MTA [84].

9.7.4.10 Comments

A paradigm shift in endodontology in the last decade has altered the traditional treatment concepts towards more biologically based regenerative research and practice. Regeneration of necrotic immature permanent teeth could be an invaluable technique to save countless numbers of anterior teeth each year; however, there are no standardised treatment protocols based on high-level evidence. There is a pressing need for prospective high-quality RCTs to develop and recommend appropriate treatment regimen for continued hard tissue formation of immature teeth.

In addition, full pulpotomy which is the most invasive form of VPT in apexogenesis treatment of vital immature permanent teeth is supported with limited number of randomised controlled trial evidence; however, there is a gap of data for other less aggressive VPT techniques.

Clinical Bottom Line

To answer the PICO question for permanent immature teeth, *GoR-A* recommendations were formulated (based on one systematic review and recent randomised controlled trials with *LoE1* evidence) as outlined below:

1. MTA vital pulp dressing placed for apexogenesis treatment has similar success rates when compared to calcium hydroxide, zinc oxide eugenol and calcium-enriched mixture cement.
2. MTA when used as apical plug for apexification has similar success rates when compared to calcium hydroxide but reduces treatment time.
3. ProRoot and Angelus MTA apical plugs have similar effects in apexification treatment.

9.7.5 Mineral Trioxide Aggregate for Vital Pulp Therapy of Mature Permanent Teeth

PICO Question

In vital pulp therapy of mature permanent teeth, how does MTA compare with other pulp protecting materials in terms of treatment outcomes?

9.7.5.1 Definition

Theoretically, dressing and protecting an exposed vital pulp in mature permanent teeth from bacterial invasion with an ideal pulp capping material would maintain pulp vitality. The general evidence-based consensus is that iatrogenic and symptom-free pulp exposures can be successfully treated by VPT [4]. For this reason, an ideal pulp capping material should be biocompatible, antimicrobial, non-toxic and specifically able to seal the path of communication between exposed dental pulp and oral microbial flora. Calcium hydroxide used to be the universal capping material in the past; however, new materials, i.e. MTA and CEM, have replaced it with a very positive trend in recent years.

The traditional school of thought recommended high-price root canal therapy for carious pulp exposures in mature permanent teeth specifically with signs of irreversible pulpitis and apical periodontitis; however recently, several clinical studies have reported that vital teeth can be treated successfully with low-price VPT [4, 16, 26, 39]. One- and two-year results of an ongoing multicentre randomised clinical trial have revealed that in comparison with root canal therapy, VPT/CEM is a cost-effective and reliable bio-method for management of permanent molars with irreversible pulpitis with/without apical periodontitis [14, 15]. Moreover, it also has an outstanding pain-reducing effect in irreversible pulpitis [10] and can be recommended for general clinical practice. This treatment modality will doubtlessly improve quality of dental care for mature vital permanent teeth.

9.7.5.2 Incidence/Prevalence

Dental caries has remained the most prevalent chronic disease of humans; the main chief complaint of patients with deep dental caries/irreversible pulpitis, seeking for dental care, is pain [7].

A recent Cochrane review stated that mean incidence of pulp exposure is 34.7 % after complete caries removal for the management of dentinal caries in previously unrestored primary and permanent teeth [92].

On the other hand, apical periodontitis is an important radiographic sign for untreated decayed teeth as well as failed root canal treated teeth. Current evidence demonstrates that an inflamed vital pulp can lead to AP and a recent study showed that CBCT can detect AP better than conventional radiography specifically in teeth with irreversible pulpitis [1]. A systematic review of epidemiological studies on more than 300,000 teeth from 33 studies mostly performed in developed countries verified that the prevalence of AP is very high, broadly equivalent to 1 radiolucency per patient [83].

9.7.5.3 Aetiology

The cause and effect relationship between the presence of microorganisms and pulpal inflammation and necrosis is well documented [56, 99]. In germ-free animal models, the pulp-periapical complex remained vital and without any inflammation/necrosis after pulp exposure. Therefore, microorganisms and their toxins play the most important role in the aetiology of pulp and periapical pathosis (e.g. pulpitis and AP) [99].

Note: There is no scientific basis on which to assess the value of markers of inflammation intended to differentiate between reversible and irreversible pulpitis [65], making clinical diagnosis of pulpal status perplexing. As a general consensus in endodontology, there is poor correlation between clinical signs/symptoms of pulpal diseases with histological features, i.e. inflammation [98]; therefore, these complicated clinico-histological terminologies need reconsideration. Added to this ambiguity is the finding that several clinical studies have proved that clinically diagnosed irreversible pulpitis can be associated with radiographically apical periodontitis [26, 116]. Immuno-histological evidence revealed that not only an infected necrotic pulp but also an inflamed vital pulp has the potential to extend the inflammation to periapical tissues at an early stage and create apical periodontitis [122]. Whilst two-dimensional periapical radiographs have limited ability to detect such lesions [24], three-dimensional cone-beam computed tomography can distinguish AP in 13.7 % of examined human teeth with established irreversible pulpitis [1].

9.7.5.4 Prognosis

Current best evidence provides inconclusive information regarding factors influencing treatment outcome of vital pulp therapy in permanent teeth [4]. A preliminary retrospective study stated that there is a statistically significant association between the clinical status of pulpotomy and quality of restoration [36]; however, a recent prognostic study reported that the type of pulp capping material (i.e. MTA) was the single most important factor influencing the tooth survival rate [30].

Surprisingly, there is also a deficit of high-level evidence for the effect of treatment factors on primary root canal treatment outcome for management of various pulpal diagnoses [93]. Besides, a high-quality cohort study revealed that the survival rate of endodontically treated teeth in comparison to their vital counterparts is alarmingly low, with molars having the worst survival rates (hazard ratio = 7.4; CI 95 %: 3.2–15.1) [27].

9.7.5.5 Aim of Treatment

Vital pulp therapy for permanent mature teeth is typically indicated after iatrogenic or carious pulp exposure as well as accidental traumatic injuries to the teeth. When no/inadequate treatment is carried out for such teeth, the dental pulp becomes nonvital, and traditionally, pulpectomy and primary root canal therapy may be indicated. Consequently, the main treatment objective of VPT is to maintain pulp vitality of a carious permanent mature tooth by protecting the remaining pulp using a pulp capping agent so that the tooth becomes symptom-free and functional.

In case of ordinary root canal therapy, the three-dimensional seal of the root canal system after appropriate root canal cleaning and shaping is the main aim.

9.7.5.6 Outcomes

The clinical outcome is based on the absence of subjective symptoms (i.e. pain) and objective observation of inflammation and/or infection, i.e. abscess, swelling, sinus tract and tenderness upon palpation/percussion. The most important radiographic outcome is when AP is prevented or when healing of existing AP.

9.7.5.7 Methods of Search and Appraisal

Studies dating back to 1966 were located by searching PubMed (Medline). The main search terms were [systematic review(s) or randomized controlled trial(s) or clinical trial(s)] and [mineral trioxide aggregate] and [pulp* or pulp cap or pulpotomy or vital pulp therapy]. We also searched The Dental ELF, UTHSCSA Dental School CAT Library, *Journal of Evidence-Based Dental Practice* as well as *Evidence-Based Dentistry* and ClinicalTrials.gov for the keywords 'mineral trioxide aggregate'. Only English-language trials were assessed. Using modified van Tulder List and AMSTAR checklist, randomised controlled trials and systematic reviews of randomised controlled trials were scored, respectively.

9.7.5.8 Efficacy

Whilst there were ten randomised controlled trial [11, 44, 53, 59, 73, 91, 97, 100, 123, 124], we found only one systematic review [4]. The review analysed nonrandomised clinical trials and therefore was not classified as LoE1. Seven histological/immunohistochemical studies (Table 9.11 [44, 53, 73, 97, 100, 123, 124]) were found that compared MTA pulp capping with calcium hydroxide ($n=4$), calcium-enriched mixture ($n=2$) and different powder/liquid ratio of itself ($n=1$) on caries-free vital teeth; only one study looked at incipient caries [53]. There are three randomised controlled trials carried out for management of teeth with deep caries or established irreversible pulpitis (Table 9.12). One study compared MTA with calcium hydroxide for partial pulpotomy of permanent molars with deep caries [91], another study compared MTA with calcium hydroxide as indirect pulp capping [59], and finally a multicentre randomised controlled trial compared the post-operative pain relief as well as clinical and radiographic outcomes of pulpotomy in human permanent molars with irreversible pulpitis using calcium-enriched mixture cement or MTA [11]. There were no statistical significances between MTA and CEM or MTA and calcium

Table 9.11 List of histological studies with RCT design regarding vital pulp therapy with MTA versus calcium hydroxide (CH) or calcium-enriched mixture (CEM) cement in mature permanent teeth

Study (year)	Teeth (no.)	MTA (no. of teeth)	Control (no. of teeth)	Follow-up
Iwamoto et al. (2006) [53]	48	24	Dycal = 24	136 ± 24 days
Nair et al. (2008) [73]	33	20	CH = 13	1 week, 1 and 3 months
Sawicki et al. (2008) [97]	48	24	CH = 24	47–609 days
Zarrabi et al. (2010, 2011) [123, 124]	32	16	CEM = 16	2 and 8 weeks
Shahravan et al. (2011) [100]	29	3 water/powder ratios	–	30 days
Eskandarizadeh et al. (2011) [44]	90	WMTA = 30, GMTA = 30	Dycal = 30	30, 60 and 90 days

Table 9.12 Results of randomised controlled trials regarding vital pulp therapy with MTA versus calcium hydroxide (CH), Dycal or calcium-enriched mixture (CEM) cement in mature permanent teeth

Study (year)	Teeth no. (dropout)	MTA no. of teeth (dropout)	Control no. of teeth (dropout)	Follow-up (month)	Final outcomes (success %)
Qudeimat et al. (2007) [91]	64 (13)	32 (3)	CH = 32[a] (10)	25.4–45.6	MTA = 93.7; CH = 91
Leye Benoist et al. (2012) [59]	60 (0)	30 (0)	Dycal = 30 (0)	3 and 6	MTA = 89.6; Dycal = 73.3
Asgary and Eghbal (2013) [11]	413 (67)	MTA = 208 (29)	CEM = 205 (38)	12	MTA = 95; CEM = 92

[a]Non-setting CH then setting layer of CH

hydroxide reported in these randomised controlled trials.

Note: Histological studies evaluating pulp response to vital pulp therapy have been mainly carried out on caries-free or incipient caries vital teeth which were candidates for extraction shortly after. This shows that the studies were undertaken in different population, i.e. normal intact teeth versus carious teeth with pulp exposure or pulpitis. According to evidence-based practice concepts, the results of these kinds of studies should be excluded because they address a different population than the one required. In addition, histological evaluation is classified as a surrogate outcome. The surrogate outcome usually allows prediction of treatment effect on the more clinically relevant outcome but does not directly measure the main clinical benefit. The surrogate outcome is considered valid for an intervention if it is statistically associated with the true clinical outcome [89]. However, the presence/absence, type and intensity of histological pulp inflammation as surrogate variables do not inevitably represent the true short- and long-term treatment outcome, i.e. pain and tooth survival. Furthermore, only a minimal association between clinical and histological findings could be established for MTA or calcium hydroxide direct pulp capping [53].

9.7.5.9 Drawbacks

Tooth discolouration caused by white MTA used for the management of a complicated crown fracture via partial pulpotomy has been reported [22]. High price and long setting time are two other main drawbacks of MTA [84].

9.7.5.10 Comments

In current dental practice, VPT has become an accepted treatment for *reversible* pulpitis, with predictable outcomes [23]. When *irreversible* pulpitis is clinically diagnosed, the common school of thought recommends removal of entire vital pulp, despite containing competent stem cells with proliferative potential [121]. In the light of recent evidences and in order to gain a better understanding of pulp healing capability, the inflammatory process and pathogenesis of the dental pulp need to be reconsidered, particularly in cases of irreversible pulpitis [14]; such a modern approach can lead to preservation of the dental pulp in mature permanent teeth and, thus by healing of the diseased pulp, can have a positive impact on improving the tooth survival rate as well as patients' quality of life.

Current dental educational system defends the correlation between spontaneous pain or lingering pain in response to cold stimuli and the existence of irreversible pulpitis that necessitates the complex/expensive process of root canal therapy. However, several talented dental students have asked a long overdue and fundamental question: *Currently pulp preservation and regeneration in endodontic procedures is being increasingly emphasised in the educational curriculum, clinicians even aim to revitalise the immature necrotic pulp; then why do endodontists intentionally extirpate inflamed vital pulps with clinical diagnosis of irreversible pulpitis?* Root canal therapy of vital teeth is currently based on a *poor correlation* between clinical signs/symptoms and histological feature of the pulp [97]. Amazingly, there are LoE1 randomised controlled trials that show the vital pulp of mature molars with irreversible pulpitis that were successfully treated with simple low-cost pulpotomy treatment using appropriate biomaterials. These trials demonstrated that full pulpotomy with MTA or CEM biomaterials, as the most invasive form of VPT, established favourable short- to long term outcomes [10, 11, 14, 15]. It seems that endodontology needs to reconsider the nomenclature of dental pulp diseases and consequently create a paradigm shift in endodontic treatment approaches.

Currently, the proportion of the population who is unable to afford dental services due to its high cost is increasing, even in developed affluent countries [13]. To solve this problem, governments should accept responsibility to increase the overall spending for dental disease prevention protocols as well as evidence-based low-cost dental services. Researchers, on the other hand, should provide evidence employing recent progresses in endodontology and constantly suggest more biologic, cost-effective and successful simple treatment alternatives.

In the future, conducting the studies that consider the effects of VPTs on the oral health-related quality of life as well as health technology assessment and evidence-based practice guidelines is recommended. Last but not least, is the need for outcome assessment of less or non-invasive forms of VPT.

Clinical Bottom Line

To answer the PICO question, randomised controlled trials with *LoE1* have led to *GoR-A* (grade A recommendations) in vital pulp therapy of mature permanent teeth that state:

1. MTA partial pulpotomy has similar success rates when compared to calcium hydroxide for management of symptom-free carious pulp exposure in first molars.
2. MTA indirect pulp capping has similar success rates when compared to calcium hydroxide in teeth with active deep carious lesion/reversible pulpitis after 6 months.
3. MTA full pulpotomy has similar pain relief effect as well as clinical/radiographic success rates when compared to calcium-enriched mixture (CEM) cement in molar teeth with irreversible pulpitis.

References

1. Abella F, Patel S, Duran-Sindreu F, Mercade M, Bueno R, Roig M. Evaluating the periapical status of teeth with irreversible pulpitis by using cone-beam computed tomography scanning and periapical radiographs. J Endod. 2012;38(12):1588–91.
2. Aeinehchi M, Dadvand S, Fayazi S, Bayat-Movahed S. Randomized controlled trial of mineral trioxide aggregate and formocresol for pulpotomy in primary molar teeth. Int Endod J. 2007;40(4):261–7.
3. Agamy HA, Bakry NS, Mounir MM, Avery DR. Comparison of mineral trioxide aggregate and formocresol as pulp-capping agents in pulpotomized primary teeth. Pediatr Dent. 2004;26(4):302–9.
4. Aguilar P, Linsuwanont P. Vital pulp therapy in vital permanent teeth with cariously exposed pulp: a systematic review. J Endod. 2011;37(5):581–7.
5. Airen P, Shigli A, Airen B. Comparative evaluation of Formocresol and mineral trioxide aggregate in pulpotomized primary molars – 2 year follow up. J Clin Pediatr Dent. 2012;37(2):143–7.

6. Al-Jundi SH. Type of treatment, prognosis, and estimation of time spent to manage dental trauma in late presentation cases at a dental teaching hospital: a longitudinal and retrospective study. Dent Traumatol. 2004;20(1):1–5.
7. Anderson R, Thomas DW. 'Toothache stories': a qualitative investigation of why and how people seek emergency dental care. Community Dent Health. 2003;20(2):106–11.
8. Ansari G, Ranjpour M. Mineral trioxide aggregate and formocresol pulpotomy of primary teeth: a 2-year follow-up. Int Endod J. 2010;43(5):413–18.
9. Asgary S, Ahmadyar M. Can miniature pulpotomy procedure improve treatment outcomes of direct pulp capping? Med Hypotheses. 2012;78(2):283–5.
10. Asgary S, Eghbal MJ. The effect of pulpotomy using a calcium-enriched mixture cement versus one-visit root canal therapy on postoperative pain relief in irreversible pulpitis: a randomized clinical trial. Odontology. 2010;98(2):126–33.
11. Asgary S, Eghbal MJ. Treatment outcomes of pulpotomy in permanent molars with irreversible pulpitis using biomaterials: a multi-center randomized controlled trial. Acta Odontol Scand. 2013;71(1):130–6.
12. Asgary S, Eghbal MJ, Ehsani S. Periradicular regeneration after endodontic surgery with calcium-enriched mixture cement in dogs. J Endod. 2010;36(5):837–41.
13. Asgary S, Eghbal MJ, Fazlyab M, Baghban AA, Ghoddusi J. Five-year results of vital pulp therapy in permanent molars with irreversible pulpitis: a non-inferiority multicenter randomized clinical trial. Clin Oral Investig. 2014 Apr 27. [Epub ahead of print].
14. Asgary S, Eghbal MJ, Ghoddusi J. Two-year results of vital pulp therapy in permanent molars with irreversible pulpitis: an ongoing multicenter randomized clinical trial. Clin Oral Investig. 2014;18(2):635–41.
15. Asgary S, Eghbal MJ, Ghoddusi J, Yazdani S. One-year results of vital pulp therapy in permanent molars with irreversible pulpitis: an ongoing multicenter, randomized, non-inferiority clinical trial. Clin Oral Investig. 2013;17(2):431–9.
16. Asgary S, Ehsani S. Permanent molar pulpotomy with a new endodontic cement: a case series. J Conserv Dent. 2009;12(1):31–6.
17. Asgary S, Motazedian HR, Parirokh M, Eghbal MJ, Kheirieh S. Twenty years of research on mineral trioxide aggregate: a scientometric report. Iran Endod J. 2013;8(1):1–5.
18. Banchs F, Trope M. Revascularization of immature permanent teeth with apical periodontitis: new treatment protocol? J Endod. 2004;30(4):196–200.
19. Barone C, Dao TT, Basrani BB, Wang N, Friedman S. Treatment outcome in endodontics: the Toronto study – phases 3, 4, and 5: apical surgery. J Endod. 2010;36(1):28–35.
20. Bayne SC. Dental restorations for oral rehabilitation – testing of laboratory properties versus clinical performance for clinical decision making. J Oral Rehabil. 2007;34(12):921–32.
21. Bayne SC. Correlation of clinical performance with 'in vitro tests' of restorative dental materials that use polymer-based matrices. Dent Mater. 2012;28(1):52–71.
22. Belobrov I, Parashos P. Treatment of tooth discoloration after the use of white mineral trioxide aggregate. J Endod. 2011;37(7):1017–20.
23. Bender IB. Reversible and irreversible painful pulpitides: diagnosis and treatment. Aust Endod J. 2000; 26(1):10–4.
24. Bender IB, Seltzer S. Roentgenographic and direct observation of experimental lesions in bone: I. 1961. J Endod. 2003;29(11):702–6.
25. Beslot-Neveu A, Bonte E, Baune B, Serreau R, Aissat F, Quinquis L, et al. Mineral trioxide aggregate versus calcium hydroxide in apexification of non vital immature teeth: study protocol for a randomized controlled trial. Trials. 2011;12:174.
26. Caliskan MK. Pulpotomy of carious vital teeth with periapical involvement. Int Endod J. 1995;28(3):172–6.
27. Caplan DJ, Cai J, Yin G, White BA. Root canal filled versus non-root canal filled teeth: a retrospective comparison of survival times. J Public Health Dent. 2005;65(2):90–6.
28. Cardoso-Silva C, Barberia E, Maroto M, Garcia-Godoy F. Clinical study of Mineral Trioxide Aggregate in primary molars. Comparison between Grey and White MTA – a long term follow-up (84 months). J Dent. 2011;39(2):187–93.
29. Chala S, Abouqal R, Rida S. Apexification of immature teeth with calcium hydroxide or mineral trioxide aggregate: systematic review and meta-analysis. Oral Surg Oral Med Oral Pathol Oral Radiol Endod. 2011;112(4):e36–42.
30. Cho SY, Seo DG, Lee SJ, Lee J, Jung IY. Prognostic factors for clinical outcomes according to time after direct pulp capping. J Endod. 2013;39(3):327–31.
31. Chong BS, Pitt Ford TR, Hudson MB. A prospective clinical study of Mineral Trioxide Aggregate and IRM when used as root-end filling materials in endodontic surgery. Int Endod J. 2003;36(8):520–6.
32. Christiansen R, Kirkevang LL, Horsted-Bindslev P, Wenzel A. Randomized clinical trial of root-end resection followed by root-end filling with mineral trioxide aggregate or smoothing of the orthograde gutta-percha root filling – 1-year follow-up. Int Endod J. 2009;42(2):105–14.
33. Cvek M. A clinical report on partial pulpotomy and capping with calcium hydroxide in permanent incisors with complicated crown fracture. J Endod. 1978;4(8):232–7.
34. Damle SG, Bhattal H, Loomba A. Apexification of anterior teeth: a comparative evaluation of mineral trioxide aggregate and calcium hydroxide paste. J Clin Pediatr Dent. 2012;36(3):263–8.
35. de Paula-Silva FW, Wu MK, Leonardo MR, da Silva LA, Wesselink PR. Accuracy of periapical radiography and cone-beam computed tomography scans in diagnosing apical periodontitis using histopathological findings as a gold standard. J Endod. 2009;35(7): 1009–12.

36. Demarco FF, Rosa MS, Tarquinio SB, Piva E. Influence of the restoration quality on the success of pulpotomy treatment: a preliminary retrospective study. J Appl Oral Sci. 2005;13(1):72–7.
37. Densen P. Challenges and opportunities facing medical education. Trans Am Clin Climatol Assoc. 2011;122:48–58.
38. Doyle TL, Casas MJ, Kenny DJ, Judd PL. Mineral trioxide aggregate produces superior outcomes in vital primary molar pulpotomy. Pediatr Dent. 2010;32(1):41–7.
39. Eghbal MJ, Asgary S, Baglue RA, Parirokh M, Ghoddusi J. MTA pulpotomy of human permanent molars with irreversible pulpitis. Aust Endod J. 2009;35(1):4–8.
40. Eidelman E, Holan G, Fuks AB. Mineral trioxide aggregate vs. formocresol in pulpotomized primary molars: a preliminary report. Pediatr Dent. 2001;23(1):15–8.
41. El-Meligy OA, Avery DR. Comparison of mineral trioxide aggregate and calcium hydroxide as pulpotomy agents in young permanent teeth (apexogenesis). Pediatr Dent. 2006;28(5):399–404.
42. El-Meligy OA, Avery DR. Comparison of apexification with mineral trioxide aggregate and calcium hydroxide. Pediatr Dent. 2006;28(3):248–53.
43. Erdem AP, Guven Y, Balli B, Ilhan B, Sepet E, Ulukapi I, et al. Success rates of mineral trioxide aggregate, ferric sulfate, and formocresol pulpotomies: a 24-month study. Pediatr Dent. 2011;33(2):165–70.
44. Eskandarizadeh A, Shahpasandzadeh MH, Shahpasandzadeh M, Torabi M, Parirokh M. A comparative study on dental pulp response to calcium hydroxide, white and grey mineral trioxide aggregate as pulp capping agents. J Conserv Dent. 2011;14(4):351–5.
45. Fallahinejad Ghajari M, Asgharian Jeddi T, Iri S, Asgary S. Direct pulp-capping with calcium enriched mixture in primary molar teeth: a randomized clinical trial. Iran Endod J. 2010;5(1):27–30.
46. Fallahinejad Ghajari M, Asgharian Jeddi T, Iri S, Asgary S. Treatment outcomes of primary molars direct pulp capping after 20 months: a randomized controlled trial. Iran Endod J. 2013;8(4):149–52.
47. Farsi N, Alamoudi N, Balto K, Mushayt A. Success of mineral trioxide aggregate in pulpotomized primary molars. J Clin Pediatr Dent. 2005;29(4):307–11.
48. Ghoddusi J, Shahrami F, Alizadeh M, Kianoush K, Forghani M. Clinical and radiographic evaluation of vital pulp therapy in open apex teeth with MTA and ZOE. N Y State Dent J. 2012;78(3):34–8.
49. Godhi B, Sood PB, Sharma A. Effects of mineral trioxide aggregate and formocresol on vital pulp after pulpotomy of primary molars: an in vivo study. Contemp Clin Dent. 2011;2(4):296–301.
50. Heintze SD. Systematic reviews: I. The correlation between laboratory tests on marginal quality and bond strength. II. The correlation between marginal quality and clinical outcome. J Adhes Dent. 2007;9 Suppl 1:77–106.
51. Holan G, Eidelman E, Fuks AB. Long-term evaluation of pulpotomy in primary molars using mineral trioxide aggregate or formocresol. Pediatr Dent. 2005;27(2):129–36.
52. Hugar SM, Deshpande SD. Comparative investigation of clinical/radiographical signs of mineral trioxide aggregate and formocresol on pulpotomized primary molars. Contemp Clin Dent. 2010;1(3):146–51.
53. Iwamoto CE, Adachi E, Pameijer CH, Barnes D, Romberg EE, Jefferies S. Clinical and histological evaluation of white ProRoot MTA in direct pulp capping. Am J Dent. 2006;19(2):85–90.
54. Jabbarifar SEKA, Ghasemi D. Success rate of formocresol pulpotomy versus mineral trioxide aggregate in human primary molar tooth. J Res Med Sci. 2004;6:55–8.
55. Jacobovitz M, de Pontes Lima RK. The use of calcium hydroxide and mineral trioxide aggregate on apexification of a replanted tooth: a case report. Dent Traumatol. 2009;25(3):e32–6.
56. Kakehashi S, Stanley HR, Fitzgerald RJ. The effects of surgical exposures of dental pulps in germfree and conventional laboratory rats. J South Calif Dent Assoc. 1966;34(9):449–51.
57. Kazem M, Eghbal MJ, Asgary S. Comparison of bacterial and dye microleakage of different root-end filling materials. Iran Endod J. 2010;5(1):17.
58. Lee SJ, Monsef M, Torabinejad M. Sealing ability of a mineral trioxide aggregate for repair of lateral root perforations. J Endod. 1993;19(11):541–4.
59. Leye Benoist F, Gaye Ndiaye F, Kane AW, Benoist HM, Farge P. Evaluation of mineral trioxide aggregate (MTA) versus calcium hydroxide cement (Dycal(®)) in the formation of a dentine bridge: a randomised controlled trial. Int Dent J. 2012;62(1):33–9.
60. Lindeboom JA, Frenken JW, Kroon FH, van den Akker HP. A comparative prospective randomized clinical study of MTA and IRM as root-end filling materials in single-rooted teeth in endodontic surgery. Oral Surg Oral Med Oral Pathol Oral Radiol Endod. 2005;100(4):495–500.
61. Liu H, Zhou Q, Qin M. Mineral trioxide aggregate versus calcium hydroxide for pulpotomy in primary molars. Chin J Dent Res. 2011;14(2):121–5.
62. Magnusson BO, Sundell SO. Stepwise excavation of deep carious lesions in primary molars. J Int Assoc Dent Child. 1977;8(2):36–40.
63. Malekafzali B, Shekarchi F, Asgary S. Treatment outcomes of pulpotomy in primary molars using two endodontic biomaterials. A 2-year randomised clinical trial. Eur J Paediatr Dent. 2011;12(3):189–93.
64. Mehrdad L, Malekafzali B, Shekarchi F, Safi Y, Asgary S. Histological and CBCT evaluation of a pulpotomised primary molar using calcium enriched mixture cement. Eur Arch Paediatr Dent. 2013;14(3):191–4.
65. Methods of diagnosis and treatment in endodontics: a systematic review. Swedish Council on Health Technology Assessment. 2012. p. 55.
66. Miyashita H, Worthington HV, Qualtrough A, Plasschaert A. Pulp management for caries in adults: maintaining pulp vitality. Cochrane Database Syst Rev. 2007;(2):CD004484.

67. Montori VM, Wilczynski NL, Morgan D, Haynes RB. Optimal search strategies for retrieving systematic reviews from Medline: analytical survey. BMJ. 2005;330(7482):68.
68. Moore A, Howley MF, O'Connell AC. Treatment of open apex teeth using two types of white mineral trioxide aggregate after initial dressing with calcium hydroxide in children. Dent Traumatol. 2011;27(3): 166–73.
69. Moretti AB, Sakai VT, Oliveira TM, Fornetti AP, Santos CF, Machado MA, et al. The effectiveness of mineral trioxide aggregate, calcium hydroxide and formocresol for pulpotomies in primary teeth. Int Endod J. 2008;41(7):547–55.
70. Nadin G, Goel BR, Yeung CA, Glenny AM. Pulp treatment for extensive decay in primary teeth. Cochrane Database Syst Rev. 2003;(1):CD003220.
71. Naik S, Hegde AH. Mineral trioxide aggregate as a pulpotomy agent in primary molars: an in vivo study. J Indian Soc Pedod Prev Dent. 2005;23(1):13–6.
72. Nair PN. On the causes of persistent apical periodontitis: a review. Int Endod J. 2006;39(4):249–81.
73. Nair PN, Duncan HF, Pitt Ford TR, Luder HU. Histological, ultrastructural and quantitative investigations on the response of healthy human pulps to experimental capping with mineral trioxide aggregate: a randomized controlled trial. Int Endod J. 2008;41(2):128–50.
74. Ng FK, Messer LB. Mineral trioxide aggregate as a pulpotomy medicament: an evidence-based assessment. Eur Arch Paediatr Dent. 2008;9(2):58–73.
75. Noorollahian H. Comparison of mineral trioxide aggregate and formocresol as pulp medicaments for pulpotomies in primary molars. Br Dent J. 2008; 204(11):E20.
76. Nosrat A, Homayounfar N, Oloomi K. Drawbacks and unfavorable outcomes of regenerative endodontic treatments of necrotic immature teeth: a literature review and report of a case. J Endod. 2012;38(10):1428–34.
77. Nosrat A, Seifi A, Asgary S. Regenerative endodontic treatment (revascularization) for necrotic immature permanent molars: a review and report of two cases with a new biomaterial. J Endod. 2011;37(4):562–7.
78. Nosrat A, Seifi A, Asgary S. Pulpotomy in caries-exposed immature permanent molars using calcium-enriched mixture cement or mineral trioxide aggregate: a randomized clinical trial. Int J Paediatr Dent. 2013;23(1):56–63.
79. Odabas ME, Alacam A, Sillelioglu H, Deveci C. Clinical and radiographic success rates of mineral trioxide aggregate and ferric sulphate pulpotomies performed by dental students. Eur J Paediatr Dent. 2012;13(2):118–22.
80. Oliveira TM, Moretti AB, Sakai VT, Lourenco Neto N, Santos CF, Machado MA, et al. Clinical, radiographic and histologic analysis of the effects of pulp capping materials used in pulpotomies of human primary teeth. Eur Arch Paediatr Dent. 2013;14(2):65–71.
81. Olivo SA, Macedo LG, Gadotti IC, Fuentes J, Stanton T, Magee DJ. Scales to assess the quality of randomized controlled trials: a systematic review. Phys Ther. 2008;88(2):156–75.
82. Orstavik D, Kerekes K, Eriksen HM. The periapical index: a scoring system for radiographic assessment of apical periodontitis. Endod Dent Traumatol. 1986;2(1):20–34.
83. Pak JG, Fayazi S, White SN. Prevalence of periapical radiolucency and root canal treatment: a systematic review of cross-sectional studies. J Endod. 2012;38(9): 1170–6.
84. Parirokh M, Torabinejad M. Mineral trioxide aggregate: a comprehensive literature review – Part III: Clinical applications, drawbacks, and mechanism of action. J Endod. 2010;36(3):400–13.
85. Peng L, Ye L, Tan H, Zhou X. Evaluation of the formocresol versus mineral trioxide aggregate primary molar pulpotomy: a meta-analysis. Oral Surg Oral Med Oral Pathol Oral Radiol Endod. 2006;102(6):e40–4.
86. Percinoto C, de Castro AM, Pinto LM. Clinical and radiographic evaluation of pulpotomies employing calcium hydroxide and trioxide mineral aggregate. Gen Dent. 2006;54(4):258–61.
87. Pihlstrom BL, Barnett ML. Design, operation, and interpretation of clinical trials. J Dent Res. 2010;89(8): 759–72.
88. Pradhan DP, Chawla HS, Gauba K, Goyal A. Comparative evaluation of endodontic management of teeth with unformed apices with mineral trioxide aggregate and calcium hydroxide. J Dent Child (Chic). 2006;73(2):79–85.
89. Prentice RL. Surrogate endpoints in clinical trials: definition and operational criteria. Stat Med. 1989; 8(4):431–40.
90. Primus CM. Comments on "arsenic release provided by MTA and Portland cement" by Duarte MA, et al. Oral Surg Oral Med Oral Pathol Oral Radiol Endod. 2006;101(4):416–17; author reply 417–8.
91. Qudeimat MA, Barrieshi-Nusair KM, Owais AI. Calcium hydroxide vs mineral trioxide aggregates for partial pulpotomy of permanent molars with deep caries. Eur Arch Paediatr Dent. 2007;8(2):99–104.
92. Ricketts D, Lamont T, Innes NP, Kidd E, Clarkson JE. Operative caries management in adults and children. Cochrane Database Syst Rev. 2013;(3): CD003808.
93. Rosenberg PA, Schindler WG, Krell KV, Hicks ML, Davis SB. Identify the endodontic treatment modalities. J Endod. 2009;35(12):1675–94.
94. Sackett DL, Rosenberg WM, Gray JA, Haynes RB, Richardson WS. Evidence based medicine: what it is and what it isn't. BMJ. 1996;312(7023):71–2.
95. Sackett D, Straus S, Richardson W, Rosenberg W, Haynes R. Evidence-based medicine: how to practice and teach EBM. Edinburgh: Churchill Livingstone; 2000.
96. Sakai VT, Moretti AB, Oliveira TM, Fornetti AP, Santos CF, Machado MA, et al. Pulpotomy of human primary molars with MTA and Portland cement: a randomised controlled trial. Br Dent J. 2009;207(3):E5; discussion 128–9.

97. Sawicki L, Pameijer CH, Emerich K, Adamowicz-Klepalska B. Histological evaluation of mineral trioxide aggregate and calcium hydroxide in direct pulp capping of human immature permanent teeth. Am J Dent. 2008;21(4):262–6.
98. Seltzer S, Bender IB, Ziontz M. The dynamics of pulp inflammation: correlations between diagnostic data and actual histologic findings in the pulp. Oral Surg Oral Med Oral Pathol. 1963;16:969–77.
99. Shabahang S. State of the art and science of endodontics. J Am Dent Assoc. 2005;136(1):41–52; quiz 89–90.
100. Shahravan A, Jalali SP, Torabi M, Haghdoost AA, Gorjestani H. A histological study of pulp reaction to various water/powder ratios of white mineral trioxide aggregate as pulp-capping material in human teeth: a double-blinded, randomized controlled trial. Int Endod J. 2011;44(11):1029–33.
101. Shea BJ, Hamel C, Wells GA, Bouter LM, Kristjansson E, Grimshaw J, et al. AMSTAR is a reliable and valid measurement tool to assess the methodological quality of systematic reviews. J Clin Epidemiol. 2009;62(10):1013–20.
102. Simancas-Pallares MA, Diaz-Caballero AJ, Luna-Ricardo LM. Mineral trioxide aggregate in primary teeth pulpotomy. A systematic literature review. Med Oral Patol Oral Cir Bucal. 2010;15(6):e942–6.
103. Song M, Jung IY, Lee SJ, Lee CY, Kim E. Prognostic factors for clinical outcomes in endodontic microsurgery: a retrospective study. J Endod. 2011;37(7): 927–33.
104. Song M, Kim E. A prospective randomized controlled study of mineral trioxide aggregate and super ethoxy-benzoic acid as root-end filling materials in endodontic microsurgery. J Endod. 2012;38(7): 875–9.
105. Sonmez D, Duruturk L. Success rate of calcium hydroxide pulpotomy in primary molars restored with amalgam and stainless steel crowns. Br Dent J. 2010;208(9):E18; discussion 408–9.
106. Sonmez D, Sari S, Cetinbas T. A comparison of four pulpotomy techniques in primary molars: a long-term follow-up. J Endod. 2008;34(8):950–5.
107. Srinivasan D, Jayanthi M. Comparative evaluation of formocresol and mineral trioxide aggregate as pulpotomy agents in deciduous teeth. Indian J Dent Res. 2011;22(3):385–90.
108. Subay RK, Ilhan B, Ulukapi H. Mineral trioxide aggregate as a pulpotomy agent in immature teeth: long-term case report. Eur J Dent. 2013;7(1):133–8.
109. Subramaniam P, Konde S, Mathew S, Sugnani S. Mineral trioxide aggregate as pulp capping agent for primary teeth pulpotomy: 2 year follow up study. J Clin Pediatr Dent. 2009;33(4):311–14.
110. Sushynski JM, Zealand CM, Botero TM, Boynton JR, Majewski RF, Shelburne CE, et al. Comparison of gray mineral trioxide aggregate and diluted formocresol in pulpotomized primary molars: a 6- to 24-month observation. Pediatr Dent. 2012;34(5): 120–8.
111. Tang Y, Li X, Yin S. Outcomes of MTA as root-end filling in endodontic surgery: a systematic review. Quintessence Int. 2010;41(7):557–66.
112. Torabinejad M, Chivian N. Clinical applications of mineral trioxide aggregate. J Endod. 1999;25(3): 197–205.
113. Torabinejad M, Parirokh M. Mineral trioxide aggregate: a comprehensive literature review – part II: leakage and biocompatibility investigations. J Endod. 2010;36(2):190–202.
114. Torabinejad M, Pitt Ford TR, McKendry DJ, Abedi HR, Miller DA, Kariyawasam SP. Histologic assessment of mineral trioxide aggregate as a root-end filling in monkeys. J Endod. 1997;23(4):225–8.
115. Torabinejad M, Watson TF, Pitt Ford TR. Sealing ability of a mineral trioxide aggregate when used as a root end filling material. J Endod. 1993;19(12): 591–5.
116. Torabzadeh H, Asgary S. Indirect pulp therapy in a symptomatic mature molar using calcium enriched mixture cement. J Conserv Dent. 2013;16(1):83–6.
117. Tuna D, Olmez A. Clinical long-term evaluation of MTA as a direct pulp capping material in primary teeth. Int Endod J. 2008;41(4):273–8.
118. van Tulder M, Furlan A, Bombardier C, Bouter L. Updated method guidelines for systematic reviews in the cochrane collaboration back review group. Spine (Phila Pa 1976). 2003;28(12):1290–9.
119. Verhagen AP, de Vet HC, de Bie RA, Kessels AG, Boers M, Bouter LM, et al. The Delphi list: a criteria list for quality assessment of randomized clinical trials for conducting systematic reviews developed by Delphi consensus. J Clin Epidemiol. 1998;51(12): 1235–41.
120. von Arx T, Jensen SS, Hanni S, Friedman S. Five-year longitudinal assessment of the prognosis of apical microsurgery. J Endod. 2012;38(5):570–9.
121. Wang Z, Pan J, Wright JT, Bencharit S, Zhang S, Everett ET, et al. Putative stem cells in human dental pulp with irreversible pulpitis: an exploratory study. J Endod. 2010;36(5):820–5.
122. Yamasaki M, Kumazawa M, Kohsaka T, Nakamura H, Kameyama Y. Pulpal and periapical tissue reactions after experimental pulpal exposure in rats. J Endod. 1994;20(1):13–7.
123. Zarrabi MH, Javidi M, Jafarian AH, Joushan B. Histologic assessment of human pulp response to capping with mineral trioxide aggregate and a novel endodontic cement. J Endod. 2010;36(11): 1778–81.
124. Zarrabi MH, Javidi M, Jafarian AH, Joushan B. Immunohistochemical expression of fibronectin and tenascin in human tooth pulp capped with mineral trioxide aggregate and a novel endodontic cement. J Endod. 2011;37(12):1613–18.
125. Zealand CM, Briskie DM, Botero TM, Boynton JR, Hu JC. Comparing gray mineral trioxide aggregate and diluted formocresol in pulpotomized human primary molars. Pediatr Dent. 2010; 32(5):393–9.

Index

J. Camilleri (ed.), *Mineral Trioxide Aggregate in Dentistry*,
DOI 10.1007/978-3-642-55157-4, © Springer-Verlag Berlin Heidelberg 2014

GPSR Compliance

The European Union's (EU) General Product Safety Regulation (GPSR) is a set of rules that requires consumer products to be safe and our obligations to ensure this.

If you have any concerns about our products, you can contact us on ProductSafety@springernature.com

In case Publisher is established outside the EU, the EU authorized representative is:

Springer Nature Customer Service Center GmbH
Europaplatz 3
69115 Heidelberg, Germany

Batch number: 10705706

Printed by Printforce, the Netherlands